Curriculum Development in Nursing Education
Second Edition

Carroll L. Iwasiw, EdD, RN, MScN
Professor
Cofounding Editor, *International Journal of Nursing Education Scholarship*

Dolly Goldenberg, PhD, RN, MA (English), MScN
Adjunct Professor
Cofounding Editor, *International Journal of Nursing Education Scholarship*

Mary-Anne Andrusyszyn, EdD, RN, MScN
Professor and Director
Cofounding Editor, *International Journal of Nursing Education Scholarship*

Arthur Labatt Family School of Nursing
Faculty of Health Sciences
University of Western Ontario
London, Ontario, Canada

D0565504

JONES AND BARTLETT PUBLISHERS
Sudbury, Massachusetts
BOSTON   TORONTO   LONDON   SINGAPORE

World Headquarters

Jones and Bartlett Publishers
40 Tall Pine Drive
Sudbury, MA 01776
978-443-5000
info@jbpub.com
www.jbpub.com

Jones and Bartlett Publishers
Canada
6339 Ormindale Way
Mississauga, Ontario L5V 1J2
Canada

Jones and Bartlett Publishers
International
Barb House, Barb Mews
London W6 7PA
United Kingdom

Jones and Bartlett's books and products are available through most bookstores and online booksellers. To contact Jones and Bartlett Publishers directly, call 800-832-0034, fax 978-443-8000, or visit our website, www.jbpub.com.Copyright © 2005 by Jones and Bartlett Publishers, Inc.

The authors, editor, and publisher have made every effort to provide accurate information. However, they are not responsible for errors, omissions, or for any outcomes related to the use of the contents of this book and take no responsibility for the use of the products and procedures described. Treatments and side effects described in this book may not be applicable to all people; likewise, some people may require a dose or experience a side effect that is not described herein. Drugs and medical devices are discussed that may have limited availability controlled by the Food and Drug Administration (FDA) for use only in a research study or clinical trial. Research, clinical practice, and government regulations often change the accepted standard in this field. When consideration is being given to use of any drug in the clinical setting, the health care provider or reader is responsible for determining FDA status of the drug, reading the package insert, and reviewing prescribing information for the most up-to-date recommendations on dose, precautions, and contraindications, and determining the appropriate usage for the product. This is especially important in the case of drugs that are new or seldom used.

Production Credits

Publisher: Kevin Sullivan
Aquisitions Editor: Emily Ekle
Aquisitions Editor: Amy Sibley
Associate Editor: Patricia Donnelly
Editorial Assistant: Rachel Shuster
Associate Production Editor: Amanda Clerkin
Associate Marketing Manager: Ilana Goddess

Manufacturing and Inventory Control Supervisor: Amy Bacus
Composition: Auburn Associates, Inc.
Cover Design: Kristin E. Ohlin
Cover Image Credit: © Markus Gann/ShutterStock, Inc.
Printing and Binding: Malloy, Inc.
Cover Printing: Malloy, Inc.

Library of Congress Cataloging-in-Publication Data

Iwasiw, Carroll L.
    Curriculum development in nursing education / Carroll L. Iwasiw, Dolly Goldenberg, Mary-Anne Andrusyszyn.—2nd ed.
        p. ; cm.
    Includes bibliographical references and index.
    ISBN 978-0-7637-5595-9 (pbk.)
    1. Nursing—Study and teaching. 2. Curriculum planning. I. Goldenberg, Dolly. II. Andrusyszyn, Mary-Anne. III. Title.
    [DNLM: 1. Education, Nursing. 2. Curriculum. WY 18 I96c 2009]
    RT71.I95 2009
    610.73071′1—dc22
                                                                                        2008029747
6048

Printed in the United States of America
13   12   11   10   9   8   7   6

Dedication

We dedicate this book to former professors who ignited our love of nursing education, and to colleagues and graduate students. You have shaped and extended our thinking about curriculum development by your comments and questions in classes, workshops, and informal discussions. We also dedicate this book to our families, colleagues, and friends, for their encouragement throughout this endeavor. In particular, we thank Zenon Andrusyszyn for his graphics and support, and Dr. Sol, Jay, and Rob Goldenberg for their everlasting wisdom and wit.

Table of Contents

Preface

This book is written for all those who engage in designing or developing nursing curricula in baccalaureate, associate degree, and diploma nursing education. As such, this includes experienced or recently appointed nurse faculty, part-time and/or adjunct faculty, graduate students, teaching assistants, and those who aspire to become nurse educators.

The second edition of this book represents our continuing dedication to the advancement of nursing education, and in particular, to the ongoing development of nursing curricula. Our experience as nurse educators and curriculum developers continues and enables us to review what was, and still is, relevant from the first edition, as well as embrace new and contemporary ideas and insights from our experience, and from students, colleagues, and other authors.

As with the first edition, our book is about the processes involved in developing a curriculum for nursing education. However, during our planning for this second edition, it became apparent to us that a major determinant in a nursing education curriculum is the context in which the curriculum is developed and offered, and which makes each school's curriculum somewhat unique. This context is the professional, societal, health, and educational situations to which the curriculum must respond. This idea was presented in the first edition, but is now described more fully. Readers will find this premise of a context-relevant curriculum pervasive throughout the book. Accordingly, the title of the curriculum model reflects this idea.

This second edition has been expanded, with new chapters added. Furthermore, the book has been realigned into several distinct parts or sections, for a clearer representation of the curriculum development process. A new chapter about curriculum considerations for flexible delivery is now included, not only in response to requests for more information, but also because of the prevalent usage of flexible delivery in nursing education.

Chapter configurations are unchanged, as we have retained helpful and relevant tables and figures, concise chapter summaries, synthesis activities, as well as questions for consideration at the conclusion of each chapter. Fictionalized case studies highlight the main ideas of each chapter; some are from the first edition and some are new. The cases, together with concluding chapter questions, assist readers in deliberations pertaining to curriculum development activities in their own setting. Chapter references have been updated, while those still recent and important remain.

As in the first edition, we do not advocate any particular curriculum philosophy, model, design, teaching approach, or evaluation strategy. Rather, we propose ideas for creating a relevant yet dynamic nursing education curriculum. This second edition continues to offer a current, accessible, and comprehensive textbook on curriculum development, and incorporates a balance of theoretical perspectives and practical applications. We have retained information about historical beginnings, which provide context for traditional, new, and emerging ideas.

It is commonly recognized that the practice of nursing is changing, due to the ongoing developments in the fields of health care, nursing education, and general education. These social, cultural, and political forces, which include a shifting global market-driven economy; shortages of practicing nurses and faculty; diverse values; and uncertainties of life, continue to impinge upon how we prepare graduates for nursing practice and educator roles. Rapidly growing amounts of information and burgeoning healthcare technologies; new and creative delivery methods; culturally, racially, and age-diverse student groups; and nursing education as a legitimate science that is evidence-based, are ongoing issues that nursing faculty must face. Obviously, these factors must be considered in the development of nursing education curricula.

In this textbook we identify, as we did before, that the term *curriculum* is used to mean the totality of the curriculum, philosophical approaches, outcomes, design, courses, teaching-learning and evaluation strategies, interactions, learning climate, human and physical resources, and curriculum policies. However, we have introduced a new term, *curriculum nucleus,* the essence of the curriculum, to encapsulate philosophical approaches and that which is derived from the contextual data: core curriculum concepts, key professional abilities, and principal teaching-learning approaches. The concept of the curriculum nucleus containing these constituents and as being a central and pre-eminent part of the total curriculum was developed by the first author. The idea germinated from teaching courses about curriculum development and evaluation, using the idea in curriculum activities, and from endorsement at faculty and curriculum development workshops. Depicted in Chapter 7 is a figure conceptualizing the curriculum nucleus and its relationship to the total curriculum.

As well, throughout the book, the term *student clinical experience* is used to refer to practice experiences in health care and community contexts: acute-care hospitals, long-term care facilities, walk-in clinics, private practitioners' offices, community health agencies, day-care facilities, people's homes, store-front clinics, and so forth. The term *clinical* is inclusive of the full range of practice experiences and sites possible in a nursing curriculum.

We continue to maintain that the process of curriculum development is iterative, with many phases taking place concurrently. Unfortunately, it is not possible to depict or fully describe the recursive and interactive nature of curriculum development, and thus each aspect of the process is presented separately.

More specifically, in Part I, readers are introduced to the premise of a context-relevant curriculum, as well as to the distinction between the terms *nursing curriculum* and *nursing program*. Part II overviews supports for curriculum development. In Chapter 2 of this section, support that faculty will need when undertaking the process of developing a curriculum is described. Chapters 3 and 4, on leading curriculum development, and organizing curriculum development, are presented consecutively since they are distinct and important initial steps in preparing for curriculum development. This is a change from the first edition where they were combined into one chapter. Readers will find this difference helpful when considering and undergoing initial preparation for the curriculum development process. Chapter 5 concentrates on faculty development for curriculum development and change, essential activities that nurse educators undergo in preparation for, and during, curriculum development. Notably, faculty development related to the particular phase of curriculum development addressed in each chapter is described throughout the book.

In Part III, highlighted are the many facets of the curriculum development process. Chapter 6 addresses the contextual factors, that is, the forces, situations and circumstances that curriculum developers must take into account when gathering data for a context-relevant curriculum. Then in Chapter 7, readers are taken from the data-gathering phase to the curriculum nucleus, a new concept about curriculum development, coined by the authors. The curriculum nucleus represents that which is derived and concluded from the contextual data, along with the philosophical approaches. Developing philosophical approaches and formulating curriculum outcomes, a central basis of the curriculum, are contained in Chapter 8. In Chapters 9 and 10, curriculum and course design, respectively, are detailed.

In Part IV, curriculum implementation and evaluation are addressed. Chapter 11 offers the logistics involved in preparing for curriculum implementation. In Chapter 12, the processes inherent in internal curriculum evaluation, as well as the preparation involved in undergoing external evaluation are described. In Part V, Chapter 13, a new chapter, is devoted entirely to curriculum considerations for flexible delivery.

Finally, Part VI represents another addition to our second edition. This 14th chapter concludes the book and offers ideas about future perspectives of curriculum development and evaluation in nursing education.

In summary, this second edition continues to be unique in its concentrated presentation of the ways and means of curriculum development in nursing education. As authors, we hope that those of you who are already involved in curriculum development will continue to reflect on your current approaches, but also consider new or additional perspectives. To those new to curriculum development, this book could enable you to become a more informed participant in this process.

PART I

Introduction to Curriculum Development in Nursing Education: The Context-Relevant Curriculum

CHAPTER 1

Introduction to Context-Relevant Curriculum Development in Nursing Education

Chapter Overview

Curriculum development in nursing education is a creative process intended to produce a unified, meaningful curriculum. It is an ongoing activity in nursing education, even in schools of nursing with established curricula. The extent of the development ranges from regular refinement of class activities and assignments to the creation of a completely original and reconceptualized curriculum. In this book, curriculum development activities are presented individually for ease of description and comprehension. However, emphasized is the idea that the curriculum development process does not necessarily occur in precisely sequential stages or phases. Rather, some work occurs simultaneously, and each new decision has the potential to affect previous ones. This chapter begins with definitions of *curriculum* and a description of curriculum development in nursing education. It contains a summary of the major aspects of the curriculum development process, serving as an advance organizer for the book. Additionally, attention is given to some of the interpersonal issues that can influence the curriculum development team, and hence, the completed work. The ideas about curriculum development presented in this chapter are discussed more expansively in succeeding chapters.

Chapter Goals

- Review definitions and conceptualizations of *curriculum*.
- Ponder the meaning of a context-relevant curriculum.
- Overview the curriculum development process in nursing education.
- Consider supports for successful curriculum development.
- Appreciate the interpersonal aspects of the curriculum development process.

Definitions and Conceptualizations of *Curriculum*

Definitions of *curriculum* have been in existence since about 1820, first used in Scotland and then professionally in America a century later (Wiles & Bondi, 2007). There have been so many definitions, often in response to social forces, that the scope and interpretation of *curriculum* have greatly expanded, creating some uncertainty and divergence of opinion about the meaning and intent of the word.

Traditional definitions include a *course of study*, or *that which is taught*. More esoteric is the definition of curriculum as *symbolic representation*: that is, "institutional and discursive practices, structures, images, and experiences that can be identified and analyzed in various ways, i.e., politically, racially, autobiographically, phenomenologically, theologically, internationally, and in terms of gender and deconstruction" (Pinar, Reynolds, Slattery, & Taubman, as cited in Oliva, 2005, p. 5). Oliva has analyzed these and other curriculum definitions, noting that some focus on *purpose*, which is what the curriculum is meant to achieve. Other definitions address the *context* in which the curriculum is implemented, revealing the underlying philosophy, such as in a learner-centered curriculum. Finally, some curriculum definitions emphasize *instructional strategies* or *terminal objectives*. Similarly, Wiles (1999) has categorized definitions of curriculum *as subject matter, a plan, experience,* or *outcome*.

Curriculum has also been conceived as *prescriptive*, referring to defined objectives, content, activities, and/or outputs, as exemplified by the following: "Curriculum is a prescribed body of knowledge and methods by which it might be communicated" (Block, as cited in Glatthorn, Boschee, & Whitehead, 2006, p. 5). In contrast, *descriptive* definitions refer to experiences or the curriculum in action, as in "The reconstruction of knowledge and experience that enables the learner to grow in exercising intelligent control of subsequent knowledge and experience" (D. Tanner & L. N. Tanner, as cited in Oliva, 2005, p. 4). In a similar vein, C. A. Tanner (2004) proposes the idea that curriculum is "stories to be heard . . . broad learning goals, and ways we engage students in authentic learning" (pp. 3–4). A recent definition combines both prescriptive and descriptive perspectives, with curriculum seen as the plan "for guiding learning . . . usually represented in retrievable documents of several levels of generality, and the actualization of those plans in the classroom, as experienced by the learners and as recorded by an observer; those experiences take place in a learning environment that also influences what is learned" (Glatthorn et al., p. 5).

Curriculum has been described as *legitimate* (sanctioned), *illegitimate* (not sanctioned), *hidden* (unacknowledged socialization process), and *null* (thought to exist, but not there) (Bevis, 2000; Eisner, 1985). Another perspective is that curriculum can be categorized into five types. The *recommended curriculum* is proposed by external policy-making groups or experts and describes skills and concepts that ought to be emphasized. The printed and distributed plan is the *written curriculum*. The *supported curriculum* is reflected in, and shaped by, available resources. That which is delivered and observable is the *taught curriculum*. The *tested curriculum* is examined through formal evaluation of student learning. Finally, the *learned curriculum* is evident in the changes in knowledge, behavior, and attitudes that result from the educational experience (Glatthorn et al., 2006).

Despite differing definitions and conceptions, a curriculum is implemented with the intention that learning occurs. The written plan usually contains philosophical statements and goals or outcomes; indicates some selection, organization, and sequencing of subject matter and learning experiences; and integrates evaluation of learning. These elements, among others, are addressed as aspects of the curriculum development process.

In this book, the term *nursing curriculum* is defined as the totality of the philosophical approaches, curriculum outcome statements, overall design, courses, teaching-learning strategies, delivery methods, interactions, learning climate, evaluation methods, curriculum policies, and resources. As such, this conceptualization aligns with ideas of curriculum as prescription and description, context, instructional strategies, a plan, experiences, terminal goals, and outcomes, as well as the written, supported, taught, tested, and learned curriculum.

A context-relevant curriculum is one that is responsive to learners; to current and projected societal, health, and community situations; to imperatives of the nursing profession; is consistent with the mission, philosophy, and goals of the educational institution; and that is feasible within the realities of the school and community. This type of curriculum is defined by, and grounded in, the forces and circumstances that affect society, health care, education, recipients of nursing care, the nursing profession, and the educational institution. Although there will be significant similarities in the nursing curricula of many programs, those that are most strongly contextually relevant will have unique features reflective of local and/or regional circumstances. Moreover, context-relevant curricula are dynamic, changing in response to altered circumstances.

Although the term *nursing curriculum* is often viewed interchangeably with *nursing program*, we view the latter as being broader in scope. The nursing program includes the nursing curriculum, as well as the administrative structures of the school; faculty members' complete teaching, research, and professional activities (all of which affect curriculum); the school's relationship with other academic units and community agencies; institution-wide support services; and institutional support for the school of nursing within and beyond the parent institution.

Curriculum Development in Nursing Education

Curriculum development in nursing education is a creative process intended to produce a unified, meaningful nursing curriculum. The ultimate purpose is to create learning opportunities that will build students' professional knowledge and skills so that graduates will practice nursing competently in a changing healthcare environment, thereby contributing to the health and quality of life of those they serve.

Curriculum development is a process that can be described as more akin to art than science. It is characterized by interaction, cooperation, change, and possibly conflict; composed of overlapping, interactive, and iterative decisions; shaped by contextual realities and political timeliness; and influenced by the personal interests, styles of interaction, philosophies, judgments, and values of stakeholders.

The complex processes that lead to a substantial revision of an existing curriculum or creation of a new curriculum provide an opportunity for faculty members to develop and implement fresh perspectives on the education of nursing students and to influence the culture of the school of nursing. As well, curriculum development provides an avenue to strengthen the school's impact on the community and gain support from members of the educational institution, community, and nursing profession.

The curriculum development process has neither a beginning nor end. Once developed, the nursing curriculum undergoes refinements and modifications as it is implemented and evaluated. This occurs because a "perfect" nursing curriculum cannot be achieved and finalized when the context in which it is being implemented is constantly changing, and because nursing faculty strive to be responsive to that context.

Model of Context-Relevant Curriculum Development in Nursing Education

Although written and schematic representations of curriculum development are generally linear and sequential, this is not how nursing curricula are actually developed. Curriculum development is a highly iterative process, with each decision influencing concurrent and subsequent choices, and possibly leading to a rethinking of previous ideas. A unified nursing curriculum results from ongoing communication among groups working on different aspects of curriculum development, review and critique of completed work, and confirmation of decisions. Scales (1985) wrote that ". . . in actual practice, development and implementation of the curriculum is an integrated phenomenon . . . developed in a very integrated and interrelating manner; one component . . . not necessarily spring[ing] full grown and naturally from another, nor will any single component usually stand without some revision after subsequent parts are developed" (p. 3). Scales' view of curriculum development as an iterative process is emphasized throughout this book.

The iterative and recursive nature of curriculum work cannot be illustrated accurately in a two-dimensional representation. Depicting all the multiple and repetitive interactions that occur between and among the individual elements of curriculum development would result in a crowded and confusing model. Therefore, like other authors before us, we present a model of the curriculum development process in nursing education that appears linear. However, chapter descriptions of each element of the model will make evident that the process is interactive. The Model of Context–Relevant Curriculum Development in Nursing Education depicts the overall process for developing a context-relevant curriculum and is illustrated in Figure 1-1. The process is summarized below.

Determine the Need for Curriculum Development   When a decision is made to open a school of nursing or to introduce a new program within an existing school, curriculum development is necessary. More typically, curriculum development begins with an acknowledgment that the existing curriculum is no longer working as effectively as desired. This recognition can arise from altered circumstances within the school (e.g., changing faculty or student profile) or outside the school (e.g., changed standards of nursing practice or accreditation standards).

Gain Support   Curriculum development requires the support of nursing faculty and educational administrators. Gaining support for the curriculum development enterprise includes describing the logical reasons for altering the curriculum and appealing to the values held collectively by members of the school and educational institution. Faculty members' support and commitment are essential for all curriculum endeavors. Additionally, administrative support, in the form of altered work assignments, secretarial assistance, and possibly promotion and tenure considerations, provides evidence of institutional encouragement for the initiative. Faculty who want to undertake curriculum development need to ensure that the means to complete the work will be available.

Plan and Implement Faculty Development   Faculty development is the core of the curriculum development process, and therefore, is a continuing activity. Although curriculum development is inherently a faculty development endeavor, some faculty members, including those on the curriculum development team, may need planned assistance to acquire the knowledge and skills necessary to engage in the work. Accordingly, deliberate faculty development is essential to prepare members to influence decisions and the progress of curriculum work through informed participation.

Organize for Curriculum Development   Attention to the logistical matters that will lead to a successful outcome is essential. Organizing for curriculum development requires consideration of, and decisions about, leadership, the decision-making processes, committee structures and purposes, and approaches to getting the work done.

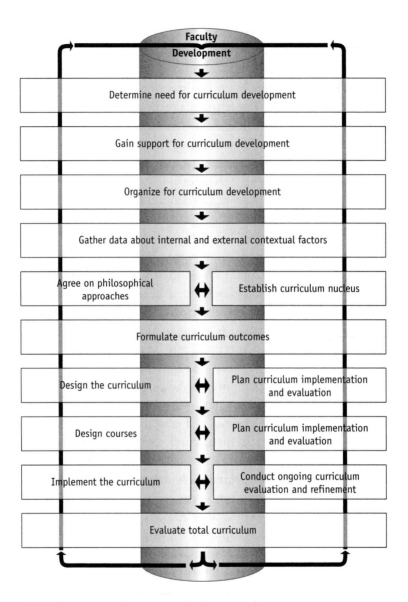

FIGURE 1-1 Model of Context-Relevant Curriculum Development

Gather Data About Internal and External Contextual Factors Systematic data-gathering about the environment in which the curriculum will be implemented and in which graduates will practice nursing is critical to ensure that the curriculum is relevant to its context. Contextual factors are those forces, situations, and circumstances that exist both within and outside the educational institution and have the potential to influence the school and its curriculum. The contextual factors are interrelated, complex, and at times, seamless, and overlapping. Internal contextual factors exist within the school and the educational institution; external contextual factors originate outside the institution.

Typically, information is obtained about internal factors of history; philosophy, mission, and goals; culture; financial resources; programs and policies; and infrastructure. Similarly, data are gathered about the external contextual factors: demographics; culture; health care; professional standards and trends; technology; environment; and social, political, and economic conditions. It is necessary to determine precisely which data are required about each contextual factor, as well as the most appropriate data sources.

Agree on Philosophical Approaches Information about philosophical approaches used in, or suitable for, nursing education, along with values and beliefs of the curriculum development team, lead to the development of statements of philosophical approaches relevant for the school and curriculum. Reaching resolution about the philosophical approaches is a critical milestone in curriculum development, since all aspects of the finalized curriculum should be congruent with espoused values and beliefs and the concepts that form the philosophical approaches.

Determine the Curriculum Nucleus The curriculum nucleus comprises the core curriculum concepts, key professional abilities, and principal teaching-learning approaches, all derived from the contextual data, as well as the philosophical approaches. The philosophical approaches are in themselves part of the nucleus, contribute to the core curriculum concepts, and influence the key professional abilities and principal teaching-learning approaches. The curriculum nucleus is simultaneously the foundation and essence of the curriculum and provides direction to its further development.

Formulate Curriculum Outcome Statements The curriculum outcome statements reflect broad abilities of graduates, each focusing on professional practice and representing an integration of cognitive, psychomotor, and/or affective actions. Curriculum outcome statements are written to incorporate the desired abilities of graduates, philosophical approaches, and core curriculum concepts. They are a public statement of what graduates will be like.

Design the Curriculum The term *curriculum design* refers to the configuration of the course of studies. In designing the curriculum, faculty determine level outcomes or competencies; nursing, non-nursing, and elective courses; course sequencing; relationships between and among courses; delivery methods; and associated policies. Brief course descriptions and course outcomes or competencies are prepared for nursing courses.

Design Courses Designing courses requires attention to the following components: purpose and description, course outcomes, teaching–learning strategies, content, classes, student learning activities, and evaluation of student learning. Each course must be congruent with the curriculum intent and clearly relate to intended curriculum outcomes.

Plan Curriculum Implementation and Evaluation Successful implementation of the curriculum is dependent on forethought as the curriculum is being designed. The essential aspects of preparing for implementation are informing stakeholders; marketing; attending to contractual agreements and logistics; and planning ongoing faculty development.

Curriculum evaluation is an organized and thoughtful appraisal of both the elements central to the course of studies undertaken by students and graduates' abilities. The aspects to be evaluated include the philosophical approaches, curriculum outcome statements, overall design, courses, teaching-learning strategies, interactions, learning climate, evaluation methods, curriculum policies, resources, and actual outcomes demonstrated by graduates. Planning curriculum evaluation should occur simultaneously with curriculum and course design.

Implement the Curriculum Curriculum implementation begins when the first course is introduced and continues for the life of the curriculum. Successful implementation is dependent on faculty adoption of the curriculum tenets and congruent teaching-learning approaches.

Conduct Ongoing Curriculum Evaluation and Refinement The evaluation plan is put into action simultaneously with curriculum implementation. Ongoing evaluation results in small refinements that smooth implementation, fill identified gaps, and/or remove redundancies.

Evaluate the Total Curriculum Once completely implemented, the curriculum is evaluated to determine if all elements are appropriate and congruent with one another, and to ascertain graduates' success. Internal curriculum evaluation is undertaken by members of the school of nursing, whereas external curriculum evaluation is generally conducted as a part of program evaluation by provincial, state, regional, or national approval or accrediting bodies.

Feedback Loops The feedback loops in the model reflect the idea that at every stage of curriculum development, implementation, and evaluation, judgments are made about the appropriateness and fit of one element with previous elements, and the possibility of change. The feedback loops signify that the curriculum is dynamic, and subject to change as information and opinion about its effectiveness and appropriateness are gathered.

Supports for Successful Curriculum Development

Curriculum development does not transpire without preceding and ongoing support. Four essential forms of support are faculty endorsement for, and sustained involvement in, the enterprise; leadership of the endeavor; effective organization of the work; and faculty development. All must be in place before the intellectual effort of curriculum development begins, and all must continue to be strongly evident throughout the process. The four supports are both pre- and co-requisites of successful curriculum development. Of the four, faculty development alone is presented as the core of the curriculum development model, because this dimension makes possible the design, implementation, and evaluation of the curriculum. The four supports are described in Part II. Readers are reminded that these supports continue to be important in the processes described in the remainder of the book.

Interpersonal Aspects of Curriculum Development

Curriculum development is not a sterile process of objective, detached decision-making. Rather, it is marked by the dynamics of all interpersonal activities. Since "Each school [of nursing] is characterized by its unique blend of persons, each with different skills, knowledge, experience, and personality" (Oliva, 2005, p. 86), the dynamics vary from school to school. In general, however, learning, conflict, cooperation, resistance, eagerness, formation of group alliances, power struggles, commitment to shared goals, sadness, and satisfaction can occur. The human dimension is a constant factor in the curriculum development process, and it must be attended to even when the tasks and deadlines of curriculum development are pressing. It is important, therefore, to ensure that all members of the curriculum development team feel valued and appreciated for ideas they offer and work they complete.

Curriculum deliberations occur in collaboration with colleagues whose values may be divergent. Since values affect perspectives and choices, they are a powerful (although sometimes unrecognized) influence on curriculum development. Consequently, it is incumbent upon curriculum developers to reflect on their ideals and beliefs, discuss them openly with colleagues, and consider how these influence their preferences about the developing curriculum. Clarification of individual and collective values is integral to curriculum development, and can be essential in times of emotional debate or apparently irresolvable conflict.

Resistance to curriculum change can occur because of differing values about nursing education, feelings of uncertainty about fitting into a new curriculum, disinterest, or a general disinclination to expend the effort necessary to create and implement a new curriculum. The opposition of some can sabotage the efforts of committed curriculum developers, and planned intervention may be necessary.

Creating and implementing a curriculum represent a significant change for faculty in which they progress from known and comfortable ways of being to uncertainty and to new understandings and practices. Collegial support and reinforcement sustain this progress. Collectively, faculty can create and institute strategies to recognize their progress, offer encouragement to each other, and celebrate their successes. In these ways, both faculty cohesion and the curriculum are strengthened.

A full review of interpersonal dynamics is beyond the scope of this book. However, diligent attention should be given to this aspect of curriculum development. The success of the curriculum is dependent on the dedication of all stakeholders, and this is most likely to develop when individuals communicate openly and supportively with one another.

Chapter Summary

Curriculum development is an endeavor that faculty and other stakeholders undertake with the goal of preparing graduates who will practice nursing competently in a constantly changing healthcare environment. The Model of Context-Relevant Curriculum Development describes a process for developing a curriculum that is relevant for the context in which the curriculum will be offered and graduates will work. Curriculum development begins with the recognition that a new curriculum is needed and may seem to be complete when the newly created curriculum is implemented. However, development of a context-relevant curriculum is really a dynamic process, since evaluation and subsequent refinement are constant features of nursing curricula, even during implementation. Successful curriculum development, implementation, and evaluation are contingent on dedicated participants whose efforts are valued and who are supported during the process.

References

Bevis, E. O. (2000). Nursing curriculum as professional education. In E. O. Bevis & J. Watson (Eds.), *Toward a caring curriculum. A new pedagogy for nursing* (pp. 67–106). Boston: Jones and Bartlett.

Glatthorn, A. A., Boschee, F., & Whitehead, B. M. (2006). *Curriculum leadership: Development and implementation.* Thousand Oaks: Sage.

Eisner, E. (1985). *The educational imagination* (2nd ed.). New York: MacMillan.

Oliva, P. (2005). *Developing the curriculum* (6th ed.). Boston: Pearson Education.

Scales, F. S. (1985). *Nursing curriculum. Development, structure, function.* Norwalk, CT: Appleton-Century Crofts.

Tanner, C. A. (2004). The meaning of curriculum: Content to be covered or stories to be heard? *Journal of Nursing Education, 43,* 3–4.

Wiles, J. (1999). *Curriculum essentials: A resource for educators.* Needham Heights, MA: Allyn and Bacon.

Wiles, J., & Bondi, J. (2007). *Curriculum development. A guide to practice* (7th ed.). Upper Saddle River, NJ: Pearson Merrill Prentice Hall.

PART II

Supports for Curriculum Development

CHAPTER 2

Faculty Support for Curriculum Development

Chapter Overview

This chapter provides insight into considerations that must precede a decision to undertake curriculum development and that can lead to faculty support for the idea of curriculum development. Although a creation of a completely reconceptualized curriculum or revision of an existing one may seem the obvious answer for rectifying identified curriculum shortcomings, it is advisable to give thoughtful consideration to faculty readiness to embark on this endeavor. Since faculty members have the main responsibility for curriculum development, their support is essential.

Reflection about the reasons for curriculum redesign, extent of the development to be undertaken, the timeframe, and strategies to gain support for the idea are addressed. A chapter summary follows. Synthesis activities include two cases: the first is followed by a critique, and the second provides an opportunity to analyze readiness for curriculum revision or development. Questions to guide thinking about preliminary considerations for curriculum development and means to gain faculty support conclude the chapter. These questions are designed to help the reader decide if circumstances are right to begin the formal process of curriculum development in individual settings.

Chapter Goals

- Consider factors and influences that precipitate curriculum development or revision.
- Reflect on the extent of curriculum development necessary.
- Propose strategies to gain faculty support for curriculum development.
- Assess faculty readiness for curriculum development or revision.
- Justify the decision to proceed with or suspend the curriculum development process.

Considerations for Curriculum Development

The idea of engaging in curriculum development generally arises among a small group of faculty members who believe that the current curriculum is no longer adequate to prepare students to practice competently in the healthcare and societal contexts they will encounter when they graduate. Identifying reasons why curriculum development is necessary, the extent of the curriculum development that might be required, and possible timelines are important ideas to present to colleagues when seeking their support for curriculum development.

Why Consider Curriculum Development?

The purpose of nursing programs is to graduate nurses who will practice competently in a changing healthcare environment, and thereby contribute to the health and quality of life of the individuals, families, groups, and/or communities they serve. Situations that impede the ability of the school of nursing to achieve this purpose, and as a consequence, threaten its stability, success, or reputation, precipitate thoughts of modifying the curriculum or creating a new one.

Alterations within the school of nursing context can influence faculty to consider the possibility of curriculum development. These might include the following:

- Availability of resources
- Faculty numbers or expertise
- Student profiles
- Introduction of new ideas by stakeholders
- General discontent with the status quo
- Results of internal curriculum evaluation
- Results of external program or school reviews.

Changing circumstances within the context of the parent educational institution might also lead to a belief that curriculum development is timely. Some examples might include changes in:

- Educational technologies
- Library resources and services
- Academic policy
- Faculty and staff union contracts
- Institutional budget.

Similarly, varying situations outside the educational institution can be important signals to faculty that curriculum development is required to ensure that the curriculum is context-relevant. Changes might occur such as those in:

- Nursing and educational paradigms
- Organization of nursing education throughout a state or province
- Competition from other schools
- Graduates' success rates on licensure or registration exams
- New graduates' ability to meet employers' expectations
- Accreditation or approval standards
- Nursing workforce
- Provision of health care
- Professional and/or governmental regulations.

A single situation, or a combination of circumstances, can result in the view that the existing curriculum is no longer working as effectively as desired, is outmoded in some way, or not as responsive to the context as it should be. The consideration of curriculum development or revision can arise gradually as new ideas and educational methods emerge. Alternately, curriculum development can be unavoidable and even urgent because of profound contextual changes within the school of nursing, parent institution, or the environment outside the educational agency.

Continuing shifts in health and healthcare systems, technologies, population profiles, expectations, and demands have led to the realization that the education of nurses, and therefore, nursing curricula, must be subjected to evaluation, revision, and maybe even dramatic change. The magnitude, intensity, and pace of societal and healthcare dynamics challenge nurse educators to develop relevant, evidence-based curricula to prepare nurses for new roles and responsibilities consistent with evolving health care and healthcare systems. A curriculum "not only reflects but is a product of its time" (Oliva, 2005, p. 27). Accordingly, as time moves on, it becomes necessary for the curriculum to reflect a new era in society and health care. The desire to create an up-to-date, progressive, and context-relevant curriculum arises from nurse educators' professional obligation to ensure that graduates will be able to practice nursing competently.

How Extensive Should the Curriculum Development Be?

Those initiating the idea of curriculum development should give thought to the extent of curriculum development they believe necessary in order to achieve a unified, context-relevant curriculum that will build students' professional knowledge and skills. Within the nursing curriculum, the philosophical approaches, curriculum outcome statements, overall design, courses, teaching-learning strategies, interactions, learning climate, evaluation methods, curriculum policies, and resources, should be related, logical, consistent, conceptually congruent, and mutually supportive. The scope of curriculum development can encompass those related to:

- The creation of a completely new and reconceptualized curriculum whose description and implementation is not based upon an existing curriculum, *or*
- A significant revision of an existing curriculum, such that many curriculum elements are substantially modified and curriculum unity is preserved or achieved.

A revision extends well beyond the ongoing curriculum refinement (i.e., fine-tuning activities such as the annual updating and improvement of courses) in which faculty members routinely engage, either singly or in small teaching groups. Because curriculum development entails dedicated effort by the total faculty group, it is wise to give careful thought to which aspects of the current curriculum are working or not. This analysis is important when trying to gain support for curriculum development from faculty colleagues.

Should the existing curriculum be revised, or should a new curriculum be created? There is no formulaic answer to this question. Rather, the answer results from a comprehensive and holistic assessment of many factors and the application of faculty judgment about the appraisal. These factors include, but are not limited to those listed below:

- The time period since the curriculum was originally created or significantly revised
- The nature and extent of altered circumstances in the school and beyond
- Faculty members' emotional and intellectual investment in the existing curriculum
- Faculty energy for change
- Results of ongoing curriculum evaluation
- Sources of student and faculty discontent with the existing curriculum.

In general, a desire for extensive change in a major element of the curriculum, such as the philosophical approaches (and the resultant curriculum outcome statements, teaching-learning approaches, and evaluation methods), will lead to the creation of a new curriculum. Similarly, significant changes in the nature and availability of clinical placements could bring forth ideas of starting anew with curriculum development.

In contrast, a conviction that, for example, altered course sequencing could yield better outcomes for learners, would likely result in curriculum revision. In the same vein, the recognition that students are not achieving a particular curriculum outcome would probably lead to revision within the existing curriculum, but not necessarily the development of a new curriculum.

What Will the Timeframe Be?

Another consideration when proposing curriculum revision or development of an entirely new curriculum is the timeframe for conclusion of the work. How urgently is the redesigned curriculum needed? When should the new or revised curriculum be implemented? There are several factors to examine when thinking about the start and completion dates for the potential curriculum development project. Each must be assessed within the context of all the other questions posed in this chapter.

First to consider is the urgency of the curriculum redesign. This is influenced by the factors that prompted consideration of curriculum development initially. If, for example, two successive groups of graduates have had a high failure rate on licensing examinations, then there is pressure to improve the curriculum quickly. Similarly, a change in clinical services in local healthcare agencies may necessitate an immediate refocusing of clinical courses. Conversely, the immediacy of altering an undergraduate curriculum to reflect a slowly changing trend in local demographics is not as great.

Another factor to review when contemplating a timeframe is the culture of the school and parent institution. Is this an organization that innovates, or is this one that is satisfied with the status quo? Are the behavioral norms and expectations constructive or defensive (passive or aggressive), leading respectively to organizational adaptability or ineffectiveness (Balthazard, Cooke, & Potter, 2006)? Does the institution operate at a measured pace, with each step clearly delineated, or is implementation expected to follow rapidly after decisions (Tappan, 2001)? Will it be necessary to gain approval from administrators for each step of the curriculum development process, or will they want only to be informed of progress? The speed at which work normally proceeds within the organization, as well as general receptivity to change (Yoder-Wise & Menix, 2007), will affect the interval allotted for curriculum development and implementation.

The annual work cycle of the school of nursing influences the schedule for beginning and completing the curriculum development process. Is there a semester when faculty members are less busy with teaching and able to devote concentrated time to curriculum development? If so, consideration should be given to the amount of work that could be achieved in those time periods. If not, the amount of curriculum development time that can be integrated into the ongoing work of the school should be assessed.

Finally, when thinking about a timeframe for curriculum development, a mindful review should be conducted of the people who might be involved in order to identify those likely to be supporters and resisters. How much time can the supporters be expected to give to curriculum development? How much time will be taken up with overcoming resistance and winning support? This too will affect the expected completion of the curriculum. Before trying to gain support for curriculum development, it is important to have a tentative schedule in mind. Participants must have some idea of the amount of time and work that is being asked of them before they can commit to a curriculum project.

Gaining Faculty Support for Curriculum Development

Although a small group of faculty members may initiate the idea of curriculum development, it is ultimately the decision of the total faculty group about whether to undertake curriculum development, and if so, the extent of development and the timelines for completion. The decision to proceed with curriculum development or not, is influenced by the depth of discontent with the existing curriculum; knowledge of nursing education, clinical practice, and research; resources available for curriculum development; and beliefs about how a redesigned curriculum could influence the success of the school and individual members. These ideas form the basis for gaining faculty support for curriculum development.

Curriculum development cannot proceed on the conviction of only a few faculty members; it requires the commitment and effort of all faculty and many other stakeholders (Hull, St. Romain, Alexander, Schaff, & Jones, 2001; Kramer, 2005). First and foremost is support from faculty colleagues, as they will assume the largest responsibility for curriculum development. Next, the dean/director's support is a prerequisite to formally starting the intensive work of curriculum development. As well, advocates should seek support from learners, clinical colleagues, educational partners, healthcare clients, and administrators. The endorsement of representatives from each group strengthens the case for proceeding with curriculum development work, since all are stakeholders in the school of nursing and its curriculum.

How Can Support Be Gained from Faculty Colleagues?

Gaining faculty colleagues' support for curriculum development involves an appeal to logic and values. Neither alone is sufficient. The precise approach will, of course, be dependent on the organization and the people involved. First, faculty proposing curriculum development must be able to clearly articulate why curriculum development is necessary. For example, it is important to present factual data about how deficiencies in the current curriculum are evident, what the consequences are, and how these led to the conclusion that the curriculum is outdated. Secondly, the perceived need for curriculum development can be linked to values held by faculty members, the school of nursing, and/or the educational institution. For example, if the institution takes pride in being innovative, responsive to diversity, and a leader in education, then curriculum development can be presented as a means to support those values. In Table 2-1, ideas are offered that could be helpful in convincing colleagues that curriculum development is needed. Innovations (or the possibility of an innovation) are most likely to be accepted if the new idea is congruent with the values of the organization and its members (Greenhalgh, Robert, Bate, Macfarlane, & Kyriakidou, 2005).

Table 2-1 Examples to Convince Faculty of Need for Curriculum Development

Appeal to Logic	Appeal to Values
Need for curriculum change or development due to: • Deficiency in current curriculum • Unsatisfactory curriculum evaluations • Trends requiring new approaches • Evidence from literature to support change	Opportunity to shape the curriculum Desire for: • Professional and personal growth of learners and faculty members • Competent graduates • Enhancement of school prestige • Status as innovators, leaders
Requirement to provide a curriculum responsive to health care and societal needs	Opportunity for: • Personal prestige • Innovation and transformation • Organizational preeminence • Enhanced reputation of individuals and school

Positive consequences of curriculum development:
• Strengthened congruence with:
  • Organizational mission and values
  • Personal and professional values
• Favorable program evaluations from external bodies
• Student satisfaction, leading to enhanced work environment for faculty
• Appeal to potential faculty members
	Consequences of avoiding curriculum development:
	• Decreased appeal and marketability of school to applicants, students, faculty
	• Decreased marketability of graduates to employers
	• Lost opportunities for funding
	• Negative implications for program approval and/or accreditation
	• Diminished prestige

Possibility of obtaining funding for curriculum development	

It is important to consider the best way to seek support. Should colleagues be approached individually or collectively? Clearly, there are advantages and drawbacks to both. (See Table 2-2 for an analysis of approaching colleagues individually or collectively.) A combination may be appropriate, first talking with colleagues individually to gain the acceptance

Table 2-2   Advantages and Disadvantages of Approaching Colleagues Individually or Collectively for Curriculum Development

Approach	Advantages	Disadvantages
Individual	Freer expression and exploration of ideas	One viewpoint; no collective ideas
	Less threatening	Lack of support for persons proposing change
	Quick response or possible decision	Time required to collect and compile ideas from individuals
	Greater willingness to share experiences	Discomfort resulting from disagreement
	In-depth, thoughtful response possible	Pressure to conform
	Personal consultation valued	
Collective	Group response more broad	Delayed response or decision (many ideas before consensus)
	Sharing of many ideas	Time required to share all experiences relative to decision
	Opportunity to use democratic or consensual process, which strengthens a decision to proceed	Potential group veto of curriculum change
	Increased awareness of others' strengths and weaknesses	Undue influence by strong group members
	Opportunity to learn from each others' feedback	Group think
	Improved faculty bonding by uniting to reach common goal	
	Shared thinking for responses, resulting in a stronger position	
	Less time-consuming	
	Opportunity for group to make more informed assessments of need for change	

of informal leaders, and then presenting ideas to a larger group. The decision will be influenced by knowledge of the interpersonal dynamics among colleagues and by the credibility of those seeking support for curriculum change.

How Can Support Be Obtained from the Dean/Director?

The support of the dean/director is necessary before curriculum work can proceed, no matter how much endorsement exists among faculty. Matters to address with the dean/director are included in Table 2-3. It is unlikely that precise information about each point will be available. However, thoughtful identification of both the academic and administrative aspects of curriculum development will increase the credibility of those proposing curriculum development to the dean/director. The initial goal is to gain support for the idea of initiating curriculum development and a commitment to examine ways to provide resources for the undertaking.

How Can Initial Objections Be Addressed?

Although some faculty members may be enthusiastic about the idea of curriculum development, others may have a different view. It can be expected that some will feel hesitant and others may resist the possibility of curriculum development, and thus, change. Overcoming initial objections is the foundation to winning faculty support. To ignore opposition will likely result in either a failure to proceed, or in slow and resentful involvement. Therefore, it is wise to anticipate, recognize, and respond to objections promptly.

First, challenges about the accuracy of information that illustrates the need for curriculum development, or the conclusions drawn, can be anticipated. This may reflect an honest, intellectual disagreement, a deeply held belief in the value of the current curriculum, a general response to change, or opposition to those proposing curriculum development.

Table 2-3   Matters to Discuss with Dean/Director

1. Need for curriculum development
2. Extent of faculty colleague support
3. Estimated time for development and implementation of redesigned curriculum
4. Effect on other work:
   - Teaching (classroom, clinical)
   - Student advisement
   - Research, publications, and presentations
   - Committee and community involvement
5. People to be involved
6. Resources needed:
   - Faculty release time
   - Support personnel
   - Materials
   - Technological equipment
   - Physical space
   - Funding
7. Positive consequences of curriculum development for the school

When reasons for curriculum development are questioned, it is tempting to invite challengers to explain their position. This is a strategy to be used with caution, since a distracting and ongoing dispute about who is right or which facts are correct is not productive. Such disagreements can annoy or even alienate others, who might then view curriculum development as a potentially endless series of conflicts. In the face of criticism about the reasons for curriculum development, it is more constructive to respond that the reasons are compelling, but, naturally, all will draw their own conclusions.

It may be that some faculty are feeling so overstretched with their current workloads that even the *idea* of curriculum development, and thus more work, is overwhelming. The time required for this endeavor can seem daunting and may be a real barrier. It is important to recognize and acknowledge that curriculum development is a large undertaking. Therefore, the reality of workloads and available time should be explored thoroughly. Competing demands may make curriculum development impossible at this time. Perhaps some responsibilities can be delayed or given up, at least for a short period, to allow the process to unfold.

To win the support of particular individuals, it is wise to identify the criticisms they have voiced about the current curriculum, as well as aspects they value. Through individual or small group meetings, they can be reminded that curriculum development is an opportunity to eliminate the weaker aspects of the current curriculum. As well, it is essential to emphasize that active involvement in the curriculum development process could lead to maintaining or updating cherished parts of the existing curriculum. Affirming that strengths of the present curriculum may be retained, if this is deemed appropriate by the curriculum development team, might induce cooperation.

Financial constraints will be a concern for the dean/director and may also be raised by other faculty members. Curriculum development takes time, and faculty and staff time is costly. It may be necessary, therefore, to enumerate the costs and potential risks of avoiding curriculum development. These can include unfavorable external reviews by approval or accrediting bodies, decreased ability to attract students and faculty, difficulty retaining faculty, and unrealized funding opportunities. A statement recognizing that resources are needed for curriculum development and an assurance that this matter will be discussed with the dean/director, will go a long way in gaining support. As well, it is helpful to identify possible funding sources for curriculum development, such as internal university funds or foundations known to be donors for nursing education innovations. Adequate system resources are needed for change to occur and be sustained (Greenhalgh et al., 2005).

Another reason for objecting to the idea of curriculum development might be that those proposing it do not have the respect of colleagues. It is essential that those advocating curriculum development have good relationships with colleagues and are seen as having credible views about curriculum. If not, the proposal for curriculum change may be rejected.

Identifying if personalities are the reason for opposition is a painful process. Those recommending curriculum development might consider whether or not their ideas are usually sought and supported by colleagues, and if others generally choose to work with them. If personality seems to be a reason for objections, it would be wise to leave the initiation of the idea to others who are respected within the faculty group. If this is not possible, some interpersonal work must be done before faculty support will be gained. Objections that may be raised to the idea of curriculum development and possible responses are summarized in Table 2-4.

Table 2-4 Responses to Initial Objections to the Idea of Curriculum Change

Nature of Objections	Responses
Challenge to reasons for curriculum change	Respond that reasons are compelling
Satisfaction with current curriculum	Emphasize the: • importance of offering a curriculum that will maximize student learning and graduates' success • opportunity to be on the cutting edge of change and transformation in nursing education • personal and professional growth potential inherent in curriculum development
Fear that treasured part of the curriculum will be lost	Affirm that as curriculum work proceeds, aspects of the current curriculum may be retained Comment that active involvement is the only means to ensure a satisfactory curriculum
Time required for curriculum development	Present possible funding opportunities for curriculum development and faculty release time Note that individuals' involvement will influence process, and thus, time required
Fear that curriculum development will negatively affect research and writing time	Underscore the opportunities for research and scholarly writing that arise from curriculum development, implementation, and evaluation State that curriculum development is a role responsibility
Lack of support for faculty proposing change	Let credible faculty initiate idea of curriculum change

Deciding to Proceed with Curriculum Development

Not all objections will be overcome, nor will all resistance melt away. Nonetheless, once faculty members individually and collectively have considered the reasons for and against curriculum development, a majority concurs, and the dean/director supports the idea, then the curriculum development process is ready to proceed. Faculty support is the foundation upon which the quality of the curriculum development process will rest, and therefore, faculty members' endorsement of the decision to proceed is essential. The decision may be reached by consensus, or it may be formalized by a motion that specifies a timeline for implementing a redesigned curriculum, depending on the typical decision-making procedures in the school of nursing.

Once a decision about moving forward has been reached, it is usual to advise stakeholders, some of whom may subsequently become involved in the process. Informing others beyond the school of nursing makes public the intention to proceed with curriculum development and creates an expectation of change.

Chapter Summary

Faculty support for curriculum development is mandatory for the process to begin and for a successful outcome to be achieved. This is gained through open and thoughtful consideration of the reasons for curriculum development and honest attention to factors that could be limiting. Attention to the values of individual and collective faculty, the extent of curriculum development that might be necessary, and the timeframe for the undertaking, will influence whether approval is gained. The impetus and decision to proceed must be thoughtfully reviewed, since curriculum development is intensive, extensive, and requires ongoing faculty dedication and involvement.

Synthesis Activities

Two case studies are presented to illustrate the ideas in this chapter. The first is critiqued. Consider whether pertinent aspects of the case have been assessed and whether there are other points to be discussed. The second case is followed by questions to guide analysis. Finally, questions are offered to guide your consideration of faculty support for curriculum development in your situation.

Charlevoix University Undergraduate Nursing Program

Charlevoix University School of Nursing has introduced a new baccalaureate nursing program. To minimize the reality and appearance of a theory-practice gap, theory and clinical courses are not separate. Rather, all nursing courses include both theoretical and clinical components. Broad outcomes and general descriptions for all courses were developed by the curriculum designers. The description of one fourth-year course, "Nursing Care of Complex Clients" was: "Through classroom and clinical experiences, students will integrate concepts from previous nursing and non-nursing courses, in high-acuity situations where individuals experience complex physiological, psychological, and/or social needs."

Tom McLean, a clinical nurse specialist in the intensive care unit of a quaternary-care teaching hospital, was hired in July, two months prior to the first offering of fourth-year courses. He was assigned to teach the theoretical aspects and manage the associated clinical experiences of the Nursing Care of Complex Clients course.

It was necessary for Tom to develop the course fully. He did so mainly by himself, consulting with the undergraduate program chair about matters related to course structure such as hours of instruction, examination regulations, and frequency of clinical evaluation. In his first year of teaching, Tom's content focus in the course was the client in the emergency room and intensive care unit.

Throughout the first offering of the course, Tom met regularly with the clinical teachers to discuss matters related to the course and to student progress. As well, he met informally with clinical staff. Tom was struck by the remarks of both teachers and staff nurses that it took the students a long time "to get up to speed" in the clinical sites. He also noted on the clinical evaluations that many learners were hesitant about the technical equipment, had difficulty attaching meaning to signs of rapidly changing physiological status, and/or felt overwhelmed by the clinical situations.

Tom discussed the situation with Sandra Greenberg, a trusted friend and pediatric intensive care advanced practice nurse who was responsible for the course in children's health, which is prerequisite to Tom's course. She said that learners reacted in a similar fashion when assigned to pediatric units of the tertiary-care teaching hospital where she is a clinical teacher.

Sandra and Tom believe they must do everything possible to ensure that students completing the program are able to provide competent, hospital-based care in situations of high acuity. They begin to consider reshaping the undergraduate curriculum to emphasize enhanced knowledge and skill development related to tertiary-level care. For example, they talked about reconfiguring the family nursing courses to address care of ICU patients' families. They would like to see curriculum revisions implemented in the next academic year so that successive classes will be "up to speed."

Knowing that they require the support of nursing faculty for curriculum revision, Tom and Sandra tested their ideas with a few faculty members whose teaching is aligned with acute care nursing, as well as with intensive care advanced practitioners. All were supportive of the idea of increasing the focus on acute and intensive care in the curriculum, and most said they will do whatever possible to help. Filled with enthusiasm for their plan, Tom and Sandra arranged a meeting with the undergraduate program chair, certain that their ideas would be welcomed and appreciated.

Critique

The reasons for the proposed curriculum revision are Tom's once-only experience in teaching the Nursing Care of Complex Clients course, learners' clinical performance evaluations, and comments from other acute-care teachers and clinicians. As well, Tom and Sandra want to ensure that graduating students would be able to provide competent hospital-based acute care. They are enthusiastic about a curriculum revision, but lack a sufficient database upon which to recommend their proposed changes.

Tom and Sandra should examine the curriculum philosophy and intent, review the original course outcomes, and determine the expected level of performance for graduating students. Was the course really meant to focus on intensive care and emergency situations? They also need more concrete information about what it meant for learners not to be "up to speed" on the units, and determine whether being "up to speed" is a reasonable expectation.

Tom and Sandra have the support of faculty and skilled practitioners with a similar clinical focus, but they have not yet explored their perspective with faculty whose teaching lies in the areas of family nursing, mental health nursing, or community health. Also, they should consider that the current curriculum represents the most recent judgment of faculty. Moreover, having just introduced a new curriculum, it is unlikely that most faculty members will be interested in revamping it significantly.

Lacking a strong rationale for a curriculum revision, Tom and Sandra cannot expect their ideas to be warmly received nor acted upon. Rather, they would be wise to examine the curriculum documents and determine if their courses and expectations of students are congruent with the curriculum intent. As well, they should consider whether allegiance to their clinical specialties has overshadowed the broader perspective of nursing that is required in undergraduate education. Tom and Sandra have gained tentative support from faculty and clinical personnel with a vested interest in acute care nursing. However, without stronger evidence of the need for revision in the current curriculum, they cannot expect widespread support.

The undergraduate program chair might consider if Tom and Sandra have been adequately oriented to the curriculum. Does the program that assists new faculty need modification? It is possible that, even if they have been oriented to the curriculum, Tom and Sandra have not fully understood its intent since they were not a part of the overall curriculum development. Alternately, might Tom and Sandra have identified a real curriculum gap? The undergraduate program chair should commend Tom and Sandra for their commitment to ensuring student success, and carefully pursue these questions.

Meadowvale University School of Nursing

Dr. Manuela Lopez is director and professor of Meadowvale University School of Nursing. Enrollment is 550 undergraduate and 85 graduate students. The teaching staff comprises 26 full-time faculty of whom 19 are doctorally-prepared, and 7 masters-prepared. There are 40 part-time faculty, 22 with a masters degree, and 18 with a baccalaureate degree. Approximately 30% of faculty members were hired in the previous 3 years.

Dr. Lopez is an active member of the university administrators group, the community health administrators association, and nursing professional organizations. She keeps abreast of changes in nursing, nursing education, and health care. She has excellent relationships with faculty members, university administrators, and clinical and professional colleagues.

The undergraduate curriculum was first implemented 15 years ago. Since then, there have been minor curriculum revisions, but the philosophical approaches, goals, and basic structure of the largely behaviorist curriculum have remained unchanged.

Although faculty have attended workshops and conferences on new and evolving educational paradigms, some are generally comfortable with the present curriculum. Others act more in accordance with a caring, humanistic-educative approach, while still others are strong feminists. Several faculty advance ideas of social justice in the courses they teach.

Members of the school of nursing were shocked when, for the first time, nearly 20% of graduates failed the NCLEX. Those graduates were public in voicing their displeasure with the school. Along with this, there has been informal feedback from a few employers that Meadowvale graduates are having difficulties beyond those experienced by new graduates of other schools. Further, there has been increasing pressure from the university's central administration to increase the number and size of research grants and the publication rate of faculty.

The school is 3 years away from an accreditation review, and Dr. Lopez thinks that the time might be right for curriculum development. She calls a special meeting to discuss this possibility.

Questions for Consideration and Analysis of the Meadowvale University Case

1. What factors or influences would propel Meadowvale nursing faculty toward curriculum development? What might be the objections and responses to these?
2. What could be the sources of support for curriculum development? Sources of resistance?
3. How would Dr. Lopez's initiation of the idea of curriculum development influence faculty members' decision about whether or not to proceed?
4. What is a suitable timeframe for curriculum revision in light of the reasons for curriculum development and the upcoming accreditation review?
5. How would Dr. Lopez assess faculty members' acceptance of the need for curriculum development and their readiness to support the process?

Curriculum Development Activities for Consideration in Your Setting

The following questions are intended to stimulate your thinking about faculty support for curriculum development in your setting.

1. Why is curriculum development necessary now? What is the evidence for proposing that we proceed with curriculum work?
2. From whom do we need to gain support for the idea of curriculum development?
3. How do we gain support? What are the advantages and disadvantages of approaching our colleagues individually or collectively?
4. How can we present evidence about the necessity for curriculum development so it is convincing to faculty colleagues?
5. How extensive do we believe curriculum development should be? Should it be a revision of the current curriculum or a completely new curriculum?
6. What might the timeframe be for completion of the work?
7. How might participation in the curriculum development process affect faculty members' other commitments?
8. What are the objections to curriculum development that we can anticipate and how should we respond?

9. In addition to the need for curriculum development, what else should we be prepared to discuss with the dean/director in a preliminary way?

10. What resources will we require to be successful? What funding sources are available outside the school of nursing?

11. What potential risks are associated with not going forward at this time?

12. What other considerations require thoughtful attention?

13. Do we have sufficient faculty support to proceed with curriculum development?

14. Is informal agreement to proceed sufficient, or would a formal motion be preferable?

15. If agreement to proceed is obtained, which stakeholders should we inform of our decision?

References

Balthazard, P. A., Cooke, R. A., & Potter, R. E. (2006). Dysfunctional culture, dysfunctional organization. *Journal of Managerial Psychology, 21*, 709–732.

Greenhalgh, T., Robert, G., Bate, P., Macfarlane, R., & Kyriakidou, O. (2005). *Diffusion of innovations in health service organizations: A systematic literature review.* Oxford: BMJ Books/Blackwell.

Hull, E., St. Romain, J. A., Alexander, P., Schaff, S., & Jones, W. (2001). Moving cemeteries: A framework for facilitating curriculum revision. *Nurse Educator, 26*, 280–282.

Kramer, N. A. (2005). Capturing the curriculum. *Nurse Educator, 30*, 80–84.

Oliva, P. (2005). *Developing the curriculum* (6th ed.). Boston: Pearson Education.

Tappan, R. M. (2001). *Nursing leadership and management: Concepts and practice* (4th ed.). Philadelphia: F. A. Davis.

Yoder-Wise, P. S., & Menix, K. (2007). Leading change. In P. S. Yoder-Wise (Ed.), *Leading and managing in nursing* (4th ed.). St. Louis, MO: Mosby Elsevier.

CHAPTER 3

Leading Curriculum Development

Chapter Overview

Insight into leadership in general, and more specifically, into formal leadership for curriculum development is provided in this chapter. Effective leadership is foundational for curriculum redesign to occur. Following information about leadership and leaders, the curriculum leader's responsibilities are delineated. A discussion of activities associated with leading curriculum redesign is succeeded by suggestions for faculty development for curriculum leadership. The synthesis activities that complete the chapter include a case study and critique to illustrate the foremost points of the chapter. A second case is offered for analysis. Finally, questions are presented to assist readers with the determination of curriculum development leadership in individual settings.

Chapter Goals

- Review conceptions of leadership and leaders.
- Overview factors important in leading curriculum development.
- Address the formal curriculum leader's role and responsibilities.
- Contemplate faculty development activities related to leading curriculum development.

Leadership

Few topics in the social sciences have attracted as much commentary, theory, and research as that of leaders and leadership. The word *leader* itself has a long history of usage, as far back as the 1300s, but it was only during the first half of the 1800s that the term *leadership* became known (Marquis & Huston, 2006). Furthermore, it is acknowledged that there is "no single definition broad enough to encompass the total leadership process" (Bednash, 2003, as cited in Marquis & Huston). Schools of thought about leadership have been evolutionary, and there is an expanding body of knowledge on the subject. Progression has occurred from the great man theory, to traits or characteristics of leaders, to behavioral theory, to a focus on the individual leader, to leaders and followers, to the situation and environment, and now on leadership styles.

Leadership is the process of influencing people to accomplish goals or to move toward group goal setting and achievement. This statement emphasizes that leadership is not a solitary activity. There is a relationship between the leader, another individual, group, organization, or community. The relationship can arise from a formal arrangement in which the leader is in a position of authority in a role that is sanctioned or assigned within an organization. Alternately, there can be a relationship of informal leadership, in which the leader "demonstrates leadership outside the scope of a formal leadership role or as a member of a group rather than as a head or leader of the group" (Searle Leach, 2003, p. 167).

Whether leadership is formal or informal, the components of effective leadership in a culture of change are moral purpose, understanding change, building relationships, and creating and sharing knowledge (Fullan, 2001, 2003). Moreover, for sustainable change, the leader must influence the group to give ongoing attention to a collective moral purpose, a commitment to changing contexts, and to lateral capacity-building, accountability, vertical relationships, deep learning by participants, commitment to short- and longer-term results, and recognition that energy for improvement is cyclical (Fullan, 2005). Leadership means working with others to create unity and shared purpose.

Leadership levels have been identified: *individual*, in which leaders mentor, coach, and motivate; *group*, where leaders build teams and resolve conflicts; and *organizational*, in which leaders build a culture (Huber, 2000). At each level, the leader must *diagnose* (understand the situation); *adapt* (match behaviors and resources to the situation); and *communicate* (advance the [curriculum] process in ways that individuals can understand and [eventually] accept) (Hersey, Blanchard, & Johnson, 1996). The leader's vision, goals, scope of influence, and complexity of strategies expand with each level.

Leadership Styles

Leadership styles have been extensively studied since the time of the ancient Greek philosopher, Plato (429–347 BCE), Socrates' most famous pupil. Former classic ideas about leadership styles, namely *democratic, autocratic,* and *laissez-faire,* have been replaced with other approaches that conceptualize styles in relation to leaders' views of followers (McGregor, 1960; Blake & Mouton, 1964), variables of task structure and position power (Fiedler, 1967), and situations (Hersey et al., 1996). One style is not necessarily better than another, as many factors affect leaders and leadership styles (Goldenberg, 1990). Each style has advantages and disadvantages, depending on the situational complexity, competing demands, and organizational culture.

Transactional and Transformational Leadership   A focus on the relationship between leaders and followers has led to the identification of *transactional* and *transformative* leadership. *Transactional leaders* function within the existing organizational culture in a care-giving role, concern themselves with day-to-day operations, set goals expected of the group, and assign rewards in an exchange posture or bargain contract, for mutual benefit. They "set strategic goals ... deal with risk-taking situations" (Polifko-Harris, 2004, p. 75) and manage-by-exception, a technique found to be an essential component of effective leadership in some situations.

Transformational leaders motivate the group to perform to their full potential over time, by influencing a change in perceptions, providing a vision and sense of direction, and involving group members in decisions about how to achieve the vision (Robbins & Davidhizar, 2007). These are charismatic leaders who use individualized consideration and intellectual satisfaction in the group, and engage with others so that they and the group members raise each other to higher levels of motivation and ethical decision-making. They focus on collective purpose and mutual growth and development; articulate a vision; behave as change agents; and empower others to expend extra effort beyond performance expectations. They develop pride and satisfaction in the work, enthusiasm, team spirit, and a sense of accomplishment. This style is better suited to the work of professionals (Bass & Avolio, 1990), and could be effective for curriculum leaders.

Attributes of transformational leaders include charisma, individualized consideration, and intellectual stimulation. These contrast with attributes of transactional leaders who focus on contingency reward and manage by exception. Hence, a transactional leader would not attempt to change a work culture, whereas a transformational leader would (Lewis, French, & Phetmany, 2000). Interestingly, Chan and Chan (2005), in a study of 510 professional employees in four different countries, found a synergy between transformational and transactional leadership, and concluded that one could augment the other in producing greater amounts of performance and satisfaction.

Quantum Leadership   This style is based on chaos theory and involves visionary and facilitative leaders and equitably involved participants. In the time before a change is completely implemented (e.g., when one curriculum is being phased out and another phased in), "the leader's role is to live fully in the role of potential reality" (Porter-O'Grady & Malloch, 2007, p. 7). This leadership style represents a way of being: showing passion and commitment to the change; relentlessly communicating the vision; being honest and direct about why the change is necessary and how it will affect people; engaging others in making changes; and being open to critique (Porter-O'Grady & Malloch).

Other Descriptions of Leadership Styles   Other current views of effective leadership styles reflect an intermingling of trait, behavior, and contingency approaches (Sullivan & Decker, 2005). Some of these leadership styles include the following:

- *Charismatic leadership* is based on personal characteristics and qualities, and involves charming, persuasive leaders and affectionate, committed participants.
- *Relational leadership* is based on the idea that connections among people, and collaboration, are the bases for achieving goals.
- *Shared leadership* is based on empowerment principles, and involves participative, transformational leaders and empowered, knowledgeable participants.
- *Servant leadership* is based on a desire to serve, and involves leaders who serve others and participants who are evolving into those who serve others.

Still other labels have been ascribed to leadership styles, primarily in the corporate culture. Examples include:

- *Ethical leadership* "incorporates integration and assignment of responsibility to people with different personal and cultural value systems in decision-making" (Schnebel, 2000, p. 86).
- *Stakeholder leadership* is based on "a nonhierarchical conceptualization [of] cooperative stakeholder relationships" to fulfill leader and stakeholder potential for effectiveness (Schneider, 2002, p. 210).
- *Paternalistic leadership* is the indigenous leadership style in some Chinese societies. It "combines strong discipline and authority," incorporates "moral integrity . . . a paternalistic atmosphere" (Cheng, Chou, Wu, Huang, & Farh, 2004, p. 91), and involves subordinates in leadership.
- *Level 5 leadership* is a style in which leaders exhibit humility, will, and unwavering resolve; select superior successors; and give credit to others while assigning blame to themselves (Collins, 2005).
- *Responsible leadership* incorporates interaction with many stakeholders inside and outside the corporation (Maak & Pless, 2006).

Appointment as a Formal Leader

Leaders can be informally chosen or formally elected by members of a group who recognize and accept the leader's influence to lead, and who view the leader as someone who is competent and trustworthy. This is referred to as *emergent leadership*. Leaders can also be appointed or elected to the position by people external to the group. This is called *imposed* or *organizational leadership*. Imposed leaders may have difficulty being accepted by the group or receiving support because of lack of trust.

Successful Leaders

To lead successfully, leaders must maintain balance, generate self-motivation, build self-confidence, listen to constituents, and maintain a positive attitude (Yoder-Wise, 2007). Leaders are most effective when they work in an environment that offers organizational, human, financial, personal, and social support. Successful leaders have a concern for others, and an ability to create a sense of presence. They are accessible and build collaborative relationships. Successful leaders support teamwork and are skilled in conflict management (Registered Nurses Association of Ontario [RNAO], 2006). Similarly, Bernhard and Walsh (1990) describe interrelated attributes for effective leaders to include awareness of self and group members; advocacy for the group; and accountability for one's actions to self, group, profession, and superiors.

So many attributes of leaders have been described that, according to Searle Leach (2003), there may not be a particular set of characteristics to determine an effective leader. However, generally ascribed qualities of effective leaders include being visionary, enthusiastic, supportive, knowledgeable, visible, responsive, flexible, caring, trustworthy, honest, and self-confident. These leaders have high standards and expectations, and integrity; they value learning, education, and professional development; they take initiative and are risk takers. Effective leaders communicate openly; have the capacity to adapt; demonstrate power and status in the organization; and inspire subordinates. They are active in professional organizations; have mastered the dream; are able to change and design organizational structure; and first and foremost, have the desire to lead (Kellerman, 2004; RNAO, 2006; Scott, Sochalski, & Aiken, 1999; Shamian, 2005; Zaleznik, 2004). These qualities have been encapsulated as being strategic, engaging people, managing the project, using self, and demonstrating leadership practices (Skelton-Green, Simpson, & Scott, 2007).

Successful leaders recognize their own shortcomings and those of others. Commenting that leadership is not a moral concept, Kellerman (2004) cautions that leaders are prone to variations in benevolent motives and integrity. Prentice (2004) suggests that leaders should learn that people are "complex and different; respond to rewards, ambition, patriotism, loss of the good and beautiful, boredom, self-doubt" (p. 104), and other desires and emotions. In other words, leaders and followers are human, and neither should expect perfection of themselves nor of others.

Curriculum Development Leadership

The curriculum development process is an ideal context in which leadership can occur (Scarborough, 2002). A formal leader is needed, and informal leadership can arise in the work of the curriculum committees, subcommittees, and task forces. Curriculum development leaders must give careful attention to the concepts of leadership described above and to the style appropriate to the stakeholders engaged in the curriculum work.

Leadership roles in curriculum development are multiple, due to the numerous environments in which the work is conducted and the levels at which leaders must operate. In fact, 10 leadership roles have been identified: expert, instructor, trainer, retriever, referrer, linker, demonstrator, modeler, advocate, confronter, counselor, advisor, observer, data collector, analyzer, diagnoser, designer, manager, and evaluator (Havelock and Associates, as cited in Wiles & Bondi, 1998).

Curriculum Development Leader

Although knowledgeable about the curriculum development process and the substance and relevance of the work to be done, the curriculum leader does not have decision-making authority about the new curriculum. That authority rests with the dean/director and the faculty. However, the curriculum leader does have responsibility for ensuring that the curriculum is developed in a timely fashion, and that it meets the changing needs of a diverse learner group, clients, community, and society. This requires working effectively with external stakeholders and members of all committees that are formed.

When working with curriculum groups, it is particularly important that the curriculum leader attend to the interpersonal dimensions of group activity. Since curriculum developers are often strongly invested in their work, the potential for conflict exists. Therefore, the leader requires skill in effective group functioning, and the ability to use a style that is appropriate to the curriculum participants and situations. In addition to the qualities of an effective leader, the curriculum leader requires expert knowledge and management or logistical skills.

Expert Knowledge   The curriculum leader must be knowledgeable about nursing education, curriculum development, and within the educational institution, academic policy and approval processes. Of course, the first two are essential. The third type of knowledge can be readily acquired through institutional documents, Web sites, and academic leaders.

The curriculum leader must also be intimately knowledgeable about the type of program for which the curriculum is being developed, such as associate, baccalaureate, or graduate degree program. An understanding of the nature of such programs, the expectations of graduates, and approval and accreditation requirements will allow this leader to guide novice curriculum developers to suitable resources, processes, and decisions. Provision of ideas for consideration or concrete suggestions for action (for example, philosophies that the group might review and compare), propel the work group forward. The leader should be thoroughly immersed in the literature, practice, and governance of nursing education in order to bring important ideas to the group and have credibility with members.

Although the ultimate responsibility for the completed curriculum rests with all faculty members, it is the leader who initiates and provides direction to the work. This requires knowledge and experience in all aspects of curriculum development, from gaining support through planning evaluation. The leader must be expert in the technical aspects, such as how to write outcomes or design a course, as well as the processes that lead to achievement of the curriculum development milestones. It is the leader who ensures that the necessary processes are in place and that important matters are addressed and decided upon in a timely fashion.

Each educational institution has academic policies and approval mechanisms that partially define the context for the redesigned curriculum. The curriculum leader must know these so that proposals that do not align with them can be readily identified and steps taken to revise or alter them. Some stakeholders may not be aware of the scope of an institution's policies; hence, it is the curriculum leader's responsibility to inform them. Similarly, the leader's familiarity with approval processes will be essential to ensure that program and institutional requirements are met.

Management and Logistical Skills   The curriculum leader's expert knowledge in management and decision-making (Marquis & Huston, 2006) should be evident in the identification of activities that must be completed and the progress made in the curriculum development endeavor. The curriculum leader:

- Initiates organization of the curriculum development work
- Proposes committees to be formed
- Ensures that curriculum development activities proceed in a timely fashion to meet agreed-upon deadlines
- Negotiates with the school leader for adequate resources for curriculum development
- Serves as an ex-officio member of the curriculum committee (if not already a member)
- Consults with subcommittees about their activities, as requested
- Provides information to speed the work of committees
- Initiates discussion (and perhaps negotiates) with other departments about non-nursing courses
- Liaises with the dean/director, advisory committee, and the nursing community
- Arranges for faculty development activities
- Prepares reports and finalizes documents for institutional approval of the curriculum
- Assists in marketing the new or revised curriculum
- Participates in planning curriculum implementation and evaluation.

Appointment of the Formal Curriculum Development Leader

Most schools will have a formal leader for the curriculum development process. The curriculum leader might be the undergraduate chair, chair of a standing curriculum committee, or another faculty member who is deemed to be appropriate. This individual could be appointed by the dean/director, or determined by faculty members. Typically, this will be an appointed position, since the inherent responsibilities will have implications for other aspects of the person's workload.

An alternative to selecting or appointing an internal leader is to seek direction from a curriculum consultant, who might be appointed for a short term. It is important to remember, however, that consultants should be chosen carefully according to their area of expertise related to curriculum development and to the needs of faculty. Typically, external consultants are short-term adjuncts to curriculum development, rather than an integral part of the daily activities.

In general, selection of the formal leader occurs in a manner congruent with usual practices in the school of nursing. Most frequently, the dean/director consults with faculty members; uses his or her own judgment about individuals' curriculum knowledge, interpersonal relationships, and capacity for leadership; and then comes to a decision about an appropriate choice. If, however, curriculum development leadership is already a part of the role description of the undergraduate chair or curriculum committee chair, ostensibly there will be no decision to be made. However, when that chair directs time and attention to leading curriculum redesign, the dean/director will have to appraise the extent of the chair's other responsibilities and perhaps make adjustments.

Career Development of Curriculum Leaders

Most leaders do not spring forth, fully confident and effective. Rather, they undergo a process of growth and maturation in the leader role. Warren C. Bennis (2004) likened an individual's development as a leader to a seven-stage process, akin to Shakespeare's *Seven Ages of Man* in *As You Like It*. Moving from the Infant Executive stage, where a beginning leader seeks to recruit a mentor for guidance, to Schoolboy, where the early leader learns how to do the job in public, subject to scrutiny; to the stage of Lover with a Woeful Ballad, struggling with the "tsunami" of problems every organization presents. In the fourth stage, Bearded Soldier, the leader becomes more effective, is willing, even eager to hire people better than him/herself, knowing talented underlings can help him or her shine. The effective leader then moves into the General stage, becoming adept at not simply allowing people to speak the truth but to actually being able to hear what they are saying. Subsequently, the superior leader, the Statesman, works hard to pass on wisdom in the interests of the organization. In the final stage, Sage, the superior leader embraces the role of mentor to young colleagues (pp. 46–53).

In contrast to Bennis's (2004) poetic view of leadership development, Carroll (2005) asserts that specific leadership competencies can be learned, and meaningful models of leadership should form part of graduate programs in nursing administration. She warns that cloning current leaders will not lead to success in an environment where complexity theory is used to manage organizations. According to Moody, Horton-Deutch, and Pesut (2007), academic leaders in nursing must monitor the complex systems of nursing education, research, and practice; respond to changing student populations and knowledge technologies; foster connections among faculty, administrators, and stakeholders; and persevere in a faculty shortage. Curriculum leaders must also function with these challenges, and, therefore, it is reasonable to conclude that planned curriculum leadership development is necessary.

Brubaker (2004) has proposed a deliberative process of development for curriculum leadership in the public school system. The elements include graduate education, developing and learning from one's professional autobiography, purposeful observations of leaders, a desire to be a curriculum leader, and engaging in activities to maintain one's motivation. All these are possible for nurse educators. For faculty without nursing education courses in their graduate programs, there are courses and certificate programs in nursing education, as well as a wealth of books about curriculum development and leadership. The desire to take on curriculum leadership will propel motivated faculty to seek opportunities to observe and consult with leaders, and to take on progressive curriculum responsibilities. Another important dimension of leadership development is having a mentor who observes the protégé, asks the protégé for self-assessment, and provides feedback. The protégé continues to practice with ongoing shared assessment (Mullen, 2007). As healthcare and nursing education systems become more complex, curriculum leaders with formal preparation for the role will be essential.

Faculty Development

Preparing leaders for the curriculum development process is essential to the success of this undertaking. If a faculty member with the necessary leadership knowledge, skill, and experience is willing to undertake this task, and is acceptable to the curriculum group, the work ahead will be expedited. However, if only a few among the faculty have sufficient preparation for curriculum development or leadership, especially curriculum leadership, faculty development preparation would be appropriate for them.

Selecting the curriculum leader, as well as those interested in being leaders for various curriculum task groups, is first and foremost. Faculty development activities for those interested could initially focus on what leadership is, leadership development and approaches, acceptance of leadership responsibilities, and importantly, specific information about what would be involved in developing the curriculum. Practicing curriculum leadership behaviors through role-playing might facilitate learning in these sessions.

If members with leadership and curriculum development experience are available, these persons could be called upon to mentor those without experience. Experienced faculty have a responsibility to nurture the next generation of curriculum leaders, and superior leaders (*Statesman* or *Sage*, according to Bennis, 2004), should feel obligated to embrace the role of mentor and to pass on their wisdom to novice colleagues. Developing leaders is especially important currently, since a large cohort of experienced faculty will soon be retiring and new faculty must be nurtured to assume curriculum leadership roles.

Chapter Summary

Effective leadership is of paramount importance in curriculum development. Determining who the formal curriculum leader will be, and the responsibilities inherent in the position, lay the groundwork for success. Curriculum development leadership requires knowledge of the curriculum process, management and organizational skills, and the ability to work collaboratively with others.

Synthesis
Activities

Two cases are presented for review and discussion. The first is critiqued to identify the key elements of leading curriculum development. Read the case carefully and analyze Dr. Romanatti's activities. Consider the analysis and propose additional ideas. The second is followed by questions to guide your critique. Finally, questions are presented about leading curriculum development in individual contexts.

Appleby University School of Nursing

The Dean of Appleby University School of Nursing, Dr. Marco Romanatti, has been in his position for 6 months, and after hearing complaints from some faculty about the curriculum, has decided that the development of a new curriculum is in order. This will be Dr. Romanatti's first experience in such a large educational undertaking, and he is eager to ensure that the process goes smoothly and quickly. He selected Dr. Louisa Ireland, a "senior" faculty member, who is friendly with many "junior" faculty, to serve as the formal curriculum development leader. He believes that Dr. Ireland would be acceptable to faculty, and after a brief conversation about Dr. Ireland's relationships with faculty, he asked her to lead the curriculum development activities. He subsequently called a meeting of all faculty members who would be expected to participate in curriculum development to inform them of his choice for the formal curriculum leader, and of his plans for developing the curriculum.

Critique

In his enthusiasm, Dr. Romanatti has taken on a transactional leadership role, in order to get the work done quickly, but this may not be suitable nor appreciated by the faculty. It would have been wise for Dr. Romanatti, before appointing Dr. Ireland, to consider if she has the necessary knowledge of nursing education, curriculum development, academic policies, approval processes, and so on. Discussion with a potential curriculum leader regarding the role and inherent responsibilities should also occur prior to making and announcing the appointment. The appointment is ultimately Dr. Romanatti's responsibility, but it must be a thoughtful appointment, and one for which he should seek faculty input.

Dr. Romanatti would be wise to ensure that his colleagues support the idea of curriculum development and that he has not responded to the wishes of only a few. He should accept that some faculty might only make a tentative commitment to engage in curriculum work until they are certain that the necessary resources have been secured. Moreover, some faculty may be unwilling to agree to participate in curriculum development simply because they do not know what the process involves. Once Dr. Romanatti is certain that there is agreement about the need for curriculum development, the curriculum leader, that person's role and responsibilities, and about the extent to which individual faculty are willing to participate, he can turn his attention to securing the necessary resources for the undertaking.

Mountainview College Department of Nursing

Mountainview Community College, an associate degree-granting college, is located in a medium-sized metropolitan city of approximately 400,000 inhabitants. Health facilities include four hospitals, several drop-in clinics staffed by physicians and primary health-care nurse practitioners, and a visiting nurse service in which all community-based health care except medical care is coordinated. The college provides business, technology, community service, and health science programs to approximately 6500 full- and part-time students. Among the programs is a 2-year, associate-degree nursing (ADN) program. Springhaven University is also located in the city and offers a 4-year baccalaureate nursing (BSN) program.

In addition to offering the 2-year ADN program, Mountainview College has entered into a collaborative partnership with Springhaven University to offer the first 2 years of the BSN program. Springhaven will offer the third and fourth years. There is agreement to develop a new curriculum together. Participants from both institutions and the health community are working collaboratively to develop the new BSN curriculum.

Questions for Consideration and Analysis of the Mountainview College Case

1. Describe matters that the dean of nursing at Springhaven University and the chair of the nursing department at Mountainview Community College should discuss about leadership of the collaborative curriculum development project.

2. What factors should be considered when deciding on leadership for the collaborative curriculum development process?

3. How might a curriculum leader be selected or appointed? Who should the leader be? Should there be two leaders, one for each institution? Why or why not? How could community nursing leaders contribute to the leadership of the curriculum development enterprise?

4. What should be included in a faculty development program to prepare potential curriculum leaders?

Curriculum Development Activities for Consideration in Your Setting

The following questions might stimulate thinking about leading curriculum development in your setting.

1. What qualities are important in a formal leader? What qualities could be important to our faculty and colleagues? Do we have such a leader?

2. Which leadership styles have been or could be effective in our school of nursing? Who has exhibited these styles?

3. Which faculty members have the expert knowledge necessary to lead the curriculum development process?

4. How can we go about appointing a formal curriculum development leader? What approach should we use? How effective would this be in selecting the best curriculum development leader?

5. Who could contribute to faculty development for curriculum leadership?

References

Bass, B., & Avolio, B. (1990). *Transformational leadership development: Manual for the multifactor leadership questionnaire.* Palo Alto, CA: Consulting Psychology Press.

Bennis, W. G. (2004). The seven ages of the leader. *Harvard Business Review, 82*(1), 46–53.

Bernhard, L. A., & Walsh, M. (1990). *Leadership. The key to the professionalization of nursing* (2nd ed.). St. Louis, MO: C.V. Mosby.

Blake, R., & Mouton, J. (1964). *The managerial grid.* Houston, TX: Gulf.

Brubaker, D. L. (2004). *Creative curriculum leadership.* Thousand Oaks, CA: Corwin Press.

Carroll, T. L. (2005). Leadership skills and attributes of women and nurse executives. *Nursing Administration Quarterly, 29*, 146–153.

Chan, A. T. S., & Chan, E. H. W. (2005). Impact of perceived leadership styles on work outcomes: Case of building professionals. *Journal of Construction Engineering and Management, 131*, 413–422.

Cheng, B. S., Chou, L. F., Wu, T. Y., Huang, M. P., & Farh, J. L. (2004). Paternalistic leadership and subordinate responses: Establishing a leadership model in Chinese organizations. *Asian Journal of Social Psychology, 7*(1), 89–117.

Collins, J. (2005). Level 5 leadership: The triumph of humility and fierce resolve. *Harvard Business Review, 83*(7–8), 136–146.

Fiedler, F. (1967). *A theory of leadership effectiveness.* New York: McGraw-Hill.

Fullan, M. (2001). *Leading in a culture of change.* San Francisco: Jossey-Bass.

Fullan, M. (2003). *Change forces with a vengeance.* London: Routledge Falmer.

Fullan, M. (2005). *Leadership sustainability. Systems thinkers in action.* Thousand Oaks, CA: Corwin Press.

Goldenberg, D. (1990). Nursing education leadership: Effect of situational and constraint variables on leadership style. *Journal of Advanced Nursing, 15*, 1326–1334.

Hersey, P., Blanchard, K. H., & Johnson, D. E. (1996). *Management of organizational behavior. Utilizing human resources* (7th ed.). Upper Saddle River, NJ: Prentice-Hall.

Huber, D. (2000). *Leadership and nursing care management* (2nd ed.). Philadelphia: W. B. Saunders.

Kellerman, B. (2004). Leadership. Warts and all. *Harvard Business Review, 82*(1), 40–45, 112.

Lewis, D., French, E., & Phetmany, T. (2000). Cross-cultural diversity: Leadership and workplace relations in Australia. *Asia Pacific Business Review, 7*(1), 105–125.

Maak, T., & Pless, N. M. (2006). Responsible leadership in a stakeholder society—A relational perspective. *Journal of Business Ethics, 66*(1), 99–115.

Marquis, B. L., & Huston, C. J. (2006). *Leadership roles and management functions in nursing. Theory and application* (5th ed.). Philadelphia: Lippincott Williams & Wilkins.

McGregor, D. (1960). *The human side of enterprise.* New York: McGraw-Hill.

Moody, R. C., Horton-Deutch, S., & Pesut, D. J. (2007). Appreciative inquiry for leading in complex systems: Supporting the transformation of academic nursing culture. *Journal of Nursing Education, 46,* 319–324.

Mullen, C. A. (2007). *Curriculum leadership development: A guide for aspiring school leaders.* Mahwah, NJ: Lawrence Erlbaum.

Polifko-Harris, K. (2004). *Case applications in nursing leadership and management.* Clifton Park, NY: Thomson, Delmar Learning.

Porter-O'Grady, T., & Malloch, K. (2007). *Quantum leadership: A resource for health care innovation* (2nd ed.). Boston: Jones and Bartlett.

Prentice, W. C. H. (2004). Understanding leadership. *Harvard Business Review, 82*(1), 102–109.

Registered Nurses Association of Ontario. (2006). Developing and sustaining leadership. *Nurse Best Practice Guidelines. Healthy Work Environment.* Toronto: Author.

Robbins, B., & Davidhizar, R. (2007). Transformational leadership in health care today. *Health Care Manager, 26,* 234–239.

Scarborough, J. D. (2002). Transforming leadership: An assessment tool. *Journal of Industrial Technology, 18*(2), 8.

Schnebel, E. (2000). Values in decision-making processes: Systematic structures of J. Habermas and N. Luhmann for the appreciation of responsibility in leadership. *Journal of Business Ethics, 27*(1), 79–88.

Schneider, M. (2002). A stakeholder model of organizational leadership. *Organizational Science, 13*(2), 209–221.

Scott, J. G., Sochalski, J., & Aiken, L. (1999). Review of magnet hospital research: Findings and implications for nursing practice. *Journal of Nursing Administration, 29*(1), 9–19.

Searle Leach, L. (2003). Leadership and management. In. P. Kelly-Heidenthal, *Nursing leadership and management* (pp. 157–180). Clifton Park, NY: Thomson, Delmar Learning.

Shamian, J. (2005). Be true to yourself and your values. *Canadian Journal of Nursing Leadership, 18*(3). Retrieved October 30, 2007, from http://longwoods.com/product.php?productid=17613

Skelton-Green, J., Simpson, B., & Scott, J. (2007). An integrated approach to change leadership. *Canadian Journal of Nursing Leadership, 20*(3). Retrieved October 30, 2007, from http://longwoods.com/product.php? productid=17227&cat=511&page=1

Sullivan, E. J., & Decker, P. J. (2005). *Effective leadership and management in nursing* (6th ed.). Upper Saddle River, NJ: Pearson Prentice Hall.

Wiles, J., & Bondi, J. (1998). *Curriculum development: A guide to practice* (5th ed.). Upper Saddle River, NJ: Merrill, an imprint of Prentice Hall.

Yoder-Wise, P. S. (2007). *Leading and managing in nursing* (4th ed.). St. Louis, MO: Mosby Elsevier.

Zaleznik, A. (2004). Managers and leaders. Are they different? *Harvard Business Review, 82*(1), 74–81, 113.

CHAPTER 4

Organizing Curriculum Development

Chapter Overview

This chapter provides practical guidelines about the first steps of curriculum development that will be helpful for organizing the work ahead. Once a decision has been made to proceed with curriculum development, it is essential that the enterprise be organized in such a way that the work can be satisfactorily completed in a timely fashion. Matters such as stakeholders to be involved, committee structure, decision-making, work plans, authorship, academic freedom, faculty development, and the acquisition of resources must be decided before the process of curriculum development can begin. Remember, there is no precise sequence for attending to these issues; in reality they are usually addressed concurrently. Agreements achieved about committee structure, membership, decision-making approaches, and so forth, are all subject to review and revision as curriculum development proceeds.

A discussion of activities associated with organizing curriculum development is followed by ideas about faculty development related to the initial organization. The synthesis activities that conclude the chapter comprise a case study and critique to illustrate the main ideas of the chapter, a second case for analysis, and questions to guide activities to organize curriculum development in readers' settings.

Chapter Goals

- Overview factors important in organizing curriculum development.
- Identify stakeholders who should be involved in curriculum development.
- Consider activities to organize curriculum development.
- Contemplate faculty development activities related to organizing curriculum development.

Organizing Curriculum Development

Development and implementation of a redesigned curriculum leads to changes in the culture of the school: what activities are undertaken, how they are completed, and how members relate to one another. Therefore, when beginning to organize curriculum development activities, it is important to select a change theory to guide the overall processes of curriculum development and culture change. Consideration is given to persons who will be involved; committees and subcommittees that will complete or facilitate the work; decision-making and approval processes; as well as the required resources to facilitate the ongoing work. It would also be prudent to consider faculty workload and academic freedom issues in order to prevent serious concerns or disagreements. Deciding on publication and authorship potential related to the development process and the finalized curriculum should be discussed early. Defining the context in which the work will proceed and bringing some order to curriculum development activities expedites the subsequent work and helps to make the process seem possible to those who are new to curriculum development.

Selection of a Change Theory

Selection of a change theory to guide the overall processes of curriculum development and implementation, and the attendant culture change, will allow curriculum developers to have a framework for their activities. A change theory can give direction to the activities that need to occur with the total faculty group and stakeholders as they undertake and complete their work.

An example of the use of a change theory is provided by King Mixon, Kemp, Towle, and Schrader (2005). In the development of a curriculum that merged three nursing programs at Boise State University, Kotter's Eight-Stage Process was used as a framework for organizing the work. This process was directed at the creation of both a curriculum and a new and unified culture:

- Stage 1: Create a sense of urgency and take control of the process.
- Stage 2: Create a guiding coalition of stakeholders; build trust and a common goal.

- Stage 3: Develop the vision, strategy, and philosophy. Create task forces to work on vision; outcomes, threads and competencies, admissions and progression; marketing; and organizational culture.
- Stage 4: Communicate the vision and strategies.
- Stage 5: Develop empowering and broad-based action through the creation of work teams to address curriculum, organizational culture and design, outcomes assessment, advisement, recruitment and marketing, student affairs, and scholarship.
- Stage 6: Generate short-term wins; celebrate curriculum approval and recruitment success.
- Stage 7: Consolidate gains to produce more change in the culture.
- Stage 8: Anchor cultural changes.

Another theory that could be used is the Transtheoretical Model of Behavior Change (Prochaska, DiClemente, & Norcross, 1992; Prochaska et al., 2004; Prochaska, Redding, Harlow, Rossi, & Velicer, 1994). In Chapter 5, the theory is described and applied to faculty development and change during curriculum development and implementation. Whichever theory is chosen, intentional use of a theoretical perspective provides a means to plan activities and understand the processes that are occurring within individuals and the total group as they develop a redesigned curriculum and experience culture change.

Determining Who Should Be Involved

Although many stakeholders should be involved, shaping the curriculum is very much the province of the *nursing faculty* as they have the most direct influence on curriculum development by virtue of their knowledge, experience, and decision-making power (Conley, 1973). Experienced faculty members offer knowledge of curriculum development, institutional policies and resources, and health care in the community. Their insights provide structure and guidance to the process. Novices bring new ideas that are not bound by traditions in the school of nursing (Hull, St. Romain, Alexander, Schaff, & Jones, 2001), and thereby help to move the group's thinking forward.

In programs with educational partners who share in offering nursing courses, the partner faculty members should also be involved, and not only the nursing members of the credential-granting institution. Indeed, curriculum development is the pivotal and ongoing point of faculty activity in the majority of nursing programs (Rush, Ouellet, & Wasson, 1991). Those who participate will likely feel most responsible and strongly invested in the curriculum and will strive to implement it in the manner envisioned.

However, accountability for revising or creating a curriculum does not belong solely to faculty members who will be teaching in the redesigned curriculum. *Faculty members from other programs in the school* have important contributions to make and should be involved, since they can bring a different perspective of nursing and nursing education, broadening curriculum discussions. As well, *faculty from other disciplines* relevant to nursing should be invited to participate, not necessarily for the direct contributions they can make, but to build support for the curriculum through their ongoing interaction with nursing faculty.

The *dean/director* participates in curriculum development through delegation of responsibilities to the curriculum leader, and/or by active involvement in the process. This involvement, however, will depend on other responsibilities and priorities in the school and institution, but such participation would signify the importance of curriculum development to the school and parent institution. Importantly, the dean/director is obligated to ensure that necessary resources are available so curriculum development can proceed.

Active participation by *institutional administrators* is unlikely to occur. Yet, they can be invited to events celebrating milestones in curriculum development. In this way, their interest and support may increase.

Student participation in curriculum development is very important (Thornton & Chapman, 2000), as they bring previous experiences and perspectives, needs, and aspirations, which, when combined, influence the curriculum. Their role should be as credible as that of other participants (Attridge, 1996). Active involvement by learners helps them understand the complexity of curriculum development, and builds support for the curriculum. As well, periodic requests for information or reaction to proposals from student groups conveys that their role in shaping the curriculum is valued and that they have a professional responsibility to improve nursing education for current and future colleagues.

The importance of collaborative interface with *colleagues from practice settings* should not be overlooked. Service agencies are affected by the curriculum and potential faculty role changes. Clinical experts and leaders can provide useful, practical input, and validate suggested practice changes. Curriculum dialogue among clinicians, faculty, students, and administrators has been described as mutually enriching, not only to themselves, but to the nursing curriculum and profession (Carmon, Hauber, & Chase, 1992). In particular, the involvement of colleagues from practice settings can lead to the development of collaborative projects to enhance clinical learning environments (Palmer, Harmer Cox, Clark Callister, Johnsen, & Matsumara, 2005).

Who else should be involved in the curriculum development process? Anyone from the larger community, according to Rentschler and Spegman (1996). This could include *program graduates, professors emeriti, healthcare leaders, educators from the school system, community leaders, and clients,* as well as *members of professional bodies.* Their knowledge, experience, and vested interests would assure that standards are maintained and expectations of preparing nurses "for the changing healthcare field, rapid proliferation of health knowledge and technology, and diverse client needs" (Rentschler & Spegman, p. 390) would be upheld. Table 4-1 presents a summary of those who could be involved in curriculum development.

Table 4-1   Persons Involved in Curriculum Development

Graduate and undergraduate nursing faculty

Nursing students

Program graduates

Professors emeriti

Educational institution administrators

Healthcare leaders

Clinicians

Members of professional nursing associations

Community leaders

Clients

Faculty from other disciplines

Educators from the school system

Deciding Committee Structure

After agreement is reached on a change theory to guide the overall curriculum development and implementation process, and about stakeholders who should be involved in curriculum development, it is necessary to determine which committees should be formed, their structure, and functions. Committees are essential for developing a curriculum, not only because the work must be shared, but also because the discussion that occurs during meetings leads to agreement and acceptance of ideas.

Organizing Committee Structure   The key to successful curriculum development is a committee structure conducive to the task, yet amenable to modification if necessary. Activities of all committees and subcommittees ought to proceed in an organized fashion, be based on realistic expectations, and be supported by adequate resources. When structuring committees, important considerations are the purposes of the committee, membership, tasks to be accomplished, methods of achieving the work, and deadlines for completion. These are the *what, how, who,* and *when* aspects of the proposed committees.

The committee structure (number, purpose, and membership of committees) should be considered carefully so that it facilitates curriculum development. This requires attention to determining the best way to accomplish the curriculum development work and associated responsibilities (such as gaining community support), while ensuring inclusion of all faculty, interested learners, and stakeholders. The types of committees that could be suitable and ideas about membership follow. Each committee or subcommittee should have a clear purpose, and its accountability and deadlines must be defined.

Organizing also requires that the designated curriculum leader and members together establish strategies to achieve the task of curriculum development expeditiously. Policies, plans, and activities to accomplish the tasks, and the best way to use available human and material resources, must be agreed upon. Committees, groups, and individuals, tied together horizontally and vertically through a common vision of the overall goal, possibly overlapping membership, facilitative relationships, shared communication, and information systems, will most likely be necessary to complete the activities. Thus, the work groups are organized in a relational design (Porter-O'Grady & Malloch, 2007).

Within the committees, it is necessary to establish member roles; define tasks; schedule meetings; arrange for the recording of minutes; and do the work assigned within the specified timeline. Leadership for particular curriculum development activities may be temporary, as leaders could be appointed, elected, or rotated, and because subcommittees will disband when their work is completed. Membership on particular curriculum committees or subcommittees is usually based on interest and expertise. In general, committee members require the following:

- A broad understanding of nursing education, the school of nursing, and the educational institution
- Knowledge of curriculum development, learning, teaching, evaluation of learning, educational and nursing philosophies, student characteristics and needs, available resources, graduation requirements, approval and/or accreditation standards, and licensing requirements
- Familiarity with healthcare issues and the community to be served.

Types of Committees   Undoubtedly, a workable committee structure includes a *curriculum committee* of dedicated, knowledgeable participants who will be responsible for the overall development of the proposed curriculum. Members of the curriculum committee will become members of subcommittees.

A possible committee structure could be one that allows all members to function as a *total faculty group*, which develops and approves all curriculum proposals. This type of structure can be effective in a small school of nursing. However, in most schools, such a structure could slow curriculum development and, therefore, it is more usual for the total faculty group to come together to discuss and approve the work of subcommittees. Use of a total faculty group at critical points in curriculum development can promote faculty buy-in.

The use of *subcommittees* or *task forces (ad hoc committees)* within the curriculum committee is another structure to consider. These facilitate optimal participation of all people involved in curriculum development. Discrete tasks such as collecting contextual data, formulating the philosophical approaches, and writing curriculum outcome statements are given to the subcommittees. These small groups enable each participant to contribute and critique the work accomplished. They are transitory, task-oriented, and their dissolution is natural when the work is done. Usually, task forces do small short-term tasks, whereas subcommittees have the total ongoing responsibility of developing their portion of the curriculum and reporting back to the curriculum committee and the total faculty group. Like subcommittees, task groups provide feedback and generate more than one alternative for every phase of their work. According to Bevis (1989), each task force or subcommittee should undertake to:

- Set its own rules.
- Announce plans.
- Provide information.
- Make vested interests explicit and intellectual conflict legitimate.
- Identify high investment areas and risks.
- Incorporate changes and acceptable alternatives.
- Agree to respond to each others' contributions.
- Suggest ways to respond to deadlocked issues.
- Offer tentative or provisional decisions.

It is important to remember that views of stakeholders and curriculum planners are to be obtained while small group members are working on specific tasks. This can be done by inviting them to become members or to attend selected committee or task force meetings, by interviews with faculty members, through survey tools for reactions to issues and ideas, and by total faculty group meetings, with materials sent out beforehand for review. Perspectives of the total student body (in addition to student representation on committees) can be obtained in a similar manner.

In addition to subcommittees with responsibility for particular aspects of curriculum development, Bevis (1989) suggests the formation of a *critique committee* to review and comment on particular curriculum elements. Subcommittee members can ask questions, recommend clarification or expansion of some points, examine incongruities, suggest revision, and provide feedback, thereby adding validity to the work. Whether or not a critique committee is formed, it is essential that all curriculum development participants be kept informed, and have opportunities to provide input into subcommittees' work on an ongoing basis.

The school might also enlist the help of an *advisory committee*, made up of members from the academic and professional communities as well as consumers. These persons could be enlisted to serve on task forces or subcommittees. Advisory bodies are a useful source of information as well as a public relations mechanism to foster understanding and promotion of the curriculum.

Finally, a *steering committee* could be formed. This occurs most frequently when a curriculum is being planned and implemented by more than one institution. Committee membership can be composed of senior administrators of the institutions, deans/directors of the nursing program(s), and the curriculum committee chair(s). The number and organizational position of members from the involved institutions are usually equal. The steering committee might assume responsibilities such as:

- Offer direction to the curriculum initiative.
- Ensure that plans are in accordance with institutional policies, or alternatively identify needed changes in policies.
- Plan for sharing of resources, if appropriate.
- Liaise with institutional governing bodies and external organizations (e.g., nursing regulatory or government) as necessary.

It is prudent to consider the inclusion of senior administrators, not only on the advisory and steering committees, but on subcommittees as well. This will keep them apprised of curriculum developments and lessen the possibility of surprises and potential vetoes (Bevis, 1989).

Whatever committee structure is used, it is important to remember that the potential for success in curriculum development is directly related to the degree of participation of stakeholders. Continued interest, willingness, cooperation, and commitment should lead to timely completion of the curriculum.

Record Keeping

Meeting minutes are essential, and these should be up-to-date and complete. Copies of working papers, documents, and minutes used or developed by the committee members should be dated and retained. It is important to inventory what has been done and what is agreed upon. These materials are a history and story of the development and unfolding of the curriculum, and how abstract ideas become operational.

Attached to the formal meeting minutes should be any substantive discussion or decisions that have occurred via e-mail between meetings. Much work is done between meetings, of course, and the e-mail discussion among group members can easily be retained as part of the "paper trail" of the group's thinking and decisions. To a large extent, the e-mails form the minutes.

Establishing a Communication System

The work of each task force and committee has an influence on the work of others, and decisions that have been reached will affect all subsequent work. Therefore, a method should be established to ensure that all curriculum developers are informed of the work that is underway or has been approved. Keeping everyone informed of progress is important.

E-mail can be used for discussion within one group, but can become burdensome if there is a multitude of e-mails from all work groups. An alternative to e-mail can be the establishment of a computer conference site for curriculum discussion. A secure, accessible, online space allows for multiple, asynchronous, threaded discussions. The use of such a program will enable those involved in curriculum development to keep abreast of the work of all subcommittees. Most importantly, messages are dated and can be reviewed and printed to accompany or serve as minutes.

In addition, it would be wise to have a central location (either virtual or real) for all approved documents. In that way, there will be no doubt about what is 'official' and what is still being developed.

Determining Decision-Making and Approval Processes

Decision-making and approval processes to accomplish the work as expeditiously and smoothly as possible should be established. Those chosen will be dependent on the usual ways of making decisions and the required approval procedures in the school of nursing. Agreement about these processes is essential: decisions must be made, ratified, and accepted as a basis for ongoing curriculum development.

Decision-making A decision is a choice among alternatives, while decision-making is more complex, as it involves the act of choosing, and converting information into action. It is a systematic process that begins with the identification of a need or problem, and ends when an evaluation of the choice is completed. Moreover, decision-making differs from problem solving in that it is influenced by emotions and intuition, is purposeful and goal-oriented, involves a choice among options, and may not always start with a problem (Huber, 2000). However, according to Little-Stoetzel (2003), both decision-making and problem solving use critical thinking, since an effective decision maker or critical thinker "generates new ideas and alternatives when making decisions [and uses] four basic skills, i.e., critical reading, critical listening, critical writing, and critical speaking [as] part of developing and using thinking for decision-making" (p. 429).

Decision-making might also be the "result of opportunities, challenges, or leadership initiatives" (Huber, 2000, p. 378). It implies responsibility and anticipation of consequences. Decision-making is considered to be the essence of leadership, and making decisions could be the most important aspect of a job, the most difficult, and the riskiest. Good decisions usually lead to attainment of goals, whereas bad decisions can impede progress, waste resources, cause harm or damage, and ultimately affect careers. Some core elements of decision-making include those listed below:

- Identifying a problem, issue, or situation
- Establishing criteria for evaluating potential solutions
- Searching for alternative solutions or actions
- Evaluating the alternatives
- Choosing specific alternatives. (Huber, 2000)

Some decision-making techniques are outlined in Table 4-2.

Table 4-2   Decision-Making Techniques

- trial and error
- pilot project
- problem critique: technique in which problem is outlined, facts determined, and potential solutions proposed
- creativity techniques: brainstorming, delphi process, and nominal group
- decision tree or critical pathways
- fish-bone (or cause and effect chart)
- group problem solving and decision-making
- cost-benefit analysis
- worst case scenario

Source: [Data from Huber, D. (2000). *Leadership and nursing care management.* (2nd ed.). Philadelphia: W. B. Saunders, pp. 384–387].

Decision-making Styles   Not only is decision-making thought of as a process with identifiable steps, there are various decision-making styles, types (models), and strategies. Decision styles, as with leadership, range from *authoritarian* or *autocratic,* in which the leader makes the decision alone; *consultative, collective,* or *participative,* where the leader seeks input before making the final decision; *facilitative,* in which the leader and group combined reach a shared decision; and *delegative,* where only the group makes the decision and the leader gives up control over the decision (Hersey, Blanchard, & Johnson, 1996).

Two types of decisions have been described: *satisfying,* which implies choosing any solution that will satisfy or minimally meet the desired goals; and *optimizing,* which involves comparing all possible solutions against the goals and choosing the one that best meets them. Satisficing decisions are easier to make since the decision maker chooses the first and quickest solution for solving the problem, while sacrificing a fuller analysis of the situation. The speed of the decision might even inspire support from the group. To find the best solution, with the potential for effectiveness and acceptability by the group, an optimizing solution would be the logical choice (Bernhard & Walsh, 1990).

Optimal Curriculum Decisions Curriculum development and design can never become a matter of routine or formulae. Curriculum development must rely on decisions determined by a variety of ideas, imagination, facts, theories, and creativity. Furthermore, curriculum decision-making is complicated as it involves people who have various levels of curriculum expertise, vested interests, private hopes and dreams, different ideas and emotions, and the desire to give the best possible education for students (Bevis, 2000).

Decisions about curriculum should not be constrained by rules or rigid formulae, but rather be guided by desired curriculum outcomes, group acceptance, and fit with internal and external contextual factors. Decision makers should acknowledge that previous decisions influence each new or subsequent decision and that new decisions may lead to a reconsideration of previous choices. Optimal decision-making, therefore, is an iterative, dynamic, and interactive process grounded in contextual reality.

Approval Processes Agreement about which decisions need formal approval, and the approval processes that will be followed, is necessary. Of course, the completed curriculum will require the formal approval mandated by the institution. However, during the development process, curricular elements may need formal approval within the school of nursing, as determined in advance. Following are questions that might help in identifying an effective approval process.

- Which aspects of the curriculum work require formal approval? By whom?
- How will the work of the task groups or subcommittees receive endorsement? Through circulation to, and feedback from, all faculty members? By the curriculum committee? By the total faculty group? All of these?

Establishing a Work Plan

When engaged in curriculum work, participants will have to redirect time and energy from other activities into curriculum development. Resources may have to be shifted from one committee to another. Assigning time to work on the curriculum during the summer when teaching responsibilities may be lighter is a usual practice. However, it is not always effective because communication can break down resulting in reduced commitment to the developing curriculum.

Curriculum development can be a slow process if groups meet infrequently. As well, the process cannot be effective if crisis-oriented approaches are used and work is begun immediately before deadlines. Accordingly, a written, realistic timetable to guide the activities of the group is important, as it places the activity in the context of its priority and the group's commitment to the entire process. Too short a time period could be self-defeating or viewed as a lack of regard for members' time and other responsibilities. In contrast, too extended a time interval can lead to discouragement, disinterest, and disenchantment with the process and progress. A written timetable, shared with all, will help to maintain participant interest and support the expectation that a revised or reconceptualized curriculum will be accomplished.

Regular meetings should be scheduled for participants to carefully assess, study, and create new ideas. If there are enough committed and qualified committee members who have expertise or who seek assistance, and who also meet on a regular basis, the goal of a developed curriculum will be achieved in a timely manner. It is neither practical nor productive to spend an extensive period of time on any one component of the curriculum. Despite the discomfort that may accompany decisions that are not firmly fixed, the group should move on to completion. As the work progresses through subsequent meetings, final decisions can be accomplished.

Critical Path Prerequisite for undertaking a project as large as curriculum development is the establishment of a detailed work plan. Initially, there must be agreement about the date when the first courses of the redesigned curriculum will be implemented. That date will be influenced by the reasons for, and extent of, curriculum development necessary. This implementation date will set the pace of the curriculum development activities and approval deadlines.

Major elements of the curriculum development process must be identified and a timeline specified, responsibility assigned for activities, procedures determined for recording meeting minutes and decisions, and the work shared. Initial decisions may need to be reviewed as the work progresses and circumstances not apparent at the outset become evident. The creation of a work plan will bring definition to the curriculum development process.

The critical path is a blueprint for action, specifying the steps to be completed, the deadlines, and the individuals or committees responsible for each phase of the curriculum development process. It provides a concrete means to assess whether the curriculum is being developed at a pace that will ensure implementation by the target date. Dates of key meetings and reporting intervals can be included as part of the critical path (Smith, 1999). As well, the start date of each activity can be included to emphasize when the work must begin to achieve the deadline (Puich, 2007). Although revisions may become necessary, the critical path explicates the work to be done and the timeframe in which it must be completed. Importantly, a detailed critical path provides the rationale for requesting resources.

Agreeing on deadlines for the major milestones of curriculum development is the first step in the creation of a critical path. Typically, the initial decision is to determine the implementation date of the first courses, by placing it first on the critical path. This highlights or gives preeminence to the implementation date of the redesigned curriculum. After deciding when the curriculum is to begin, the next step is to calculate back to the date the educational institution must approve the curriculum design. The total time available to finalize the curriculum will be evident. Major activities that should occur before final approval and their associated deadlines must be identified. It is helpful to note which individual or committee will have responsibility for each aspect of the process, as well as the approval procedures necessary throughout curriculum development. In addition, subcommittee members may find it helpful to develop critical paths for their work.

Table 4-3 provides an example of a critical path, beginning with the implementation date of the curriculum and working backward in time to when the curriculum development process actually begins. A 2-year period for the development of a typical 4-year undergraduate program is presented in consideration of the time needed for the change process among faculty (Mawn & Reece, 2000), various levels of approval that may exist in some institutions, and realities of faculty members' other responsibilities. Once the reverse ordering is completed, the chart can be rotated so that it starts with the most immediate activities and ends with curriculum implementation. This is the critical path. Alternately, a Gantt chart could be devised. The advantage of the Gantt chart is that it illustrates the duration of activities. A Gantt chart to match Table 4-3 is presented in Table 4-4, with the shaded areas representing the time period to work on each activity.

Table 4-3   Example of a Critical Path for Curriculum Development

Activities to Be Completed	Deadline (Time from Curriculum Start Date)	Individual or Group Responsible for Activity
Implement 1st year of new curriculum	24 months	School director
Prepare detailed syllabi of 1st year courses	22 months	Course professors
Interpret curriculum to clinical agencies, professional bodies	22 months	Curriculum leader Curriculum committee
Mount Web site	21 months	Curriculum leader Curriculum committee Marketing consultant Web designer
Prepare necessary documents for approval of curriculum by university governing body	21 months	Curriculum leader School director
Present curriculum to advisory body	21 months	Curriculum leader
Prepare and present motions for curriculum approval by total faculty group	20 months	Curriculum leader
Present curriculum to steering committee	20 months	Curriculum leader
Finalize curriculum design and policies	20 months	Total faculty group
Refine and negotiate courses and policies	19 months	Curriculum committee Designated subcommittees

continues

Table 4-3 continued

Activities to Be Completed	Deadline (Time from Curriculum Start Date)	Individual or Group Responsible for Activity
Present program policies to curriculum committee	17 months	Program policy subcommittee
Present course descriptions, outcomes and major content areas to curriculum committee	16 months	Course development teams
Establish course development teams	13 months	Curriculum committee
Finalize curriculum matrix	12 months	Total faculty group
Negotiate non-nursing courses	12 months	Curriculum leader
Develop curriculum matrix with nursing and non-nursing courses	10 months	Curriculum committee
Finalize curriculum philosophical approaches and outcome statements	8 months	Total faculty group
Present draft curriculum outcome statements to curriculum committee	6 months	Goals subcommittee
Present draft philosophical approaches to curriculum committee	5 months	Philosophical approaches subcommittee
Agree on curriculum nucleus	5 months	Total faculty group
Present synthesis of contextual data	4 months	Data collection subcommittee
Collect contextual data	3 months	Data collection subcommittee
Establish subcommittees and task forces	Immediately	Curriculum committee
Initiate faculty development	Immediately and ongoing	Curriculum leader
Identify major steps of curriculum development process and create critical path	Immediately	Curriculum committee
Form advisory committee	Immediately	School director Curriculum leader
Form steering committee	Immediately	School director, and/or nominations and elections committee
Appoint curriculum leader	Immediately	School director with faculty input

Table 4-4 Gantt Chart for Curriculum Development

Task/Activity	Accountability	0	1	2	3	4	5	6	7	8	9	10	11	12	13
Appoint curriculum leader	School director	■													
Form steering committee and advisory body	School director and curriculum leader	■													
Identify major steps; create critical path; establish subcommittees	Curriculum committee	■													
Plan, implement faculty development	Curriculum leader	■	■	■	■	■							■	■	■
Collect and synthesize contextual data and present to curriculum committee	Data collection subcommittee	■	■	■	■	■									
Agree on curriculum nucleus	Total faculty group						■								
Prepare draft philosophical approaches and outcome statements and present to curriculum committee	Philosophical approaches and goals subcommittees					■	■	■							
Finalize philosophical approaches and outcome statements	Total faculty group							■	■	■					
Develop curriculum matrix	Curriculum committee										■	■			
Negotiate nonnursing courses	Curriculum leader											■	■	■	
Finalize curriculum matrix	Total faculty group													■	
Establish course development teams	Curriculum committee														■

Time in Months from Start Date

Table 4-4   continued

| | | Time in Months from Start Date | | | | | | | | | | |
Task/Activity	Accountability	14	15	16	17	18	19	20	21	22	23	24
Plan, implement faculty development	Curriculum leader	■										■
Prepare course goals, descriptions and major content areas and present to curriculum committee	Course development teams	■	■	■								
Prepare program policies and present to curriculum committee	Policy subcommittee			■	■							
Refine and negotiate courses and policies	Curriculum committee and subcommittee				■	■						
Finalize curriculum design and policies	Total faculty group					■	■	■				
Present curriculum to steering committee	Curriculum leader								■			
Present curriculum to advisory body	Curriculum leader								■			
Prepare documents for curriculum approval by governing body	Curriculum leader							■				
Mount Web site	Curriculum leader, curriculum committee, Web designer							■	■			
Interpret curriculum to clinical agencies, professional bodies	Curriculum committee									■	■	
Prepare detailed syllabi for first courses	Course professors									■	■	
Implement curriculum	School director											■

Many other activities and meetings could be added to the critical path. For example, meetings of the total faculty group and the curriculum committee might be included, as well as regular meetings with the dean/director. It is important to find a comfortable balance such that the critical path can specify the major work to be done without being overly detailed. Committees or individuals can develop other critical paths to ensure that their work will be completed to match the major deadlines.

Approaches to Sharing the Work Inherent in all group work is the need to determine how activities will be completed. *Who will do what, and to what standard?* This determination is partly accomplished by decisions about committee structures. Yet, within each committee, the matter of how to share the work will arise, and the approach is unlikely to be identical in each committee and subcommittee. In some, all members may prefer to work together as much as possible, to explore ideas and achieve consensus before much writing is done. For others, there may be a desire to divide tasks among individuals or dyads, who would then bring back draft work to the group for discussion, revision, and consensus. Likely, some combination of these approaches will be agreed upon, depending on the nature of the task and the imminence of deadlines. Although it is beyond the scope of this book to describe all aspects of successful group functioning, some elements are worthy of review when considering how curriculum development can be accomplished:

- Agree on the goals to be achieved, including the task to be accomplished, the deadline for completion, and the standard of the work.
- Obtain commitment from each member to achieve the goals.
- Identify how much time each member can give to the task.
- Discuss how the group will work together.
- Consider the value of preparing a critical path for the group's work.

Because the quality of interpersonal relationships is given considerable attention in nursing education, novice curriculum developers may have high expectations that curriculum work will lead to close personal connections and personal affirmation. However, it is important to recognize that not all work groups will become cohesive teams whose synergy is intrinsically motivating (Wylie & Smith, 1999), and that, nonetheless, high-quality work can be accomplished.

Schedule of Meetings Developing a schedule of meetings for committees and task forces will both expedite the work of curriculum development and keep the groups on track for completing their tasks. These can be included in the critical path, or a separate listing of meeting dates can be prepared to coincide with the critical path. In either case, early development of a meeting schedule with a notation about the major task to be achieved will help to ensure that curriculum developers reserve the time for meetings and that curriculum work proceeds in a timely fashion.

Securing Resources

As the overall plan for curriculum development is shaped, the necessary resources will become apparent. Concrete requests for resources should be made. The requests could include release time from teaching for key curriculum developers; a specific budget for data collection activities, faculty development, or curriculum consultation; and secretarial support. Although alterations in work assignments may be subject to collective agreements, they are worthy of exploration, since it is primarily the faculty who must develop, accept, and implement the curriculum.

Identifying the Relationship of Curriculum Development to Academic Freedom

The contributions of all faculty members to curriculum development are essential for a successful outcome. Academic freedom is "the free search for truth and its free exposition" (American Association of University Professors, n.d.). This includes freedom in teaching, research, publication, and criticism of the institution. Writing about academic freedom and scientific inquiry in nursing, Kneipp, Canales, Fahrenwald, and Taylor (2007) state, "... with academic freedom comes academic duty . . . the duty to argue persuasively and logically for theoretical perspectives, areas of research and new methodological approaches, that you as a member of the scientific community, believe hold merit for advancing science in your field" (p. 8). The same duty applies to nursing curriculum development. Each faculty member has the obligation to argue logically for preferred curricular perspectives, advance a position about the nature and content of the curriculum, and propose how the suggested perspective will advance the curriculum.

Larson (1997) suggests that faculty sometimes perceive academic freedom as giving each nursing faculty member the right to plan courses independently, without attention to how these conform to the entire curriculum. She contends that this is not realistic nor should it be supported. "Academic freedom is a qualified right . . . a privilege enjoyed in consequence of incumbency in . . . an academic role and it is enjoyed conditionally in conformity with certain obligations to the academic institution and its rules and standards" (Shils, 1993, p. 189). The standards for the nursing curriculum are established by the nursing faculty and each member is obligated to plan courses in accordance with those standards.

Faculty are granted freedom in the classroom in discussing their subject (American Association of University Professors, n.d.; Canadian Association of University Teachers, 1979). Yet, teaching must be undertaken "with due respect to what is thought by qualified colleagues" (Shils, 1993, p. 190). It is for this reason that curricula are created collaboratively: the curriculum represents the consensus of colleagues.

There must be unity and progression within professional curricula. Therefore, creating courses in isolation from one another, or without reference to agreed-upon philosophical approaches or curriculum outcome statements, is neither acceptable nor sound. Curriculum development, however, should not be so constrained that creativity, pedagogical preferences, and expertise of faculty are stifled. There should be a balance between faculty autonomy and curriculum intent. A frank discussion among faculty and the dean/director would ensure resolution of the latitude possible within courses.

Contributing to curriculum development by all faculty members is essential for a successful outcome. Because this requirement may compete with other scholarly activities, such as research, some faculty may feel their academic freedom is restricted. If this is the case, open discussion about academic rights and responsibilities is warranted. Accordingly, it may be reasonable to adjust the work assignments of some faculty.

Determining Potential for Publication and Authorship

The possibility of publication arising from the curriculum development, implementation, and evaluation process should be discussed and agreed to in advance by all participants. Dialogue about this must occur early, since many expository and research articles could be generated as part of curriculum development.

Publications about the curriculum development process itself are important to consider. There may be aspects of the process that are unique, or insights attained that are worthy of sharing through journal articles and conference presentations. Often the lessons learned are relevant to curriculum developers in other settings. If it is decided that there are some researchable questions or other new knowledge that could add to the body of curriculum development scholarship, the topic of authorship should be addressed.

Many issues should be resolved at the onset. Among these are: Will one person or a team be responsible for writing proposals and articles? How will contributors be acknowledged in publications? Will primary authorship rotate among faculty or be dependent on who takes the leadership role in specific publications? Perhaps there are faculty on the curriculum development team who would thrive if involved in research and writing, and this could be an added incentive for their participation in curriculum development.

Faculty Development

Once a decision has been made to proceed with curriculum development, it is worthwhile to have a faculty development session about the curriculum development process itself. Specifically, a summary of the entire process will help novices appreciate that curriculum development is an iterative process, replete with concurrent and recurrent sub-processes. However, to ensure that faculty members do not feel overwhelmed, it is wise to identify the concrete tasks that ensure timely completion of the work. The goal is for faculty to comprehend the process and believe that it is manageable. An overview of the logistics of getting organized is essential so faculty will believe that the work is achievable.

Chapter Summary

Getting organized for curriculum development activities comprises attention to both the processes of working together and the logistics of getting the work done. Effective decision-making procedures are of paramount importance. Determining committee structures and establishing a work plan provide a concrete basis for progress. Inclusion of people beyond the nursing faculty will assist with completion of the work and broaden the perspectives of nursing faculty, and ultimately, the curriculum. Attention should be given to issues of academic freedom and publication possibilities at the beginning of the curriculum development process, since these are directly relevant to the careers of nursing faculty.

Synthesis Activities

Two cases are presented for review and discussion. The first is critiqued to identify the key elements of organizing for curriculum development. Read the case carefully and analyze Dr. Kirakova's activities. Consider the analysis and propose additional or alternative ideas. The second case is followed by questions to guide your critique. Finally, questions are presented about organizing for curriculum development.

Bevis University School of Nursing

The undergraduate chair of Bevis University School of Nursing, Dr. Svetlana Kirakova, has been appointed curriculum development leader as the school undertakes the creation of a reconceptualized curriculum. The school director appreciates Dr. Kirakova's knowledge of curriculum and organizational ability, and believes that she is the most suitable person to lead the endeavor. Dr. Kirakova immediately begins to think about the committees that will need to be formed, the time that faculty will require for curriculum work, stakeholders to include, and the interim deadlines that will have to be achieved so the curriculum implementation can begin in 24 months. She intends to begin by meeting with the curriculum committee to discuss the committee's role in the curriculum development process, possible subcommittees and their membership, and to present her proposed critical path.

Critique

Dr. Kirakova has made an excellent start to her task. It is evident that she intends to lead the process, but not to dictate it. She is seeking the collaboration of the curriculum committee by allowing them opportunity to define their role in the curriculum development process and consider the subgroups that might be necessary. In so doing, she is demonstrating her knowledge of the curriculum development process and effective leadership. As well, her consideration of subcommittees, membership, and a critical path demonstrate her commitment to getting the work done. As the time commitment of faculty becomes more apparent, Dr. Kirakova will have to return to the director to negotiate release time for some faculty. As well, she will have to assess what other resources, such as secretarial support, are needed and request these.

Old Ivy University College of Nursing

Old Ivy University College of Nursing offers BSN, BSN completion, MS, and PhD programs. It is located in a large metropolitan city of approximately 2,500,000 inhabitants. Health facilities include 12 hospitals, nurse practitioner clinics, home health services, and drop-in clinics. The university provides graduate and undergraduate programs to 52,000 full- and part-time students in a full range of programs.

The College of Nursing has approximately 1300 students, of whom nearly 60% are full-time, and these mainly in the BSN program. The BSN program is accredited. Although the curriculum content and teaching-learning approaches have been updated periodically, the overall structure of the curriculum and the location of clinical experiences have undergone little change. Most faculty members believe that the curriculum has lost its unity and that it is time to develop a new curriculum with more progressive philosophical approaches and learning experiences.

Most faculty teaching classroom courses in the BSN program have a PhD degree; some have a master's degree. Some clinical instructors have master's degrees, although the majority have a BSN. Doctorally-prepared faculty teach in the MS and PhD programs, although most without an undergraduate teaching assignment do guest lectures in the BSN program.

Dr. Lumella, the dean of the College of Nursing, is supportive of the undergraduate faculty's proposal to design a completely new curriculum. She has appointed Dr. Beverly Eme, an experienced and long-time faculty member, as the curriculum leader. Dr. Eme is a popular choice since she teaches in the BSN program and is highly supportive of faculty colleagues. Dr. Eme begins to plan how to proceed with her colleagues.

Questions for Consideration and Analysis of the Old Ivy University College of Nursing

1. How can Dr. Eme help the faculty choose a change theory to guide their overall process?

2. What committees could be struck in order to facilitate curriculum development? What purposes would they serve? How should committee members be selected or appointed? Who should the members be?

3. If some of the faculty teaching in the MS and PhD programs are reluctant to participate in undergraduate curriculum development, how could Dr. Lumella and Dr. Eme encourage them to do so?

4. What decision-making approaches would be effective for the curriculum developers?

5. What could be a practical work plan for developing the curriculum? What are the logistical factors associated with curriculum planning?

6. What potential is there for publication arising from curriculum development? How might faculty determine authorship?

7. What resources might be needed for the curriculum work to be achieved?

8. What faculty development activities would be helpful?

Curriculum Development Activities for Consideration in Your Setting

The following questions might stimulate thinking about organizing for curriculum development in your setting.

1. What approaches to decision-making do we most commonly use? How effective are they in achieving goals? Should we consider alternate approaches?

2. What committee structure(s) for curriculum development might be most efficient and successful in our situation? Who should participate?

3. When do we want to implement the new curriculum? What is the best way to develop a critical path, and who will assume responsibility for developing it? What implications will curriculum development have for current faculty?

4. What are faculty's thoughts about academic freedom and the desire for publication?

5. What sources of funding are available to support curriculum development?

6. How is faculty development received in our situation? What strategies have been most effective in moving the group forward? How can we plan the faculty development activities we need now?

7. What types of resources to support curriculum development should be discussed with the administrator?

References

American Association of University Professors. (n.d.). *Statement of principles on academic freedom and tenure with 1970 interpretive comments.* Retrieved June 6, 2007, from http://www.aaup.org/AAUP/pubsres/policydocs/1940statement.htm

Attridge, C. B. (1996). Factors confounding the development of innovative roles and practices. *Journal of Nursing Education, 35,* 406–412.

Bernhard, L. A., & Walsh, M. (1990). *Leadership. The key to the professionalization of nursing* (2nd ed.). St. Louis, MO: C.V. Mosby.

Bevis, E. O. (1989). *Curriculum building in nursing. A process* (3rd ed.). New York: National League for Nursing.

Bevis, E. O. (2000). Clusters of influence for practical decision-making about curriculum. In E. O. Bevis and J. Watson (Eds.), *Toward a caring curriculum: A new pedagogy for nursing* (pp. 107–152). Boston: Jones and Bartlett.

Canadian Association of University Teachers. (1979). Policy statement on academic freedom. Retrieved June 6, 2007, from http://www.caut.ca/ en/policies/academicfreedom.asp

Carmon, M., Hauber, R. P., & Chase, L. (1992). From anxiety to action. Facilitating faculty development during curricular change. *Nursing and Health Care, 13,* 364–368.

Conley, V. (1973). *Curriculum and instruction in nursing.* Boston: Little Brown & Co.

Hersey, P., Blanchard, K. H., & Johnson, D. E. (1996). *Management of organizational behavior. Utilizing human resources* (7th ed.). Upper Saddle River, NJ: Prentice-Hall.

Huber, D. (2000). *Leadership and nursing care management* (2nd ed.). Philadelphia: W. B. Saunders.

Hull, E., St. Romain, J. A., Alexander, P., Schaff, S., & Jones, W. (2001). Moving cemeteries: A framework for facilitating curriculum revision, *Nurse Educator, 26,* 280–282.

King Mixon, D., Kemp, M. A., Towle, M. A., & Schrader, V. C. (2005). Negotiating the merger of three nursing programs into one: Turning mission impossible into mission possible. *Annual Review of Nursing Education, 3,* 187–203.

Kneipp, S. M., Canales, M. K., Fahrenwald, N., & Taylor, J. Y. (2007). Academic freedom: Protecting "liberal science" in nursing in the 21st century. *ANS Advances in Nursing Science, 30*(1), 3–13.

Larson, E. (1997). Academic freedom amidst competing demands. *Journal of Professional Nursing, 13,* 211–216.

Little-Stoetzel, S. (2003). Decision-making. In P. Kelly-Heidenthal (Ed.), *Nursing leadership and management* (pp. 429–445). Clifton Park, NY: Thomson, Delmar Learning.

Mawn, B., & Reece, S. M. (2000). Reconfiguring a curriculum for the new millennium: The process of change. *Journal of Nursing Education, 39*(3), 101–108.

Palmer, S. P., Harmer Cox, A., Clark Callister, L., Johnsen, V., & Matsumara, G. (2005). Nursing education and service collaboration: Making a difference in the clinical learning environment. *Journal of Continuing Education in Nursing, 36,* 271–276.

Porter-O'Grady, T., & Malloch, K. (2007). *Quantum leadership: A resource for health care innovation* (2nd ed.). Boston: Jones and Bartlett.

Prochaska, J. O., DiClemente, C. C., & Norcross, J. C. (1992). In search of how people change: Applications to addictive behaviors. *American Psychologist, 47,* 1102–1114.

Prochaska, J. M., Prochaska, J., Cohen, F. C., Gomes, S. O., Laforge, R. G., & Eastwood, A. L. (2004). The transtheoretical model of change for multi-level interventions for alcohol abuse on campus. *Journal of Alcohol and Drug Education, 47*(3), 34–50.

Prochaska, J. O., Redding, C. A., Harlow, L. L., Rossi, J. S., & Velicer, W. F. (1994). The transtheoretical model of change and HIV prevention: A review. *Health Education Quarterly, 21,* 471–486.

Puich, M. (2007). The critical path. *Biopharm International, 20*(3), 28–29.

Rentschler, D. D., & Spegman, A. D. (1996). Curriculum revolution: Realities of change. *Journal of Nursing Education, 35,* 389–393.

Rush, K. L., Ouellet, L. L., & Wasson, D. (1991). Faculty development: The essence of curriculum development. *Nurse Education Today, 11,* 121–126.

Shils, E. (1993). Do we still need academic freedom? *American Scholar, 62,* 187–207.

Smith, D. L. (1999). Project management. In J. M. Hibberd & D. L. Smith (Eds.), *Nursing management in Canada* (2nd ed., pp. 471–485). Toronto: W. B. Saunders Canada.

Thornton, R., & Chapman, H. (2000). Student voice in curriculum making. *Journal of Nursing Education, 39,* 124–132.

Wylie, D., & Smith, D. L. (1999). Leading and participating in workgroups and teams. In J. M. Hibberd & D. L. Smith (Eds.), *Nursing management in Canada* (2nd ed., pp. 195–218). Toronto: W. B. Saunders Canada.

CHAPTER 5

Faculty Development for Curriculum Development and Change

Chapter Overview

This chapter addresses ideas about faculty development, an essential component of curriculum development activities. Faculty development is core to curriculum development, with both activities occurring simultaneously. Accordingly, there is no ideal placement of this chapter in the book. It is included here to allow chapters devoted to the curriculum development elements to flow without interruption.

Although faculty development is inherent to curriculum development, ongoing and planned faculty growth and evolution are necessary to bring a curriculum to fruition. In this chapter, attention is given to the meaning of, need for, and goals of faculty development, followed by a description of some useful implementation activities. Change theories are presented next, with application to faculty development specifically for curriculum development. Then, strategies to support faculty during curriculum change, and ideas for responding to resistance to change are offered. Synthesis activities include a case study and critique to exemplify important ideas, a second case for analysis, and questions to guide faculty development.

Chapter Goals

- Appreciate the necessity of faculty development as part of curriculum development.
- Relate change and empowerment theories to faculty development.
- Reflect on strategies to support faculty during change.
- Ponder ideas for responding to resistance to curriculum and faculty development.

Faculty Development for Curriculum Development

The Meaning of Faculty Development

Faculty development can be conceived of as "the theory and practice of facilitating improved faculty performance" (Halliburton, Marincovich, & Svinicki, 1988, p. 291). Traditionally, faculty development programs have concentrated on the development of faculty as teachers. More contemporary perspectives focus on the individual as a teacher, scholar, professional, person, and member of an organization. Therefore, development activities are aimed at all of these (Bartels, 2007; Foley, Redman, Horn, Davis, Neal, & Van Riper, 2003). However, faculty development specifically for curriculum development is not usually addressed.

With a more specific focus on nurse educators, faculty development is "the process of cultivating scholarly growth" (Raff & Arnold, 2001). This may include "resocialization for faculty into educative processes that are liberating for both the educator and student" (Rush, Ouellet, & Wasson, 1991, p. 123). Although some faculty may perceive the term as "discounting their level of knowledge or expertise, or as [unfavorable] commentary on the decisions they make about teaching, content, structure, or relationships" (Bevis, 2000, pp. 117–118), faculty development is intended to enhance knowledge and skills. Bartels (2007) has extended this idea to propose that faculty must also be able to "develop coherent curriculum designs, methods for the assessment of student learning, [and] evidence-based program evaluation . . ." (p. 157).

Faculty development should evolve naturally as part of the curriculum development process, and be congruent with the institutional philosophy, considerate of faculty needs, and supported by administrators and resources. Planned and purposeful faculty development related to curriculum development is far-reaching, and encompasses all aspects of the development, implementation, and evaluation processes, including specific teaching-learning methods and ways of interacting with learners, clinicians, and colleagues.

Necessity of Faculty Development for Curriculum Development

Faculty development has been described as the "essence of curriculum development" (Rush, Ouellet, & Wasson, 1991). It is foundational to the creation, implementation, and evaluation of a curriculum that reflects a new perspective and is true to the espoused philosophical approaches.

A core competency of the academic nurse educator is to "participate in curriculum design and evaluation of program outcomes" (National League for Nursing [NLN], 2005, p. 19). Among the tasks of this competency is knowledge of curriculum development: identifying program outcomes, developing competency statements, writing learning objectives, and selecting learning experiences and evaluation strategies (NLN).

However, few recent graduates of master's and doctoral programs have academic preparation in this aspect of the nurse educator role because of the emphasis on advanced practice roles and research in graduate nursing programs. As well, faculty development about the curriculum development process itself, and the creation of a unified curriculum, is rarely planned, perhaps because of an unexamined assumption that teachers implicitly know how to develop curricula, or because curriculum development activities have traditionally received little (if any) credit toward promotion and tenure decisions. The result is that knowledge about nursing curriculum may be limited to personal experience, and knowledge of curriculum development may be absent (Goldenberg, Andrusyszyn, & Iwasiw, 2004). Thus, many nursing faculty may not be equipped to undertake curriculum development or to fulfill their educator role other than in the way that they experienced it as students (Bartels, 2007).

Competence in all aspects of curriculum design and evaluation is basic to the creation of an educationally sound curriculum. As it cannot be assumed that faculty members know how to develop curriculum, it is incumbent on deans/directors to provide opportunities so that relevant knowledge and skills can be acquired. Through faculty development activities, novices can be guided to think beyond their areas of clinical expertise and their own educational experiences, to the possibilities for an entire curriculum. The interactions and synergy occurring in development sessions may prompt seasoned faculty to consider new approaches to nursing curriculum. Faculty development is the core of curriculum development and is a catalyst for the creation and operationalization of a new vision for the curriculum.

Curriculum redesign requires faculty members to look beyond their own clinical and teaching areas. They need to consider which philosophical approaches and concepts should underpin the curriculum, what the curriculum outcomes should be, and how learners can achieve the outcomes. As well, they must examine how all aspects of a curriculum interact, and the options for curriculum design. To develop a meaningful curriculum in a timely fashion, faculty and other stakeholders might require assistance with the curriculum development process itself, as well as with curriculum implementation and evaluation. Accordingly, faculty development must occur in tandem with curriculum development.

Faculty development related to all aspects of curriculum development, implementation, and evaluation is particularly timely because of the impending retirement of a large cohort of faculty (Bartfay & Howse, 2007; Canadian Nurses Association & Canadian Association of Schools of Nursing, 2007; Kaufman, 2007). Over time, there will be fewer faculty experienced in curriculum development, and the mentoring or guidance they could offer will not be available. Therefore, opportunities should be created to develop or enhance the curriculum skills of novice and mid-career nurse educators.

Goals of Faculty Development Related to Curriculum Development

There are at least four goals for faculty development related to curriculum development, implementation, and evaluation. Other goals can emerge in accordance with the learning needs of individuals or groups of faculty. For example, some may need development activities related to curriculum leadership.

The goals include enhancing knowledge and skills about curriculum development and evaluation, in which, as Bevis (2000) describes, includes changing views about curriculum, roles and relationships, and teaching approaches. All are of equal importance and are achieved synergistically.

Enhancing Knowledge and Skills About Curriculum Development and Evaluation Knowledge about curriculum development and evaluation processes varies among faculty members and other stakeholders. Some will know a great deal; others will be familiar with details of course planning, but not with the larger process. Likely, many will have learning needs related to the developing curriculum. To make certain that the curriculum development process is smooth, faculty development focused specifically on developing a curriculum is necessary. Knowledge of the total process will lead to an appreciation of the time required for curriculum development, work accomplished by task groups, and importance of shared understandings and consensus. Moreover, detailed information about each aspect of curriculum development and evaluation will allow task groups to develop their critical paths and ensure work is completed in the manner required.

Changing View of Curriculum Another goal for faculty development is acceptance of a different perception of curriculum and possibly, learning, based on the philosophical approaches chosen. Traditionally, learning was generally accepted as simply a change in behavior, dependent on content. Currently, learning is seen as knowledge construction that evolves from transactions and interactions between and among learners, clients, clinicians, and teachers. This latter process is less reliant on content, more oriented to the processes of learning and nursing practice, and is a more egalitarian view of curriculum. The intent is to develop strategies to promote learners' understanding of concepts relevant to nursing and advance their development of thinking skills necessary for successful nursing practice, rather than on detailed content linked to diseases. Although many nurse educators have enthusiastically endorsed this perspective, faculty could consider other approaches. For example, curricula could be conceived phenomenologically, ethically, narratively, contextually, or clinically. Whichever approach to curriculum is adopted, it is important to facilitate faculty members' understanding about the selected view and provide faculty development opportunities such as workshops, conferences, and mentoring to assist them in designing, implementing, and evaluating a curriculum reflecting the new view.

Changing Roles and Relationships A change in faculty roles could be a consequence of curriculum redesign. This would require altered relationships with learners, colleagues, clients, and administrators. The role change might involve a shift in activities, power, equity, and authority, depending on the curricular philosophical approaches and goals.

Changing Teaching-Learning and Evaluation Approaches A realistic goal of faculty development is to encourage nurse educators to become more aware of the teaching-learning and evaluation strategies they use, and how these might be altered. To help them do so, activities (e.g., role playing, case studies, practice teaching and critiques, or videos or films with discussion), as well as psychological support and encouragement could be employed. The purpose is to assist novice faculty to acquire the necessary skills, and to enable experienced faculty to revitalize their current practices and courses (Davis, 1993) to be congruent with the new curriculum. Faculty development activities to support changed teaching-learning and evaluation approaches should be consistent with the curriculum nucleus and should support faculty members' ability to assist learners to achieve curriculum outcomes.

Benefits of Faculty Development for Curriculum Development

Faculty development has the potential to empower faculty and benefit the school of nursing in ways that extend beyond the tasks of developing, implementing, and evaluating a curriculum. Rosabeth Moss Kanter (1977, 1993) asserts that power (ability to get work done) in organizations is derived from both formal positions and from alliances with superiors, peers, and subordinates. Alliances form the basis of cooperation to accomplish work. Formal and informal power give access to opportunity, resources, information, and support. These, in turn, influence employees in positive ways, leading to increased self-efficacy, motivation, organizational commitment, perceived autonomy, perceptions of participative management, and job satisfaction. Accordingly, burnout is decreased. Employees derive a sense of achievement, respect, and cooperation. As well, clients of the organization are satisfied. This theory is relevant for faculty development in schools of nursing.

Access to opportunity has been found to be the most empowering factor for clinical and college nurse educators (Davies, 2002; Sarmiento, Laschinger, & Iwasiw, 2004). Among college educators, empowering environments lead to decreased burnout and increased job satisfaction (Sarmiento et al.). Unfortunately, college educators view their work environments as only moderately empowering (Erwin, 1999). Formal development activities might enhance educators' perceptions of their workplace.

From a curriculum development context in schools of nursing, those with formal power are the nursing dean/director, possibly the curriculum leader, and to a lesser extent, those chosen to chair committees. However, many alliances form as work progresses, and faculty members obtain informal power from these. More directly, faculty development is a means to provide opportunity, resources, information, and support to faculty, so they can achieve a redesigned curriculum and realize its benefits.

Planned faculty development demonstrates the school's commitment to faculty and their professional growth, empowers faculty, enhances job satisfaction, and is a method to support personal and curriculum development. Additionally, formalized, systematic development activities can enhance faculty recruitment and retention when competition for new faculty is strong (Foley et al., 2003).

Steinert et al. (2006) reviewed 53 papers from 1980 to 2002 related to faculty development activities designed specifically to improve medical education. Among their conclusions were that:

- Overall satisfaction with faculty development was high.
- Participants reported positive changes in attitudes toward faculty development and teaching.
- Self-reports of increased knowledge were supported by results of formal testing.
- Changes in teaching were reported by participants and students.
- Greater educational involvement and establishment of collegial networks resulted.

It seems reasonable that similar outcomes might accrue for nursing faculty from planned faculty development activities related to the processes of curriculum development, implementation, and evaluation.

Participants in Faculty Development Activities

Faculty members are the key players in the curriculum development and implementation processes: in decisions to be made, in committee work to be accomplished, and in teaching according to the tenets of a new or revised curriculum. Consequently, the success of curriculum redesign and implementation is largely dependent upon a knowledgeable and willing faculty, and faculty development activities are planned with and for them.

Importantly, stakeholders such as students, clinicians, and administrators, who are part of the curriculum development process, should also be included in faculty development activities. Participation in these learning opportunities will expand stakeholders' knowledge and skills about curriculum processes, and strengthen their connection with, and deepen their understandings about the school of nursing.

Responsibility for Faculty Development

The school of nursing dean/director has the responsibility to invest in and support the development of faculty in order to minimize knowledge gaps in curriculum development, teaching, and research. Formal leadership confers the responsibility on the dean/director to act as a change agent and to operationalize professional development to "foster the future of the organization" (Kenner & Pressler, 2006, p. 2). Deans/directors are the primary force in initiating change, assisting faculty in their development (Smolen, 1996), creating an empowering work environment, and ensuring that stakeholders are involved in the school's activities. Identification of specific faculty development needs can be undertaken by the dean/director, the curriculum leader, a faculty development committee, or individual faculty members. Typically, it is a combination of these.

Faculty members have a professional obligation to ensure they are competent in their role functions. Therefore, they have a responsibility to:

- Attend faculty development activities.
- Be open to new ideas.
- Participate fully in faculty development.
- Commit to employing new knowledge, skills, and perspectives as they develop, implement, and evaluate the curriculum.

Responsibility for creating formal faculty development opportunities could rest with knowledgeable and experienced faculty members who have a solid foundation in nursing education theory and practice. Their development needs may be slight, so that their participation could be to provide leadership in faculty development. They might lead formal and informal sessions, provide guidance to novices, or purposefully mentor those involved.

Faculty Development Activities for Curriculum Development

Faculty engaging in curriculum development might require additional knowledge and skills about the process they are undertaking. From their literature review, Steinert and her colleagues (2006) concluded that "effective faculty development . . . included the use of experiential learning, provision of feedback, effective peer and colleague relationships, well-designed interventions following principles of teaching and learning, and the use of a diversity of educational methods within single interventions" (p. 497). Moreover, effective programs were designed to match the needs of a particular group and sustainability was linked to an extended series of related offerings (Steinert et al.).

Learning about curriculum development, implementation, and evaluation can be facilitated through planned faculty development activities such as workshops, mentoring, group discussions, and attendance at conferences. See Table 5-1 for examples of formal and informal

Table 5-1   Strategies for Formal and Informal Faculty Development

Strategies	
Formal	**Informal**
• Center for faculty development	• One-on-one
• Inservice workshops	• Dialogue and feedback
• Lectures and formal conferences by experts and/or experienced colleagues	• Meetings with department heads
	• Handbooks
• Post-graduate courses	• Mentorship
• Forums	• Preceptorship
• Seminars	• Buddy system
• Learning studies laboratory	• Learning circles
• Faculty meetings	• Luncheon meetings
• Practice teaching	• Support groups
• Integrative partnerships	• Readings
• Group meetings	• Audiovisual and computer programs
• Tours, visits	• Modeling
• Retreats	• Shadowing
	• Tutoring

strategies for faculty development that could be relevant for faculty development related to curriculum development.

Faculty development programs should be ongoing, but quite naturally assume more importance when a new curriculum is envisioned. Whether faculty development activities are formal or informal, the focus should be on the curriculum process itself. It begins with an overview of the entire process and includes organizing for curriculum development; committee leadership; collection and interpretation of contextual data; establishment of the curriculum nucleus and outcomes; curriculum and course design; and curriculum implementation and evaluation.

Curriculum developers should meet initially in faculty development sessions to gain an overview of the curriculum development process. It is incumbent upon all stakeholders to reach shared understandings about nursing education, nursing and health care, teaching-learning processes and student-teacher-practitioner relationships. Faculty discussions of this nature serve the added purpose of moving the curriculum development process forward.

Because faculty development is ongoing, a schedule must be agreed upon. Each session's topic, format, time, location, and leader need to be decided early. However, schedules and topics should not be so fixed that changes cannot be instituted to meet participant obligations, newly identified or urgent needs, and other contingencies. Nonetheless, what must be kept in mind is that in order to design and develop a curriculum that will be acceptable to all stakeholders and relevant at the time of curriculum implementation and beyond, faculty development is necessary.

When engaging in curriculum development, faculty must come together, learn and grow together, accept that change is inevitable, and take ownership and pride in the future. Faculty development can increase individuals' personal investment in the curriculum. They can feel:

- Competent in curriculum development because of attainment of new abilities and progress toward goal achievement.
- Valued in an organization that provides professional development.
- Empowered by the institution's provision of opportunities, resources, information, and support.
- Secure in group learning and interaction.
- Connected to colleagues through shared learning, acceptance, appreciation, support, and respect.

Faculty Development for Change

Curriculum development, and ultimately implementation of a redesigned curriculum, is an example of planned change: from a familiar curriculum to one that is initially undefined. Because faculty members have extensive involvement in curriculum development and implementation plans, and in opportunities to introduce aspects of the redesigned curriculum into the existing one, transition to a new curriculum might be expected to occur easily and with full faculty support. Unfortunately, the change is not always smooth.

Successful curriculum change is generally dependent upon the acquisition of new skills and perspectives by those who will implement the reconceptualized curriculum. This requires personal adjustment, which does not happen in a scheduled, orderly fashion, and is determined by individual readiness. Faculty development is a way to support stakeholders during curriculum change and should occur concurrently with developing the curriculum. Accordingly, curriculum development requires faculty development and change. In turn, faculty development supports:

- Curriculum development and change
- Personal development and change

Similarly, faculty evaluation typically leads to some curriculum modification, and this necessitates change by faculty members. Figure 5-1 depicts the intertwining and infinite nature of curriculum development, faculty development, curriculum evaluation, and change.

Creation and implementation of a completely new or revised curriculum involves phasing out and terminating the existing curriculum. This process includes change for faculty members in their perspectives, teaching-learning and evaluation approaches, interactions, course content, and possibly, sites for clinical teaching. Also, there may be altered interpersonal dynamics within the school of nursing and a realignment of teaching colleagues.

These changes can lead to feelings ranging from anticipation to resistance as the existing curriculum ends and the transition to the new or revised curriculum takes place (Kupperschmidt & Burns, 1997). Faculty development is intended to support faculty members' personal and professional growth when a new curriculum is envisioned, curriculum work begins, and a reconceptualized curriculum is introduced. Therefore, consideration of how faculty might undergo change, and appropriate activities to support them during a curriculum change, merit attention. Strategies to respond to resisters in order to enhance their participation in faculty development and acceptance of the new curriculum direction are also important. The following brief section on change theories is foundational to understanding how to support faculty and respond to resistance to curriculum change.

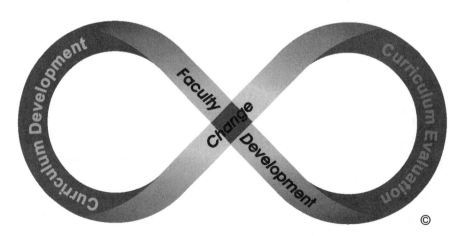

Figure 5-1 Synchronous, Intertwining, and Infinite Nature of Curriculum Development, Faculty Development, Curriculum Evaluation, and Change

Source: Iwasiw, Goldenberg, & Andrusyszyn, 2008. Used with permission.

Change Theories

Diffusion of Innovations   According to Rogers (2003), *Diffusion* is "a kind of social change, defined as the process by which alteration occurs in the structure and function of a social system" (p. 6). An *innovation* is an idea or practice that is viewed as new, and this is communicated over time among the members of the social system. Acceptance follows an S-shaped curve within a social group, with some members being slow to accept the change and others rejecting it completely. The rate of adoption is related to the following characteristics of the innovation:

- *Relative advantage* of the new idea over current practice.
- *Compatibility* with existing values and past experiences of potential adopters.
- *Complexity* of the new idea or practice.
- *Trialability* or the ability to test the innovation on a limited basis.
- *Observability* of the results of the innovation to others.

The interpersonal channel of communication is most important in the diffusion of the innovation, i.e., face-to-face interaction between and among individuals of similar status. Similarly, most people depend on a subjective evaluation of an innovation that is conveyed to them from like individuals who have adopted the innovation.

Time is a dimension of the theory: the length of time for the innovation-decision process to occur; the time for an individual to adopt the innovation; and the rate of adoption within a system.

The innovation-decision process spans the time from when knowledge of the innovation is first known; persuasion activities occur; a decision to accept or reject the innovation is made; implementation occurs; to confirmation of the decision (or discontinuance). Greenhalgh, Robert, Bate, Macfarlane, and Kyriakidou (2005) comment that this time period can be shortened by *dissemination*, i.e., "a planned and active process intended to increase the rate and level of adoption above that which might happen by diffusion alone" (p. 29).

Individuals adopt the innovation at different times during a change (Rogers, 2003):

- *Innovators* seek change and are the first to adopt the idea.
- *Early adopters* facilitate change.
- *Early majority members* prefer the status quo, but provide a support system for change and accept it.
- *Late majority members* accept the change after most others.
- *Laggards* strive to maintain the status quo.
- *Rejecters* actively oppose and may sabotage the innovation.

The *social system* is an important dimension of the theory. Communication channels, status of individuals, decision-making processes, and so forth, all influence the diffusion of innovations. Again, Greenhalgh et al. (2005) extend this idea. They comment that sustainability of an innovation in health service organizations requires systems changes.

This theory is useful for understanding individuals' acceptance of the need for curriculum change, their commitment to it, and their readiness to engage in faculty development and curriculum development activities. It points to the importance of involving respected opinion leaders in faculty development activities so they can persuade peers of the value of these endeavors, share positive evaluations of the activities, and make visible the learning they have gained. Their diffusion of the knowledge and skills they have acquired will improve the quality of the curriculum.

Transtheoretical Model of Behavior Change This model addresses behavior change of an individual as the desired outcome, and incorporates changes in attitudes, intentions, and behavior. The model incorporates four theoretical concepts central to change: stages, processes, self-efficacy, and decisional balance (Prochaska, Prochaska, Cohen, Gomes, Laforge, & Eastwood, 2004).

Behavioral change is conceptualized as a spiral, and this pattern represents the reality that people do not change in a straightforward, linear manner. Rather, at certain times, individuals can revert to former stages, and then proceed again toward the desired change. Relapse to previous stages is considered a natural part of the change cycle. The following stages represent a continuum of motivational readiness (Prochaska, DiClemente, & Norcross, 1992; Prochaska et al., 2004; Prochaska, Redding, Harlow, Rossi, & Velicer, 1994).

- Precontemplation: Person sees no need to change.
- Contemplation: Person thinks about the benefits and losses of change and admits to desiring change, but there is no intent to act.
- Preparation: Person plans to make a specific change soon, and may make small attempts at change.
- Action: Person makes an overt commitment to change and practices the new behavior over time.
- Maintenance: Person is able to avoid relapses to former stages for 6 months or more, although the temptation to relapse can persist for several years.

Participation in faculty and curriculum development can be conceptualized as encompassing a change in faculty attitude toward the current curriculum, an intention to create a new curriculum, and a change in behavior to include curriculum development activities. Curriculum implementation, then, requires a change in attitude toward learners, other faculty, and roles; an intention to behave and interact in new ways; and a change in teaching and evaluation strategies, approach to content, and interactions. Faculty development activities provide the knowledge, skills, and environment that support individual and collective change. Participation in faculty development represents action to change attitudes and behavior.

Supporting Faculty During Curriculum Development and Change

Development of a new curriculum, while faculty are concurrently fulfilling teaching and research responsibilities, requires their dedication to a new vision, and tangible organizational support. Faculty development is one form of substantive support. In Table 5-2, the Transtheoretical Model of Behavior Change (Prochaska et al., 1992; Prochaska et al., 2004; Prochaska et al., 1994) is applied to curriculum change and faculty development, with activities proposed to match the stages of the model. Activities that are matched to the stage of the majority can have a strong impact, even if some participants are not prepared to take action (Prochaska et al., 2004).

Incorporated into the strategies, and indeed within the curriculum development process itself, are factors that are inherently empowering: publicity about activities; a strong relationship between activities and a central issue in the organization; high interpersonal contact; and participation in programs, meetings, and problem-solving groups (Kanter, 1993). The school must invest in the faculty, and the faculty members, in turn, will invest themselves in the school and its future.

Responding to Resistance to Change

Some ideas were presented in Chapter 2 about responding to initial objections to curriculum change through an appeal to values and logic, in accordance with the Diffusions of Innovations theory (Rogers, 2003). Even though a school of nursing proceeds with curriculum development, there may be some members who do not agree with the necessity for curriculum change or faculty development. Although a minority group, laggards and resisters have the potential to undermine the momentum of the majority. This cannot be ignored. Every effort should be extended to help the resisters feel that their contributions are needed and valued, and to counteract the negativity that they might project. There is a diplomatic balance to be achieved between sensitivity to individual readiness for change and the requirement to progress with faculty and curriculum development.

Forms of Resistance   *Active resistance* to curriculum change and faculty development is easy to identify. Examples of active resistance include:

- Open criticism of curriculum change and faculty development.
- Refusal to acknowledge shortcomings of the present curriculum or need for faculty development.
- Predictions of dire consequences of curriculum change.
- Direct refusal to participate in faculty and curriculum development.

Table 5-2   Application of Transtheoretical Model of Behavior Change to Faculty and Curriculum Change

Stage of Change	Process of Change for Faculty	Activities to Support Faculty and Curriculum Change
Precontemplation: no intention to change	Consciousness-raising (increasing level of awareness and more accurate information-processing)	• Present data about need for curriculum change • Engage faculty in discussion about the possibility of curriculum change
	Dramatic relief (experiencing and expressing feelings)	• Stimulate faculty discussion about frustrations and disappointments experienced within the current curriculum
	Environmental re-evaluation (affective and cognitive re-experiencing of one's environment and problems)	• Initiate faculty discussion to identify features of the current curriculum they dislike
Contemplation: seriously considering a curriculum change within a specified time	Consciousness-raising	• Continue discussion about the need for curriculum change • Engage faculty in consideration of the benefits of curriculum change
	Dramatic relief	• Use guided imagery for faculty to imagine how they will feel when an up-to-date, well-received curriculum is in place
	Environmental re-evaluation*	• Share ideas about the effects of avoiding curriculum change on students, graduates, school of nursing, and educational institution • Initiate deliberations among faculty and dean or director about the possibility of removing barriers to faculty involvement in curriculum development
	Self-re-evaluation (affective and cognitive re-experiencing of one's self and problems)	• Review school and university mission and goals and how strongly the current curriculum supports mission and goals

Table 5-2 continued

Stage of Change	Process of Change for Faculty	Activities to Support Faculty and Curriculum Change
Preparation: a commitment has been made to change the curriculum	Environmental re-evaluation*	• Plan discussion about faculty values related to education, nursing practice, profession • Identify initial faculty development needs • Minimize barriers and maximize resources for faculty and curriculum development • Obtain agreement from the Total Faculty Group to proceed with curriculum development • Declare administrator support publicly • Announce curriculum development plans to stakeholders • Appoint curriculum leader
	Self-liberation (belief in one's ability to change and commitment to act on that belief)	• Form Steering and Advisory Committees • Initiate faculty development activities • Establish committees and obtain agreement from members to achieve goals • Develop critical path • Institute mentorship
Action: active engagement in: • curriculum development • faculty development • testing of new faculty behaviors in the current curriculum	Reinforcement management (reinforcing more positive behaviors and punishing negative ones)	• Provide positive feedback to individuals and committees • Provide rewards for faculty and curriculum development activities (e.g., public acknowledgment and praise, credit toward promotion and tenure)

continues

Table 5-2   continued

Stage of Change	Process of Change for Faculty	Activities to Support Faculty and Curriculum Change
	Self-liberation*	• Celebrate achievement of major milestones of critical path • Continue formal and informal faculty development and support (e.g., teaching circles, lunch discussions, on-line discussion groups, peer feedback) • Use new terminology • Introduce aspects of new curriculum into old curriculum • Mentor novices • Continue faculty development activities focused on faculty self-identified needs • Identify and acknowledge experts in school of nursing • Conduct a funeral for the old curriculum

Maintenance: sustained behavior	Counter-conditioning (substituting more positive behaviors and experiences for problem ones)	• Continue faculty development based on experiences in testing new behaviors and implementing new curriculum
		• Structure formal evaluation of faculty and courses to be congruent with new curriculum
		• Disseminate information about the new curriculum to:
		   • academic and professional communities
		   • prospective students

	Stimulus control (restructuring environment or experiences so that problem stimuli are less likely to occur)	• Launch new curriculum with a public celebration • Ask for counter-examples of effective strategies if objections arise or reversion to former curriculum occurs

Table 5-2   continued

Stage of Change	Process of Change for Faculty	Activities to Support Faculty and Curriculum Change
		• Encourage peer groups to support new faculty behaviors and curriculum implementation
	Helping relationships (relationships involving openness, caring, trust, genuineness, and empathy)	• Continue peer faculty development and support activities through group activities and mentorship
		• Schedule formal faculty development for aspects of curriculum implementation that are problematic. Focus on shared problem-solving
	Self-re-evaluation*	• Share stories abut "how far we've come" and identify new values, beliefs, and aspirations
		• Use teaching portfolios for faculty evaluation (self, peer, and administrator)

*processes not identified in these stages in original Transtheoretical Model
Source: Some data from: Prochaska, J.O., DiClemente, C.C., & Norcross, J.C. (1992). In search of how people change: Applications to addictive behaviors. *American Psychologist, 47,* 1102–1114; and Prochaska, J.O., Redding, C.A., Harlow, L.L., Rossi, J.S., & Velicer, W.F. (1994). The transtheoretical model of change and HIV prevention: A review. *Health Education Quarterly, 21,* 471–486.

Passive resistance is subtler. Although opposed to participation in faculty or curriculum development, the passive resister lacks the courage to openly state disagreement. Behavior typical of passive resistance can be:

• Lateness for, or absence from, meetings.

• Failure to meet commitments to complete work.

• Minimal participation in activities attended.

• Diverting attention from the main purpose of meetings to trivial, peripheral, or historical matters.

Passive-aggressive resistance is sabotage. The resister may publicly support faculty development and curriculum change, and is likely physically present but mentally uninvolved at these activities. The endorsement is coupled with behind-the-scenes attempts to undermine faculty development plans, the proposed curriculum, and/or those participating in faculty and curriculum development.

Responding to Resistance There are many possible sources of resistance to curriculum change, and although colleagues may attribute motivation to those opposing it, the precise reasons may never be revealed. However, it is not necessary to know the underlying rationale before confronting the unacceptable behavior. To ignore the resistance is to condone it (Chambers, 1998).

The goal of the dean/director is have the resister agree to replace the unacceptable behavior with actions that are supportive of the group's effort. The behavior should be confronted as soon as it is known, and appropriate strategies have been described by a number of authors (Chambers, 1998; Patterson, Grenny, McMillan, & Switzler, 2002; Sullivan & Decker, 2005). The dean/director should employ some or all of these measures:

- Invite the resister to a private meeting, so that the resistance can be addressed directly.
- Employ exemplary listening skills so the resister feels heard and safe.
- Describe the unacceptable behavior without attributing motivation.
- Explain the invisible consequences of the present behavior, such as diminished respect from colleagues or damage to the school's reputation.
- Clearly state expectations about the desired behavior.
- Link the desired behavior to shared values.
- Explain the benefits of a behavior change (e.g., renewed respect, acceptance).
- Obtain a commitment to behave differently.

The focus of the discussion must be the person's behavior, not the curriculum change or the reasons for it.

Particularly troubling are reports of a faculty member's public criticism of faculty development and curriculum change. The dean/director should be precise, objective, and unemotional in describing the reports and their effects on colleagues, clinical partners, and the image of the school. The goal of the interaction is to obtain the resister's agreement to refrain from further public criticism. Some reasons for resistance to faculty development and curriculum change, and possible responses, are presented in Table 5-3.

An Alternate Perspective To lessen the stress often experienced when resistance is prolonged or unrelenting, it may be helpful for faculty members to reframe the situation to make the discord or dissent seem less personal. Viewing resistance as a conflict of values, beliefs, rights, and obligations could lead to changed understandings and reactions by all involved.

In Table 5-4, presented are possible perspectives on conflict areas about the need for faculty and curriculum development. A different view and emotional distance could make the situation more tolerable, and lessen the tendency to attribute malicious motives to the resister. Explicit use of conflict resolution strategies may be in order.

Faculty members are responsible for their own reactions and behaviors. Some might choose to reject faculty and curriculum development and curricular changes, content to be miserable and out of step with colleagues, despite efforts to support them through change. It is wise to remember that changing another person's behavior may not be achievable. However, it is possible and may be necessary to change one's reaction so as not to be consumed with anxiety, anger, and the endless creation of appeasement tactics. It is preferable to focus on the task at hand and prepare for a new curriculum with motivated, growth-seeking colleagues.

Table 5-3   Possible Responses to Reasons for Resistance to Faculty Development and Curriculum Change and Possible Responses

Reasons for Resistance to Faculty Development and Curriculum Change	Possible Responses of Administrator, Curriculum Leader, and/or Faculty Majority
Belief in value of current curriculum and way of being	• Explore which aspects of curriculum and role are valued and why. • Suggest that involvement in faculty and curriculum development is the best way to ensure continuation of what is valued. • Make evident how aspects of current curriculum might be taken into account in developing curriculum.
Skepticism about quality of envisioned curriculum	• Explore concerns. • Be open to possibility that resister is correct. • Acknowledge that the resister's input has assisted in the examination of the issue, along with others' views.
Interpretation of change as personal criticism	• Validate the progressive nature of current curriculum at the time it was developed. • Explain in detail the need for a changed curriculum. • Emphasize what will be gained by changed curricular and faculty approaches. • Listen actively to resister's issues (e.g., losses, fears), and if possible, attempt to lessen the frequency of verbalization of concerns. • Emphasize that the resister's strengths are needed for faculty and curriculum development activities.

continues

Table 5-3   continued

Reasons for Resistance to Faculty Development and Curriculum Change	Possible Responses of Administrator, Curriculum Leader, and/or Faculty Majority
	• Validate the resister's past contributions and express confidence in ability to be successful.
Belief in own curriculum development expertise; hence no need for faculty development	• Acknowledge experience and knowledge that resister has accumulated.
	• Propose that resister share expertise by leading some faculty development sessions. Assign this as part of workload, if possible.
	• State consequences of non-participation.
Fear of reduced status or not fitting into new curriculum	• Emphasize that all faculty are uncertain about their place in the changed curriculum, particularly in the early stages when the future curriculum is undefined.
	• Encourage participation in faculty and curriculum development as a means of ensuring that a place can be identified and developed in the future curriculum.
	• Stress that faculty development activities will prepare all faculty for the envisioned curriculum.
Fear that inadequate skills and knowledge will be revealed	• Relate anecdotes from school or personal history when faculty felt that they could not succeed in changed circumstances, yet did achieve.
	• Propose the idea that many faculty may wonder if they "have what it takes" to function in the future curriculum.
	• Assure that school director attends faculty development activities to underscore that everyone has learning needs and to give importance to attendance.
Lack of confidence in colleagues' ability to develop acceptable curriculum	• Agree that not all faculty are equally experienced in nursing education generally, and in curriculum development particularly.
	• Underscore that the curriculum development process is inherently a form of faculty development, and therefore colleagues will enhance skills as the project unfolds.
	• Emphasize that formal and informal faculty development will occur concurrently with curriculum development, thereby expanding colleagues' skills and knowledge.
	• Indicate that curriculum development is an opportunity for the resister to share particular expertise in nursing education, thereby becoming a model for less-experienced faculty.

Table 5-3 continued

Reasons for Resistance to Faculty Development and Curriculum Change	Possible Responses of Administrator, Curriculum Leader, and/or Faculty Majority
Lack of confidence in own ability to contribute meaningfully	• Emphasize that all faculty are uncertain about undertaking curriculum development. • Remind resister that ongoing faculty development is intended to ensure that all faculty will have access to pertinent perspectives and be able to contribute to curriculum work. • Relate strengths that resister can bring to curriculum development.
Lack of interest or disinclination to expend effort required for faculty development, curriculum change, and implementation	• Explore reasons and remove barriers if possible. • Remind resister that faculty and curriculum development are shared responsibilities of all faculty. • Discuss how resister expects to be effective in future curriculum if not involved in its creation and in faculty development. • Employ all strategies to help resister feel that contributions are needed and valued. • Consider an alternate assignment in the school of nursing, as a last resort.
Concern that faculty and curriculum development will interfere with research and publication and/or progress towards tenure	• Acknowledge that faculty and curriculum development require intensive effort. • Discuss research and publication potential of curriculum development and implementation. • Describe how curriculum development can contribute to promotion and tenure. • Consider the feasibility of some faculty "opting out" of curriculum development for short periods at critical points of research activity or career progress.
Heavy workload	• Examine how workload could be altered to include participation in faculty and curriculum development activities.
Misoneism (fear of newness, innovation, or change)	• Provide as much support as possible to enhance motivation for change.
Unrevealed personal reasons	• Accept that no one can cause another to change. • Accept that it is not possible to respond constructively to what is unknown.

Chapter Summary

Faculty development is an essential component of curriculum development. Identifying learning needs and planning activities that will enhance knowledge and skills as stakeholders move through the curriculum development process will maximize opportunities

Table 5-4   Possible Perspectives on Conflict Areas about Need for Faculty and Curriculum Development

Possible Conflict Areas	Possible Perspective on Conflict Areas	
	Resister	**Faculty Majority**
Values	• Stability	• Change
	• Experience	• Personal growth
	• Personal values	• Shared values
Beliefs	• Quality education = current curriculum, teaching, and evaluation methods	• Quality education = new curriculum, teaching, and evaluation methods
	• Personal value as a teacher and nurse is expressed in current curriculum	• New curriculum will enhance growth as teachers and nurses
	• Faculty development and curriculum change are a repudiation of current practices	• Faculty development and curriculum change will expand and enhance knowledge and skills
	• Criticism	• Critique
Interpretation of the right of academic freedom	• Individual decision-making about curriculum	• Collegial decision-making and adherence to curriculum decisions made by Total Faculty Group
	• Maintenance of present programs	• Planning and implementation of a relevant and progressive program
Obligations	• Adherence to current (correct) way of doing things	• Openness to new ideas
	• Preparation of graduates for existing nursing practice	• Preparation of graduates for future nursing practice

for successful change. A wide spectrum of faculty development activities should be considered and the most suitable, selected. However, it is realistic to acknowledge that not all faculty may welcome empowerment and change; some might be very comfortable with maintaining the status quo. Change theories help to explain the processes that can occur during the curriculum development, implementation, and evaluation. Although it is likely that some faculty members will resist change, proceeding with a planned faculty development program as it relates to curriculum development and change is important and should not be delayed.

Synthesis Activities

Two cases are presented to illustrate the main ideas of the chapter. The first is critiqued, and the second is followed by questions to help with analysis. Questions at the end of this section of the chapter are intended to assist with faculty development related to curriculum development.

Copernicus University School of Nursing

Copernicus University, a mid-size university with a long history, houses several world-renowned programs. Of these, astronomy and nursing are held in high esteem for their progressive ideas. Over the last few months, and after much deliberation, the nursing faculty came to the realization that a curriculum revision would be in order. They agreed that the curriculum, as currently designed, was too structured and no longer reflected their evolving beliefs about teaching, learning, and the nursing profession.

Under Dr. Korsan's leadership, the faculty had many discussions about how the current philosophical basis of the curriculum does not match their desire for a more phenomenological approach to teaching nursing and providing patient care. They believe that the essence of lived experiences of learners and clients, along with faculty views, should shape the curriculum. All faculty were supportive of this direction, and many ideas were shared about how to proceed. Two task forces were struck. The responsibility of the first was to thoroughly research the concept of phenomenology and what implications this philosophical approach would have on revising the existing curriculum. The second was to search for and examine existing curricula grounded in phenomenology, as well as other approaches that incorporated lived experiences. These committees were to report back to the total faculty group in 2 months.

The task forces did their research on phenomenology, examined other programs that used this and other approaches, and held small focus groups with faculty in each year of the program. Findings were shared, and many issues were raised at a faculty meeting. The predominant concern was whether it was premature to select the philosophical approach without having a thorough understanding of other options. After considerable deliberation, faculty concurred that although a change was desirable, they would benefit from some planned faculty development sessions about several philosophical approaches, and an examination of what engaging in curriculum revision of this nature would mean to them.

The faculty decided that a retreat would be the best way to proceed. Dr. Korsan agreed to hire an expert for a 1-day, off-campus retreat for faculty and other stakeholders. Another faculty member thought it wise to strike a faculty development committee to plan future learning opportunities in an organized and strategic fashion. There was overall agreement for this idea, and the dean asked faculty to consider who would like to serve on this committee.

Critique

Copernicus University School of Nursing has a cohesive faculty committed to revising the undergraduate curriculum. Motivation for change came from the total faculty, who are willing to participate in task forces and focus groups, and complete literature searches. Faculty involvement is valued. Their concerns about a new direction as well as suggestions about how to proceed are respected. It is likely that the collective strength of faculty will support them through their desired revision and facilitate feelings of ownership of the proposed changes as the process unfolds.

The collective decision to proceed carefully by learning more about several philosophical approaches for nursing curricula is sensible. Faculty members recognize that a change is desirable. They believe the focus should be on lived experiences of clients, learners, and themselves; however, they do not fully understand what this change may imply or how to go about introducing it. Consideration will have to be given to faculty members' knowledge about the process of curriculum redesign. Other issues, such as how the curriculum should be developed to assure congruence with the curriculum outcomes, have not yet been identified. Whether curriculum revision is a process with which they are familiar or one with which they have had little experience, this assessment is required. It is likely that as faculty progress with curriculum development, many learning needs will arise related to roles and relationships, curriculum implementation, teaching, and evaluation. It will be important to assess their understanding about how to implement the proposed changes in the curriculum and what implications these could have for all stakeholders.

Dr. Korsan is demonstrating commitment to the process by supporting a formal faculty development opportunity facilitated by an expert, so faculty can gain a more complete understanding of philosophical approaches as these apply to nursing curricula. This is a good start. As well, the faculty of Copernicus University School of Nursing has wisely decided to form a faculty development committee. Striking this committee will maintain momentum and continue to move the process forward. The group will be able to use the data collected to plan further learning opportunities. It will be prudent for the committee to ascertain faculty needs and preferred strategies, as well as resources available to implement the plans they propose. The school's approach to adopting a new philosophical direction and the plan to proceed is being carefully executed.

Rosemount University School of Nursing

Rosemount University School of Nursing has offered baccalaureate and masters programs in nursing for 40 years. Most faculty have kept abreast of current curriculum paradigms and teaching-learning methods in order to deliver the "best" nursing program to qualified students. Faculty development through attendance at occasional in-house meetings or attendance at local, national, or international conferences has been considered important to most of the faculty. However, an ongoing faculty development program was not implemented due to resistance from a few "senior" faculty members.

Recently, Dr. Angela Fabatini, director of the school, attended a national meeting of baccalaureate nursing program deans/directors. One recommendation, among many others developed by the group, was that faculty development include activities intended to facilitate knowledgeable participation in curriculum development.

On returning from the conference, Dr. Fabatini called a faculty meeting. A review of faculty development activities was undertaken. The results revealed a fragmented approach to faculty development, sporadic faculty attendance, and very little attention to the specifics of the curriculum process. Inexperienced faculty members wanted an ongoing faculty development program to assist them in revising the present baccalaureate-nursing program. Two senior experienced faculty members voiced their resistance to this activity, claiming that the past practice of ad hoc meetings was satisfactory and that there was no necessity for change, since the program is accredited.

Questions for Consideration and Analysis of Rosemount University Case

1. What are the strengths and limitations in the present faculty development system?
2. What strategies might be instituted to encourage participation in faculty development?
3. When agreement is reached to undertake faculty development for curriculum change, what would be the goals of this activity? What development activities could be instituted?
4. What responses might be appropriate for those faculty members resisting change?
5. If the Rosemount University faculty decide to proceed with curriculum development, which change theory would be useful, and how could it be used?

Curriculum Development Activities for Consideration in Your Setting

To plan for faculty development related to curriculum development in your setting, consider the questions below:

1. Who could best champion the faculty development process in your institution?
2. What might be the anticipated and unanticipated benefits and challenges associated with initiating faculty development activities in your setting?
3. Which faculty development activities do faculty currently accept or reject?
4. How can faculty be supported to view curriculum development as an engaging and empowering process?
5. Consider the elements of the Transtheoretical Model of Behavior Change. According to these elements, which activities do you believe would be most constructive in helping faculty move smoothly through the transition from the current to the envisioned curriculum? Why?
6. What resources (human, physical, material, fiscal) can the school access to support faculty development initiatives during curriculum development?
7. What are the key elements of a faculty development program to support faculty and curriculum development and change in your school?
8. Design a faculty development program for your school of nursing.

References

Bartels, J. E. (2007). Preparing nursing faculty for baccalaureate-level and graduate-level nursing programs: Role preparation for the academy. *Journal of Nursing Education, 46,* 154–158.

Bartfay, W. J., & Howse, E. (2007). Who will teach the nurses of the future? *Canadian Nurse, 103*(7), 24–27.

Bevis, E. O. (2000). Clusters of influence for practical decision making about curriculum. In E. O. Bevis, & J. Watson (Eds.), *Toward a caring curriculum: A new pedagogy for nursing* (pp. 107–152). Boston: Jones and Bartlett.

Canadian Nurses Association & Canadian Association of Schools of Nursing. (2007). *Nursing education in Canada statistics 2005–06.* Retrieved November 12, 2007, from http://www.cna-nurses.ca/CNA/documents/pdf/publications/Nursing_Education_Statistics_2005_2006_e.pdf

Chambers, H. E. (1998). *The bad attitude survival guide.* Reading, MA: Addison-Wesley.

Davies, M. A. (2002). *Perceived workplace empowerment, job tension, and job satisfaction of clinical educators in hospital settings: Testing Kanter's theory.* Unpublished master's thesis, University of Western Ontario, London, Ontario, Canada.

Davis, B. (1993). *Tools for teaching.* San Francisco: Jossey-Bass.

Erwin, E. M. (1999). The relationships between perceptions of workplace empowerment of college nurse educators and an organizational climate for caring in the workplace. Unpublished master's thesis, University of Western Ontario, London, Ontario, Canada.

Foley, B. J., Redman, R. W., Horn, E. V., Davis, G. T., Neal, E. M., & Van Riper, M. L. (2003). Determining nursing faculty development needs. *Nursing Outlook, 51,* 227–232.

Goldenberg, D., Andrusyszyn, M. A., & Iwasiw, C. (2004). A facilitative approach to learning about curriculum development. *Journal of Nursing Education, 43,* 31–35.

Greenhalgh, T., Robert, G., Bate, P., Macfarlane, R., & Kyriakidou, O. (2005). *Diffusion of innovations in health service organizations: A systematic literature review.* Oxford: BMJ Books/Blackwell.

Halliburton, D., Marincovich, M., & Svinicki, M. (1988). Strengthening professional development. *Journal of Higher Education, 59,* 291–304.

Kanter, R. M. (1977). *Men and women of the corporation.* New York: Basic Books.

Kanter, R. M. (1993). *Men and women of the corporation* (2nd ed.). New York: Basic Books.

Kaufman, K. (2007). Introducing the NLN/Carnegie national survey of nurse educators: Compensation, workload, and teaching practice. *Nursing Education Perspectives, 2,* 164–167.

Kenner, C., & Pressler, J. I. (2006). Successfully climbing the academic leadership ladder. *Nurse Educator, 31*(1), 1–3.

Kupperschmidt, B. R., & Burns, P. (1997). Curriculum revision isn't just change: It's transition! *Journal of Professional Nursing, 13,* 90–98.

National League for Nursing. (2005). *The scope of practice of academic nurse educators.* New York: Author.

Patterson, K., Grenny, J., McMillan, R., & Switzler, A. (2002). *Crucial confrontations: Tools for resolving broken promises, violated expectations, and bad behavior.* New York: McGraw-Hill.

Prochaska, J. O., DiClemente, C. C., & Norcross, J. C. (1992). In search of how people change: Applications to addictive behaviors. *American Psychologist, 47,* 1102–1114.

Prochaska, J. M., Prochaska, J., Cohen, F. C., Gomes, S. O., Laforge, R. G., & Eastwood, A. L. (2004). The transtheoretical model of change for multi-level interventions for alcohol abuse on campus. *Journal of Alcohol and Drug Education, 47*(3), 34–50.

Prochaska, J. O., Redding, C. A., Harlow, L. L., Rossi, J. S., & Velicer, W. F. (1994). The transtheoretical model of change and HIV prevention: A review. *Health Education Quarterly, 21,* 471–486.

Raff, B. S., & Arnold, J. (2001). Faculty development: An approach to scholarship. *Nurse Educator, 26,* 159–162.

Rogers, E. M. (2003). *Diffusion of innovations* (5th ed.). New York: Free Press.

Rush, K., Ouellet, L., & Wasson, D. (1991). Faculty development: The essence of curriculum development. *Nurse Education Today, 11,* 121–126.

Sarmiento, T., Laschinger, H. K. S., & Iwasiw, C. (2004). College educators' workplace empowerment, burnout, and job satisfaction: Testing Kanter's theory. *Journal of Advanced Nursing, 24,* 134–143.

Smolen, D. (1996). Constraints that nursing program administrators encounter in promoting faculty change and development. *Journal of Professional Nursing, 12*(2), 91–98.

Steinert, Y., Mann, K., Centeno, A., Dolmans, D., Spencer, J., Gelula, M., et al. (2006). A systematic review of faculty development initiatives designed to improve teaching effectiveness in medical education: BEME Guide No. 8. *Medical Teacher, 28,* 497–526.

Sullivan, E. J., & Decker, P. J. (2005). *Effective leadership & management in nursing* (6th ed.). Upper Saddle River, NJ: Pearson Prentice Hall.

PART III

Development of a Context-Relevant Curriculum

CHAPTER 6

Data-Gathering for a Context-Relevant Curriculum

Chapter Overview

A context-relevant curriculum is responsive to the educational and societal environment in which it is offered. To create such a curriculum, contextual factors within and beyond the school of nursing must be investigated. The contextual factors are the forces, situations, and circumstances that curriculum developers must take into account as they plan a curriculum. Although the contextual factors can be viewed in many ways, the typology presented in this chapter is a reasonable way to conceptualize them. Following a definition of a *context-relevant curriculum* and discussion about the influence of the factors on the curriculum, important internal and external contextual factors are described. Next, approaches to data-gathering are outlined, including considerations to determine essential data and data sources to pursue. The term *data-gathering* is used to differentiate the activity of obtaining information for curriculum development from the data collection of research projects. Additionally, faculty development pertinent to gathering data about contextual factors is described. A case study and critique exemplify the important points of the chapter. A second case is presented for analysis. Finally, questions are included to determine readiness to undertake data-gathering activities.

Chapter Goals

- Appreciate how examination of the environment is foundational to the creation of a context-relevant curriculum.
- Identify internal and external contextual factors that influence curriculum directions.
- Determine essential data to gather about the contextual factors.
- Explore data-gathering methods and data sources relevant to curriculum development.
- Consider faculty development activities related to data-gathering about contextual factors.

The Context-Relevant Curriculum and Contextual Factors

A context-relevant curriculum is one that is responsive to learners; to current and projected societal, health, and community situations; and to imperatives of the nursing profession. It is consistent with the mission, philosophy, and goals of the educational institution, and it is feasible within the realities of the school and community. To create such a curriculum, it is necessary to have organized, comprehensive, and accurate information about the environment in which the curriculum will be offered.

The environment of the curriculum can be conceptualized as being composed of interrelated contextual factors. *Contextual factors are those forces, situations, and circumstances that exist both within and outside the school of nursing and have the potential to influence the school and its programs.* The factors are complex, and ever-changing; yet, form and boundaries must be given to them so that the concept of contextual factors is understandable and useful for curriculum development.

For the purposes of curriculum development, *internal contextual factors are those forces, situations, and circumstances that originate within the school and educational institution, that is, within the internal environment of the educational institution. External contextual factors are those forces, situations, and circumstances that originate outside the educational institution in the community, region, country, and world.* A typology of internal and external contextual factors is described in subsequent sections of this chapter.

Although differentiated for the purpose of descriptive clarity, in reality, some internal and external contextual factors blend, intermingle, and overlap. As well, some factors exist in both internal and external environments. For example, culture can be seen as an internal contextual factor when described in relation to the school of nursing, and as an external contextual factor when reviewed in relation to the community.

Because the contextual factors (e.g., social, political, and economic) can be large and nebulous, curriculum developers must define precisely what the essential data are for each factor. The data necessary for curriculum development are the specific facts and information about the contextual factors deemed most likely to shape the curriculum. These data might be as intangible as the ethos of the community's main healthcare agency and/or as concrete as the school's budget. Clearly, the more definitive the data, the stronger the basis for designing the curriculum.

An examination of the contextual factors within and across the internal and external contexts provides curriculum developers with current information and patterns and trends about the following:

- Characteristics of learners
- Learning expectations and environments
- Professional practice expectations and environments
- Clients of nursing care
- Major health problems and risks
- Health care
- Societal characteristics and needs.

Purposeful data-gathering about the contextual factors and the subsequent analysis that are proposed in the following chapter, will yield the "big picture" of the current and future environment in which the curriculum will be offered, and result in curriculum concepts that will remain relevant into the future. Thorough data-gathering and analysis provide a means for nurse educators to ensure that the curriculum "reflects [the] institutional philosophy and mission, current nursing and healthcare trends, and community and societal needs so as to prepare graduates for practice in a complex, dynamic, multicultural healthcare environment" (National League for Nursing, 2005, p. 19).

The emphasis on the contextual factors is most aligned with ideas of strategic thinking and strategic planning, whereby programs are developed for current and anticipated opportunities in the external context. This is not synonymous with a needs assessment, which connotes a gap between the present state and a desired state. A needs approach is generally based on predetermined ideas about the desired state, or what should be, and could result in a curriculum with a relatively short life span. Our approach is intended to result in a curriculum that will be relevant not only for the present, but for the future.

Internal Contextual Factors

As stated previously, the internal contextual factors are those forces, situations, and circumstances that originate within the school of nursing and educational institution. These include the mission, vision, philosophy, goals, culture, history, financial resources, programs, and infrastructure of the educational institution and school of nursing.

Mission, Vision, Philosophy, and Goals

Every organization has a mission, which is a succinct statement that captures the institution's distinctive character. It is a "broadly defined and enduring statement of purpose that distinguishes one . . . institution from other organizations of its type . . ." (Swayne, Duncan, & Ginter, 2006, p. 188). The uniqueness of the institution and the scope of its activities are evident in the mission statement. As such, the mission informs those within and outside the organization of its ultimate raison d'être. The educational institution's mission shapes the nature, scope, and boundaries of the goals, activities, and curricula of the school of nursing.

The educational institution and the school of nursing also have a vision, an "expression of hope" (Swayne et al., 2006, p. 198). It is a description of what the organization will be like when it fully meets its purpose.

The mission, vision, and purpose of the educational institution and school of nursing are articulated most directly in the strategic plan. Curriculum developers must give this plan considerable attention. The long- and short-term goals, objectives, timelines, and critical outcomes for the institution and school will give insights about institutional priorities. Data from the strategic plan give direction to recommendations about the curriculum. Conversely, knowledge of the strategic plan can signal potential roadblocks to curriculum development or particular preferences about the curriculum.

Institutions of higher education also have clearly articulated guiding principles, or beliefs and values, about the services offered, the community served, and the fundamental activities that take place within them. Statements about education, learning, knowledge development, scholarship, and so forth form the philosophy. In addition to understanding the institution's philosophy or guiding principles, it is important to identify those that operate within the school of nursing.

The nursing curriculum must be congruent with the educational institution's mission, vision, philosophy and fundamental guiding principles. Faculty members require a solid understanding of these before initiating curriculum development.

Culture

Organizations have a culture or "way of being" that may not be directly evident. The culture is a pattern of shared values, assumptions, and behaviors that are taught either implicitly or explicitly to new members (Whitehead, Weiss, & Tappan, 2007). Adjectives (e.g., progressive or traditional; friendly or hostile; bureaucratic or participatory) or metaphors (e.g., like a family; a snake pit) are often used to encapsulate prominent aspects of the culture.

Organizational culture evolves over time and is slow to change. The culture is formed by determinants such as the people in the organization, how these people interact and make decisions, the endeavors and decisions pursued or avoided, and the consequences of these actions. A significant aspect of the culture is whether change is welcomed or avoided. If a new curriculum is premised on a changed culture in the school, curriculum developers must strategize carefully, since culture change is difficult to accomplish.

History

Examining the institution's history will reveal past values, successes, and challenges, as well as the school's processes for curriculum development. Much can be learned about how past challenges have been met and successes achieved. This information may still be pertinent for decisions about the curriculum. For example, if the educational institution is one that has built an international reputation, curriculum developers might examine the way this was done, and ask how the nursing curriculum could contribute to, or capitalize on this renown. Answers to the following questions may provide some insight into the history of the institution and the school of nursing.

- When were the educational institution and the school of nursing founded, and why?
- Have the institution's and school's purposes changed over time? If so, why and how?
- How does the school's history influence current programs and operations?
- What programs are offered? How have these evolved? Over what time frame?
- Were programs developed for a niche market?
- What are the unique features that have developed within the institution, the school, and the programs?

When preparing a new curriculum, faculty members are creating the school's ongoing history. Accordingly, the processes and decisions should be recorded for future curriculum developers, so they will not be dependent on a few faculty members who are the custodians of the institutional memory, and whose recollections are lost when they leave the school.

Financial Resources

Financial resources, possibly more than any other internal contextual factor, influence the curriculum design. Knowledge of the operating costs of a school, budget planning, and budget allocation is essential.

Careful attention should be given to the cost that would be created by a redesigned curriculum. Funding limits can constrain the curriculum design, and adequate financial resources are essential for successful implementation. For example, if there are tentative thoughts about changing from a 4-year generic baccalaureate program to 1 or 2 years of pre-nursing courses, followed by intensive study in nursing, then it is essential to ascertain what this would mean for the school's income. Such knowledge would signal whether the idea is worthy of exploration or whether it should be abandoned.

Programs and Policies

The programs and policies of the educational institution and the school of nursing form an important factor of the internal environment. Within the school, the type and number of programs, physical and human resources dedicated to those programs, and the relationship of the developing curriculum to other programs, will influence curriculum design. For example, if caring for vulnerable populations is a theme of the graduate program, it would be reasonable to expect some emphasis in this area in a redesigned undergraduate curriculum.

The range of courses offered by other departments could be an asset to the curriculum designers or could limit the scope of what they can propose. Knowledge from the physical, biological, and psychosocial sciences, as well as from the arts and humanities, contributes significantly to nursing knowledge and well-rounded graduates. Hence, courses from these disciplines are essential in a nursing curriculum. The availability of courses, prerequisites, and scheduling should be ascertained. The possibility of negotiating new non-nursing courses may exist. These are typically called *support courses*. They are called *non-nursing courses* in this book because they do not merely support the nursing curriculum, they are an integral part of it.

Additionally, programs in other health science disciplines should be surveyed. Previously unused interdisciplinary or interprofessional learning opportunities may exist, or may be negotiated if the curriculum developers consider them important.

Curriculum development must be considered in light of existing policies and guidelines. Institutional and school policies and guidelines should be available and understood by the curriculum development team. Revising or adding school policies as part of curriculum development can be a complicated process and must be accomplished within the context of existing institutional regulations. Requests for policy changes that might affect the educational institution are more complex and can be expected to take a longer period of time to achieve.

Infrastructure

The term *infrastructure* refers to those elements that form the structure of the educational institution and school of nursing, and serve as the foundation of educational programs. Elements of the infrastructure include human and physical resources, as well as those to support teaching and learning. Data can be secured and scrutinized to obtain a comprehensive picture of the infrastructure.

Human Resources   Human resources form the core of the curriculum and are the most important resource of the institution. It is largely through interactions between and among students and faculty that the curriculum is experienced, and therefore, people are the center of the curriculum. Indeed, as European universities were developing in the 10th and 11th centuries, professors and students (human resources) were more than the curriculum. They were the university, meeting wherever they could because university buildings did not exist.

Faculty are key contributors to curriculum development and implementation, and represent a vital part of the internal infrastructure. They are critical sources of insight and information about what to include in the curriculum, because they know what works, what doesn't, and why. They bring the curriculum to life, execute all its dimensions, and have a vested interest in learner and program success.

Information about current nursing and non-nursing faculty and the pool of potential faculty is an important determinant of curriculum development decisions. Data about areas of specialty, educational preparation, possible retirement dates, preferences for teaching area, and so forth, will be valuable. Additionally, adjunct faculty, guest lecturers, clinical experts, preceptors, and healthcare leaders form part of faculty resources. They need to be considered when shaping the curriculum, not only for the contributions they might make to the future curriculum, but also for the involvement and perspectives they can offer to curriculum development, implementation, and evaluation.

Students are an essential human resource, as important as faculty members. Schools of nursing would not exist were it not for learners; without them, there is no need for curriculum. Student data form the basis of much internal contextual information critical to curriculum development, since the curriculum is designed for them. Table 6-1 lists student data that could be obtained to enhance understanding of the internal contextual environment.

The amount and nature of information that can be obtained about current and potential students and faculty is governed by institutional policies and human rights and privacy legislation. As an example, in some jurisdictions it is possible to ask about race; in others, it is not.

Support staff represents another important human resource. Programs could not function without people such as secretaries, admissions officers, caretakers, information technology specialists, and others. They make possible the smooth day-to-day operations of the school. Gathering data about this group, such as numbers and skill sets, is mandatory.

Information about human resources includes details about contracts that govern the working life of faculty and staff. A review of faculty and staff collective agreements provides insights into matters such as job expectations, holiday entitlement, hours of work, and so forth. These all influence the curriculum. For example, if it is not possible to assign full-time

Table 6-1   Student Data

Number of applicants

Number of admissions

Numbers meeting and exceeding admission requirements

Demographics:

- previous education
- age
- marital status
- number of dependents
- employment status

Catchment area

Proportion of full- and part-time students

Grade point average

Grades in nursing and support courses

Attrition rates and rationale

Success rate on registration or licensure examinations

Follow-up data about graduates

- employment positions
- employer evaluations
- numbers admitted to graduate programs

faculty to teach on weekends, then curriculum designers would have to weigh the educational value of weekend clinical experience against the effects of inaccessibility of full-time faculty.

Physical Resources   Availability and quality of materials and space for classrooms, offices, and laboratories must be considered as they influence what is possible in the curriculum. Knowledge of these resources can also be a basis for negotiating for new or additional facilities to match developing ideas about curriculum design and student learning needs.

Technology is an important part of the physical resources. Availability and adequacy of office computers, student computer labs, audiovisual and clinical equipment, smart classrooms, distributed learning technology, high-fidelity mannequins, and the like should be determined. Technologies assist faculty to fulfill their roles efficiently, are necessary for effective teaching, and facilitate student learning.

Resources to Support Teaching and Learning   Resources that support teaching and learning should also be examined. Knowing what is available will assist in making curriculum decisions, planning, and negotiating for additional resources.

Library resources are essential for teaching and learning. Facilities and collections should be reviewed with respect to the strengths and gaps in the library's collection. Online databases extend the library's holdings, and their availability has implications for curriculum and course designs, student assignments, and faculty research. Knowledge about shortcomings in library holdings provides a basis for negotiating altered or expanded materials and services.

Faculty development services are another element of the internal infrastructure. School and institution-wide programs related to teaching and research development can be sources of ideas and support for the new curriculum. If, for example, institution-wide programs for developing online courses are provided, then curriculum developers will know that distributed learning courses could be planned or expanded. However, if there are no programs relevant to teaching or evaluation in the envisioned curriculum, then curriculum developers will have four choices as they plan the curriculum and its implementation:

- Create and offer the faculty development program themselves.
- Hire a consultant.
- Negotiate for an institution-wide program that will not be specific to nursing.
- Avoid particular teaching and evaluation approaches in the new curriculum.

Teaching support, such as graduate teaching assistants, or other university-employed or university-sponsored students, can extend faculty teaching. Typically, graduate students contribute to curriculum implementation through teaching, grading assignments, and leading tutorial sessions. As well, sources of funding for curriculum innovation should be explored.

Student services related to assessment and development of academic skills, personal support, health, recreation, and financial assistance are integral aspects of the institutional infrastructure. These services can mean the difference between success and failure for many learners.

An inventory of available resources, knowledge of future plans for resources and services, and the possibility of negotiating new ones, are influential when shaping and bringing vitality to the curriculum. Curricularists must understand the infrastructure in which the redesigned curriculum will operate so they can plan a feasible curriculum with conviction, secure in the knowledge that the resources will be available to bring their plans to fruition.

Summary of Internal Contextual Factors

In summary, internal contextual factors are those forces, situations, and circumstances that originate within the school and educational institution and have potential to influence the curriculum. These should be examined in two ways: a macro view to capture the contextual data relevant to the institution and a micro view to focus more specifically on the school of nursing.

External Contextual Factors

As described previously, external contextual factors are those forces, situations, and circumstances that originate outside the educational institution and also have the potential to influence curriculum. They originate in the community, region, country, and world, that is, the environment beyond the educational institution.

Interestingly, as early as the 1970s, Conley (1973) urged curricularists to pay attention to social forces when planning or changing curricula. She referred to population mobility as one social factor in which persons are continually changing jobs, resulting in people lost on a medical landscape and becoming medically disengaged. She also cited the general sophistication of the public, a commercialization of the professions, wherein professionals are no longer altruistic but more interested in career ladders; and a change from a religious and philosophical orientation to a more scientific and research-based outlook. She observed the growth and spread of organized interest groups in the community, government, and unions, as well as in other conglomerates. Finally, she remarked on the shift in age composition and disease prevalence in the population. Her observations still hold true today, and are consistent with the external factors of relevance to current nursing curriculum developers.

An examination of external contextual factors is crucial to understanding the needs and characteristics of society and their application to contemporary nursing curricula. A brief survey of the most influential external contextual factors follows. Chapter 7 contains further examples of contextual data and their relationship to a context-relevant nursing curriculum.

Demographics

Demography is "the scientific study of populations that focuses on their size, distribution, age structure, fertility, marital patterns, migrations, mortality, and the social, cultural, economic, and other determinants of variations in any or all of these features" (Last, 2007). Demographic data, which have a significant influence on healthcare delivery and nursing education, should be obtained. Information pertaining to population characteristics assists curriculum developers to know about the people who are and will be clients of the healthcare system. The nursing curriculum can then be designed to align with the attributes of those who are recipients of nursing care. Local, regional, and national data should be obtained. Pertinent census data and vital statistics include the following:

- Birth, death, and fertility rates
- Distribution according to age, sex, location, and combinations of these
- Population diversity
- Employment rates and income levels by age and sex
- Ethnicity

- Residence patterns (e.g., proportion of aged living alone, in nursing homes)
- Morbidity rates and patterns
- Family structures
- Immigration and emigration patterns

Assessing population demographics is germane to developing relevant nursing curricula. Obviously, characteristics of human populations (i.e., the people nurses serve) must be included in the data that curricularists examine in order to construct a relevant curriculum.

Culture

Further to assessing the demographics of the human populations nurses serve, curriculum developers direct attention to the culture(s) within the external environment. *Culture* refers to "the way of life of a people, including their attitudes, values, beliefs, arts, sciences, modes of perception, and habits of thought and activity. Cultural features of forms of life are learned but are often too pervasive to be readily noticed from within" (Blackburn, 1996). Included in the concept are a common history, sense of destiny, value system embedded in a particular religion or mythology, as well as shared traditions, rituals, a language with a distinctive vocabulary, and "narratives that give [express] norms, and models of behavior" (Sitelman & Sitelman, 2000, p. 12). This depiction of culture is extensive and captures many of the subtleties inherent in the individuals, groups, and communities that comprised the external environment in which the nursing program is situated.

Race and *ethnicity* are often equated with a particular culture that has its own practices, rituals, and beliefs, but this is not always the case. People of the same ethnic or racial origin may represent a unified subculture, or they may have been assimilated into the dominant culture.

Each community has a number of subcultures that may not be immediately obvious, but which contribute to the tapestry of the community and, therefore, are relevant for curriculum planning. The cultures of youth, poverty, family violence, homelessness, gender, aging, work environments, and the culture of the healthcare system are some examples.

The culture of the healthcare system is worthy of note: how clients are treated, the degree of acceptance of complementary and alternative practices, the languages in which printed information is available, and the quality and nature of provider interactions. These influence nursing care and work life, clients' responses to healthcare providers, and consequently, some aspect of nursing curriculum.

Respect for the traditions, shared beliefs, values, attitudes, and norms of the distinctive cultures is prerequisite when designing a curriculum. This is particularly important in this century when cultural diversity in most regions and countries continues to increase because of immigration, emigration, and even technological advances linking individuals, groups, and communities within cyberspace.

Health and Health Care

Demographics influence the health profile of the population and health care, another external factor relevant for curriculum planners. The health of people clearly influences nursing care, and thus, curriculum. The healthcare system is a prime determinant of the clinical learning context. Both the health status of the population and the nature of services may provide previously unexamined opportunities for clinical education. Pertinent information related to *health and the healthcare system* might include the following:

- Most prevalent local and national health problems
- Nature of healthcare agencies and their services
- Nature and availability of public health and other community-based healthcare services
- Adequacy of funding for health care
- Availability of healthcare insurance
- Costs to clients and families
- Availability of healthcare resources (i.e., healthcare services, equipment, healthcare providers, health educators)
- Profile of clients receiving care
- Gaps in service.

Relevant information related to *nursing education* might include:

- Potential clinical placement sites and experiences
- Receptiveness of clinical agencies to learners
- Willingness of healthcare providers to participate in student education
- Opportunities for clinical education with students from other health professional programs.

Curriculum developers ought to gather data pertaining to settings and opportunities for student clinical learning experiences, as well as data about changes in prominent health problems, care services, and facilities. They should be current about healthcare delivery patterns, escalating costs, and available resources. Furthermore, they should be mindful of the needs and demands of more sophisticated healthcare consumers.

Professional Standards and Trends

Health care, nursing practice standards, and nursing education standards affect the practice and education of nurses. Accordingly, trends in these influence curriculum development.

Data to obtain include:

- Professional, regulatory, licensing, and accreditation requirements
- Entry-to-practice, nursing practice, legal, and ethical standards
- Self-assessment and quality assurance guidelines or requirements
- Evidence-based practices and best practice guidelines
- Research on nursing education and practice
- Contemporary nursing education models, frameworks, philosophies, and teaching-learning approaches
- Current and future roles and the scope of practice that nurses will assume
- Position statements from professional organizations, nursing leaders and experts, administrators, researchers, graduates, and the public

Technology and Informatics

Advances in technology influence the content, teaching-learning strategies, and course management of nursing curricula. Curricularists should gather data about technology and informatics for health care and education, as well as expected developments.

Technology is changing the nature of nursing education, and will continue to do so. For example, the utility of PDAs is becoming apparent (Greenfield, 2007) and use of high-fidelity mannequins is common in nursing education. Neuman (2006) describes how learning technologies are changing nursing education, through methods such as Web-based distributed learning, and proposes innovations for the future. Similarly, educational management systems can alter the roles of nursing faculty (Nelson, Meyers, Rizzolo, Rutar, Proto, & Newbold, 2006).

The e-health paradigm of health care has important implications for nursing curriculum and curriculum developers; hence, attention must be given to this. Booth (2006) asserts that "information literacy, emphasis on interdisciplinary collaboration, and patient-focused systems are invaluable inclusions in any nursing informatics content and should be mandatory in all curricula" (p. 8). Further, "topics of confidentiality, access, reliability, and quality assurance provided by e-health technology, and the relationship of these topics to patient care and nursing practice" (p. 6) should be addressed. Additionally, the wide use of the Internet by clients seeking health information, the emergence of virtual support groups, and variable reliability of online health information, also influences nursing curricula.

In spite of the seemingly all-pervasive nature of information technology, student exposure and skill in information technology seems to be limited, according to Ornes and Gassert (2007), who evaluated one undergraduate curriculum. In a larger study of how Canadian nursing schools were integrating informatics into the curriculum, no responses were received from some schools because there were no faculty members with appropriate expertise. As well, some respondents indicated that informatics was not relevant content for their curricula (Infoway, as cited in Nagle, 2007).

Environment

Environment is a broad contextual factor that refers to the atmospheric, physical, and psychological milieu of a community. The influence of the environment might not be limited by geographic and political boundaries, and therefore, must be considered in curriculum planning. For example, chemical, biological, physical, sociological, and psychological hazards and stressors can pose threats to individual, family, and community health, locally, nationally, and internationally. Data about national and international events and possible threats are important, although curriculum developers will likely focus on information about their immediate community. These data could include some or all of the issues listed below, in particular those that seem most relevant to the locale of the school of nursing:

- Weather patterns such as severe blizzards, extremely hot summers, tornadoes, or hurricanes
- Effects of climate change
- Air and water quality
- Presence of local industries known to produce environmental pollutants and hazards
- Environmental disasters, such as oil spills, volcanoes, forest fires
- Decreased energy supplies
- Nuclear and chemical spillage and warfare
- Terrorism
- Newly emerging diseases and their spread.

Social, Political, and Economic Conditions

Social, political, and economic conditions form another broad contextual factor that encompasses forces, situations, or circumstances in the external environment. Because social, political, and economic events and issues are strongly interconnected, with each affecting the others, they are presented as one contextual factor. Information about this factor is important for curriculum planning.

Data about each of the previously identified external contextual factors (demographics, culture, healthcare system, professional standards and trends, technology, and environment) are related to social, political, and economic conditions, and some data pertinent to this factor may be obtained while collecting information about the others. Examples of pertinent data are provided below.

Social behaviors and issues that affect health can include:

- Drug use in the community
- Sexual behavior of adolescents
- Unemployment rates and patterns
- Housing availability, affordability, and quality
- Nature and rate of crime in the community.

Political and legislative (local, regional, provincial/state, and national) influences affect:

- Higher education and nursing education
- Health care and social services
- Eligibility for health care and social services
- Support for nursing and nursing education from elected political parties, government officials, and community representatives
- Public concern about nursing shortages and access to health care
- Projections for a comprehensive healthcare system.

Economic conditions that affect health can include:

- Governmental financial support for higher education and nursing education
- Private, community, or public funding for the following:
  - Curriculum innovation
  - Program development
  - Faculty and student grants or scholarships
  - Present and projected local, provincial/state, and national economies.

Curriculum stakeholders should carefully assess these and other social, political, and economic issues that can have a direct bearing on the curriculum to be developed.

Summary of External Contextual Factors

In summary, external contextual factors are those forces, situations, and circumstances that originate outside the educational institution in the community, region, country, and world. Nursing curriculum developers must carefully consider data about the external contextual factors so that a future-oriented, context-relevant curriculum can be created. This type of curriculum is developed in response to demographic trends, culture, health and healthcare trends, professional standards, technology and informatics, the environment, and social, political, and economic conditions. Knowledge of these will make it possible for nurse educators to prepare professional nurses capable of caring for culturally diverse individuals, families, and groups within a dynamic society and healthcare system.

Approaches to Data-Gathering for Curriculum Development

In this book, the term *data-gathering* is used instead of *data collection* to differentiate the activities of obtaining information for curriculum development purposes, from the acquisition of information for research purposes. Although some of the methods may be the same, the purposes and rigor vary. Some differences are identified in Table 6-2.

Table 6-2 Differentiation of Information Acquisition for Curriculum Development and Research

Characteristics	Data-Gathering for Curriculum Development	Data Collection for Research
Purpose	Obtain information that will influence curriculum development	Obtain information to answer specific research questions and/or test hypothesis
Scope of information	Very broad	More limited
Procedures to obtain information	Planned, but open to change Quantitative and qualitative methods used	Formalized and limited by research design
Procedures to analyze information	Planned, but less prescribed than data analysis for research	Planned data analysis, in accordance with research design
Instruments	Quantitative and qualitative data-gathering tools or guides specific to school and curriculum context Pilot-tested with convenience sample for comprehensiveness and comprehension	Quantitative tools: • Psychometric testing with each use • Instruments with known psychometric characteristics preferred
	Quantitative tools generally are not assessed for psychometric properties and may not be reused	Qualitative questionnaires or interview guides specific to the research project
Anonymity of data sources	Usually permission to reveal source required	Yes
Requirement for approval by ethics review board	Generally no, unless data are also being used for research purposes	Yes

A thorough understanding of the context in which the curriculum will be offered can be gained only through planned data-gathering. Although some faculty members may believe that they know what the contextual situation is, and therefore, that only a small amount of effort is required for data-gathering, this perspective should not prevail. General knowledge about the context is an insufficient basis for curriculum development. The accumulation of detailed information, and the curriculum decisions that flow from analysis of the information, ground the curriculum in the context and assure its relevance.

Planning for data-gathering requires agreement about the contextual factors requiring investigation, and identification of relevant data, data sources, and methods to obtain the information. Data-gathering represents a strong public statement that a redesigned curriculum will be forthcoming, as the activities are dependent on interactions between nursing faculty and other members of the educational institution, key personnel in healthcare agencies, and community members. Although the intention to develop a curriculum is known to stakeholders involved in the planning that precedes data-gathering, it is at this time that expectations for curriculum change are raised in the wider community. Moreover, external data-gathering conveys the message that the curriculum will be relevant to its context. Because of the public nature of data-gathering activities, curriculum developers are obligated to present themselves in a credible manner, and this requires planning and organization.

The scope of data-gathering about contextual factors, and the subsequent interpretation of the data, are foundational to the nature, relevance, and longevity of the curriculum. When deciding on the data to be collected, data sources, and methods for gathering data, curricularists must strive to achieve a reasonable balance between a desire to acquire a breadth and depth of data on the one hand, and to progress in a timely manner on the other.

Deciding on Necessary Contextual Data and Data Sources

The contextual data required for curriculum development must be agreed upon so that suitable sources can be identified, and if necessary, data-gathering tools developed. There should be openness to the acquisition of data that is not initially identified but subsequently recognized as important. For example, it might be decided that data about the intended programmatic directions of the major healthcare agencies in the community would be essential, that particular healthcare leaders are appropriate data sources, and that interviews would be the most expedient method of acquiring the data. If, in the course of an interview, an administrator comments that in order to introduce new programs, some clinical units will be closed for renovations, it would be prudent to ask for more information immediately, since there are clear implications for the curriculum. In making decisions about which data to collect, curriculum developers could consider the following:

- Which contextual factors seem most germane to their situation?
- What are the precise data required?

- What is the potential utility of the data for the curriculum development process?
- Which data will truly influence the curriculum?
- What is "nice to know," but not absolutely imperative for curriculum development?
- How might the data identified influence curriculum?
- How accessible and available are the data?
- How quickly can data be obtained?
- Is acquisition of any data so important that a delay in curriculum development is justified?
- What are the consequences of failing to collect these data?

When curriculum developers decide upon the necessary data for each contextual factor, the inter-related nature of the factors will be apparent: data gathered could be pertinent to more than one factor. It is best to record the information for all the factors to which it pertains, rather than spending time on discussions about where it belongs.

A host of individuals, groups, organizations, and documents can be used as data sources to provide information that may influence curriculum decisions. Determining which sources would be most useful is dependent on the situation within each school of nursing and the community. The decision requires judgments about information such as:

- Richness of data likely to be obtained
- Accessibility and availability of data sources
- Purpose of data gathering (solely as a basis for curriculum development or also for research)
- Resources available (time, people, finances, materials).

Data-Gathering Methods

Knowledge that shapes the curriculum is generally not collected according to the rigorous standards of a formal research study. However, attention must be given to the institutional research ethics approval procedures if research is conducted along with curriculum development. If there is overlap or ambiguity about what is research and what is simply data-gathering for curriculum development, it is imperative that institutional definitions of research are clarified and policies about collecting information are heeded.

When decisions are being made about appropriate methods to gather data about the internal and external contextual factors, the main considerations are time, expertise, and resources:

- Time available for data-gathering in the curriculum development plan
- Time to locate extant documents, develop interview questions and surveys, and gather and analyze data

- Expertise of curriculum developers in data-gathering methods and data analysis
- Resources to support data-gathering, such as secretarial help.

Many methods could be employed to gather data about internal and external contextual factors. Those that will yield valuable data as expeditiously as possible, and for which the curriculum designers possess the required skills, should be used. The most common methods of data-gathering for the curriculum development process are reviewed below.

Literature Reviews and Internet Searches Ideas about curricula, trends, philosophical approaches, and strategies for nursing education, along with significant directions for health care, can be acquired from literature reviews and Internet searches. Information about other nursing programs is available on the Internet. Knowing about the current state of nursing education beyond the local situation, and learning about the convictions and opinions of experts, will expand the views of those involved in curriculum development and provide a national and international perspective for curriculum development. Ideas from beyond national borders can furnish new and relevant insights, even though the origins of the concepts, or the implementation, are geographically, and perhaps politically, distant.

More specifically, published curriculum designs and examples of courses can serve as models for new curricula. Many authors provide suggestions arising from the successes and difficulties they have encountered with curriculum design and implementation. Particularly valuable can be research reports about the outcomes of specific teaching-learning strategies or programs, since they provide evidence that can guide future educational practices. Authors whose ideas are particularly appealing, or faculty from a school with a successful curriculum, might also serve as consultants if resources permit.

Document Review A review of existing documents can be an inexpensive means of acquiring data identified as necessary to the curriculum development process. Some documents may be readily available, such as professional practice and educational program accreditation standards, or the institutional mission, vision, philosophy, and strategic plan. Conversely, others may require a more protracted effort to obtain. These might include government or clinical agency reports. Those documents that are judged to have particular relevance for future curriculum directions should be reviewed and pertinent data extracted.

Key Informant Interviews Key informants are people known to have information relevant to the purpose of the data-gathering. Individual interviews (face-to-face, telephone, or e-mail) can be an effective and inexpensive method to acquire pertinent data quickly. The interview questions should be carefully planned so that maximum relevant information can be acquired without unduly imposing upon an informant's time. Providing the questions in advance of the interview can help the informant prepare. Responses should be recorded (usually by taking notes) so that information is not forgotten. As the interview is ending, it is wise to confirm that it would be acceptable to follow up, either in person, by telephone, or e-mail, if clarification or additional data are required.

Focus Group Interviews These are planned discussions intended to obtain information about a specified topic in a non-threatening environment. They capitalize on group inter-action to explore attitudes and perceptions about a particular topic or issue. Online focus group interviews are a means to expand the geographical location of participants (Kenny, 2005). The focus group typically comprises 6 to 12 individuals with a common set of inter-ests. A facilitator whose role is to assist the group to explore the topic in depth, generally within a loose structure, guides the discussion. Although the structure is not fixed, open-ended ques-tions are prepared in advance. According to Kreuger and Casey (2000), questions should be developed to match the following sequence of categories: *opening, introductory, transition, key,* and *ending.* Ideas are recorded (often on flipcharts in addition to audio-taping) and pe-riodically reviewed to ensure accuracy of recording and comprehension. The goal is not con-sensus; rather, it is a full exploration of the topic.

Farrell, Wallis, and Evans (2007) conducted focus group and individual interviews to de-termine and compare views held by the communities of interest of two nursing schools. Each community of interest provided information about:

- Aspects of the program's past that should be brought forward into the future
- Its vision for the future of the nursing program and how the vision could be realized
- The role of the community of interest in realizing the vision.

Focus groups for the purpose of obtaining data for curriculum development can be used productively with faculty, students, staff nurses, and other stakeholders. The interview can be broad in its focus, such as the one described by Farrell et al. (2007), or narrow, examin-ing one aspect of curriculum, such as the nature of clinical learning experiences or online learning.

Surveys Face-to-face, telephone, mail, e-mail, or Web-based surveys are used to obtain data from a large number of people in a relatively short period of time. Questionnaires re-quire time to construct so that the items are understandable to respondents and data can be readily analyzed. Examples of information that could be obtained with surveys are opinions about health care and curriculum directions, the nature of future nursing practice, and pref-erences of nurses about graduate programs.

Delphi Technique The Delphi technique is a structured forecasting survey that provides a means of obtaining input from stakeholders who may be geographically distant, but whose ideas are deemed essential. A panel of experts is asked to complete an iterative series of ques-tionnaires that address their opinions, judgment, or predictions about a particular topic. Each set of responses is summarized and another questionnaire sent to the same individuals for confirmation. The iterative process is repeated until consensus is achieved about the issue of interest (Polit & Beck, 2008). Selection of the experts, diminishing return rates with each round, and the total time for the process to be completed (Keeney, Hasson, & McKenna, 2006) would be of concern to curriculum developers.

An example of the use of the Delphi technique for curriculum development occurred when a faculty panel and a panel of advance practice nurses (APNs) were surveyed three times to determine role components germane to APNs in managed care, as well as topics reflecting those role components in the curriculum. Considerable consistency existed between the panels, and this information had implications for the volume and nature of curriculum content (Hawkins, Burke, & Steinberg, 2006).

Consultations Consultations with experts and/or peers at other institutions can provide valuable knowledge, insights, and guidance about particular aspects of the curriculum (such as current philosophical approaches), as well as future directions for nursing practice and education, and implementation challenges of particular curricular designs. Frequently, the counsel they offer is gained from experience that has not yet been committed to publication. The contributions of consultants and peers from other institutions can be substantial when considered within local realities. Cost is likely a factor, and therefore, when a consultant is employed, it is wise to ensure that the purpose of the consultation has been explicated and as many stakeholders as possible are able to participate in discussions.

The Work of Data-Gathering

There is no formula for deciding which data to obtain about the contextual factors, data sources to contact, or data-gathering methods to employ. Rather, curriculum developers should give attention to the questions and considerations posed in the sections above. Then, using their knowledge of the school, their experience, and their judgment, they can reach consensus about what is reasonable and realistic. The conclusions will likely be different for each school. A work sheet could help focus thinking about data-gathering, and when posted, serve as a visual reminder of work to be completed.

Table 6-3 presents examples of data, data sources, and data-gathering methods for the internal contextual factors of mission, vision, philosophy, and goals; culture; financial resources; and infrastructure. Table 6-4 presents similar information about the external factors of culture, healthcare systems, and professional standards and trends.

The work of gathering data may be given to a task force or shared more widely among stakeholders. Sufficient time should be allowed for this aspect of the curriculum development process to ensure that a full picture is obtained of the internal and external contexts. If the new curriculum is to endure into the future, it must be based upon accurate and comprehensive data.

It is helpful to have a central repository for the data so that it will be readily accessible for subsequent analysis. Moreover, methods that will speed analysis (such as immediate computer entry of returned questionnaire responses by a secretary or research assistant, or use

Table 6-3 Examples of Data, Data Sources, and Data Gathering Methods for Internal Contextual Factors

Internal Contextual Factors	Data	Data Sources	Data Gathering Methods
Philosophy, Mission, and Goals	Published philosophy, mission, goals, strategic plan	Institutional and school documents, Web sites	Document review
	Values and guiding principles	Key informants, e.g., senior academics, current and former faculty, school dean or director	Interviews
Culture	People	Organizational charts	Document review
	Interaction styles	Key informants, e.g., senior academics, chair of institutional planning committee, administrators	Interviews
	Decision-making and processes (formal and informal)		
	Aspirations		
	Values		
	Openness to change		
	Relationship with other organizations		
Financial Resources	Priorities for institutional budget	Institutional planning documents	Document review
	School budget (current and projected)	Key informants, e.g., senior academics and administrators, faculty, staff	Interviews
	Projected budget for curriculum planning and implementation	School dean or director	
Infrastructure	Employment agreements	Collective agreements	Document review
Human resources	Nursing Faculty		
	Number of part- and full-time	School of Nursing director	Interviews
	Credentials and expertise	Faculty	
	Expected retirements and resignations		
	Characteristics of adjunct faculty		

Table 6-3   continued

Internal Contextual Factors	Data	Data Sources	Data Gathering Methods
	Pool of potential faculty	Chairs of graduate programs	Interviews, surveys
	Pool of potential clinical preceptors	Clinical agencies	Survey, focus groups
	<u>Non-Nursing Faculty</u>	Department Chairs	Interviews
	Availability and interest of non-nursing faculty to teach (and possibly develop new) support courses		
	<u>Students</u>		
	Characteristics and number of applicants	Registrar, Chair of school admissions committee	Interviews
	Demographics of current students		Document review
		Admissions committee reports	
	Attrition and completion rates	School records	
	<u>Support Staff</u>		
	Numbers	School dean or director	Interview
	Skill sets	Support staff	
Physical resources	Office space	Physical plant documents	Document review
	Classroom space and facilities		Observation
	Labs		
	Technology	Information technology group	Interviews
Resources to support teaching and learning	<u>Library</u>		
	Nature of holdings	Library staff	Interviews
	Computerized resources	Listing of current holdings	Document review
	<u>Faculty Development Services</u>		
	Nature and availability of services	Director of institution-wide services	Interviews

continues

Table 6-3   continued

Internal Contextual Factors	Data	Data Sources	Data Gathering Methods
	Possibility of creating new services	School director	Document review
		Published information (print- and web-based)	Web search
	Teaching support		
	Availability of graduate teaching assistants	Program chairs School director	Interviews
	Access to institutional funding	Funding announcements	Web search
	Student Services		
	Nature and availability of services	Director of student services	Interviews
	Possibility of creating new services if warranted by changed curriculum	Published information (print- and Web-based)	Document review

Table 6-4   Examples of Data, Data Sources, and Data Gathering Methods for External Contextual Factors

External Contextual Factors	Data	Data Sources	Data Gathering Methods
Culture	Values, beliefs, and practices of dominant culture	Key informants of ethnic, cultural groups	Interviews
	Ethnic and other groups in community	Publications of major ethnic and cultural organizations	Document review
	Values, beliefs, and practices of subcultures		
	Values, beliefs, and practices of healthcare system and providers	Mission statements of healthcare agencies	Document review
		Published codes of ethics, political positions of professional organizations	

Table 6-4   *continued*

Enternal Contextual Factors	Data	Data Sources	Data Gathering Methods
Health Care	Services provided by hospitals, community health agencies, and private providers	Promotional materials, Web sites, agency leaders	Document review, Web search
	Plans for changes in healthcare services	Healthcare executives, leaders	Interviews
	Identified gaps in service	Government policy statements	Document review, Web search
	Sources of healthcare payments	Local or provincial/state reports (print or web-based)	
	Ratio of registered to non-registered staff in major agencies	Annual reports, human resource personnel	Document review, interview
	Receptiveness of nursing staff to students	Nursing staff	Interviews
		Nursing executives	Survey, focus groups
Professional Standards and Trends	Practice regulations	Licensing and accrediting bodies	Document and Web site review
	Licensure requirements	Professional bodies	
	Scope of practice requirements and restrictions	Legislation	Document review
	Nursing care priorities and trends	Professional bodies, literature, practicing nurses	Document review, focus groups
	Professional ethics and ethical issues		Delphi technique
	Approval and accreditation standards	Approval and accrediting bodies	Literature and Web searches
	Nursing education trends	Nursing education leaders, literature, and internet resources	Survey, interviews
	Teaching-learning models	Experts (peers and consultants)	Interviews

continues

Table 6-4   continued

Enternal Contextual Factors	Data	Data Sources	Data Gathering Methods
Socio-politico-economics	Government policies and regulations Institutional, local, national and international policies Public finances	Government reports (written and web-based)	Document review, Web search
	Grants, scholarships, and other funding for students, faculty, and school	Alumni associations, professional bodies, foundations	Document review, Web search
	Political support for nursing education	Newspapers, government and political reports	Web search, document review
		Influential community and political representatives	Interviews
	Public messages about nursing and nursing education by nursing leaders	Publications by professional organizations	Document review, Web search
		Nursing leaders	Interviews

of Web-based questionnaires hosted on sites such as SurveyMonkey) should be employed whenever possible.

During data-gathering, ideas will arise about possible concepts, processes, or learning experiences that could be included in the curriculum. It is natural to begin to extrapolate these possibilities from the data. These ideas should be recorded with the understanding that they are only tentative and based on incomplete knowledge. However tempting it may be, caution should be exercised to avoid drawing premature conclusions from partial data about what the curriculum should be like. It is only when all data are assembled, interpreted, and synthesized that well-founded, context-relevant curriculum ideas will emerge.

Faculty Development

The overall goal of faculty development in relation to data-gathering about contextual factors is to expand members' appreciation and knowledge of the influence these have on context-relevant curriculum development. Faculty development can include a session in which internal and external contextual factors are reviewed. Discussion about which factors are significant and how these factors can influence curriculum development will help novice curriculum developers understand the importance of systematic data-gathering. During such a discussion, some pertinent data, data sources, and data-gathering methods can be identified, with further decisions being reserved for a task force or committee.

Likely, some attention will be given to differentiating between data-gathering for curriculum development and data collection for research. It may be appropriate to include information about, and practice in, interviewing key informants if this will be a new activity for some. These faculty development activities can be readily facilitated by those members with expertise in data-gathering and curriculum development.

Chapter Summary

Data-gathering about internal and external contextual factors that have the potential to influence curriculum is fundamental to the creation of a context-relevant curriculum. This public activity heralds a forthcoming curriculum change. Stakeholders must first identify those factors that are most relevant to the school of nursing and curriculum development. Then, decisions can be made about pertinent data, data sources, and methods. Adequate time must be given to gathering this information, since the strength and longevity of the revised curriculum will rest upon the quality of the data-gathering and the subsequent analysis. Faculty development prepares members for the decisions and activities of data-gathering essential to a context-relevant curriculum.

Synthesis Activities

Below are two case studies. The Poplarfield University School of Nursing case will be continued in Chapter 7, where the data provided below will contribute to the determination of the curriculum nucleus. Consider the critique of the case and whether additional ideas merit discussion. The second case is followed by questions to guide examination of the case. Questions to determine faculty readiness for data-gathering in your setting conclude this section of the chapter.

Poplarfield University School of Nursing

Poplarfield University is a 50-year-old institution that began as a federally funded agricultural college to support the farming community that surrounds the town. The college was located in this rural area to provide direct assistance to farmers by agricultural experts, opportunities for local higher education, and a site for crop research relevant to the area. Over time, the focus of the institution expanded to include forestry, science, arts, and 15 years ago, nursing. The intent was that local students prepared in nursing would remain in the community after graduation.

Poplarfield is a town of 60,000 people, largely supported by the farming economy and by a military base approximately 10 miles away. The original stands of poplar trees have given way to family farms and large agri-business operations.

The 85-bed Poplarfield Hospital provides emergency care, non-critical in-patient care, and rehabilitation. Ambulatory services support in-hospital care. Critically ill individuals are sent to a large medical center 100 miles away. The local public health unit has a mandate to provide health promotion and maintenance programs to individuals, families, and communities. The university provides non-emergency health services for students; the military offers the same type of health care to its members and their families. Two occupational health nurses are responsible for the work-related health concerns of employees of a large meat packing plant.

The school of nursing offers two undergraduate programs: a 4-year BSN program (total enrollment 150) and a post-RN degree completion program. Enrollment in the latter program increased markedly 6 years ago when baccalaureate entry-to-practice was mandated, but there have been only 10–12 applicants to the program in each of the past 2 years. All classroom courses in the school of nursing are taught by 10 masters-prepared faculty. These full-time faculty are also responsible for clinical teaching, together with part-time, baccalaureate-prepared faculty.

The original nursing faculty were members of the Poplarfield Hospital School of Nursing, which closed as the university program began. The two remaining original faculty members will retire within the next 2 years. Other faculty have been recruited, generally directly out of master's programs. They tend to stay for 2 or 3 years and then leave the community. Only the director, Dr. Mary Werstiuk, has a PhD, and she is expected to remain at the school as long as her husband continues his deanship in the faculty of agriculture.

Under Dr. Werstiuk's leadership, the faculty are undertaking curriculum development. A consultant has helped them to understand the influence of contextual factors on the curriculum, curb their tendency to make premature decisions about the new curriculum, and plan their data-gathering activities. They have decided that the most important external contextual factors are demographics of the community and the nursing workforce, the healthcare needs and resources of the community, and competing institutions and programs. They intend to review the mission, priorities, resources, and policies of the university and school. Careful attention was given to identifying data sources, methods of obtaining the data, and individuals to complete the tasks. They have given themselves 3 weeks for gathering contextual data.

Critique

The faculty of Poplarfield University School of Nursing have taken important steps to be systematic and focused in their data-gathering activities. They have identified important contextual factors, data sources, methods of obtaining the data, and individuals to undertake the work. However, it is necessary for them to be precise about which data are important and to match data-gathering methods with the type and sources of desired data.

For example, when considering demographics, the faculty are correct in being concerned about the profile of people in the community. They need to specify that they are interested in knowing the age profile, the birth and death rates, whether young and elderly people typically stay in the area or move elsewhere, the rate of immigration, and so on. Past and current information of this type can be obtained from government agencies responsible for tracking the population, or perhaps the local public health unit. By defining and obtaining the desired information, faculty will develop a picture of the community that subsequently will allow them to make inferences about potential students and healthcare clients. The faculty should be equally diligent in specifying the data for each of the contextual factors they have identified.

Faculty would be wise to consider other contextual factors, such as professional and accreditation standards. These, along with trends in nursing education, are essential for faculty to know as they develop the curriculum to ensure that the new curriculum will conform to required standards and will either be in line with, or ahead of, current curriculum thinking.

Similarly, faculty should review the full range of internal contextual factors and relevant data. For example, when assessing human resources, they could determine why nursing faculty stay for only 2 or 3 years, and why doctorally prepared nurses have not sought employment in the Poplarfield University School of Nursing. Within the university, strategies to attract and retain faculty, as well as retention patterns, would be valuable information to acquire.

Members of the Poplarfield University School of Nursing should further consider their plans for data-gathering. They must review the contextual factors and determine which others are relevant to them. Then, it would be important to define the data about each factor that could be of value to curriculum development, ascertain the appropriate sources, and specify the best means to obtain the data from those sources. Data collection will likely extend beyond 3 weeks. Incomplete data collection will eventually hamper curriculum design, and faculty will likely have to return to this aspect of the curriculum development process.

Bellemore University School of Nursing

Bellemore University, an accredited, long-standing institution of some 150 years, with approximately 10,000 full- and part-time students, is located in a midwestern industrial city of 350,000 inhabitants. University departments offer programs in liberal arts, social, physical, and health sciences. The 4-year baccalaureate nursing program is one of three others within the College of Health Sciences. Eighty students are admitted annually to the nursing program, which has a total complement of 290 students in the 4 years. The majority is female and enrolled on a full-time basis. Approximately 25% of students study part-time, are mature, and have taken jobs in the community in order to meet tuition costs.

Thirty full- and part-time faculty, 15 with doctoral degrees, 12 with masters preparation, and 3 with baccalaureate degrees, teach classroom and clinical courses in the school of nursing. The nursing program received full accreditation 4 years previously.

The main industry of the city of Bellemore, for which the university is named, is automobile manufacturing. The largest auto plant, which employs approximately 2000 workers, offers health services to all employees. There is concern that general downsizing of North American auto manufacturing will soon lead to downsizing of the local auto plant.

In addition to the university, the city of Bellemore boasts a 3000-student technological community college, as well as the following health facilities and services: a 450-bed acute care general hospital; a 275-bed long-term and chronic care facility; three physician-serviced medical clinics; two walk-in emergency clinics; three nurse practitioner clinics, many physicians' offices, and a county community health department.

Bellemore University School of Nursing is preparing for a reconceptualization of its 4-year baccalaureate program. Examining the contextual factors that will affect nursing practice, and hence the curriculum, is recognized as integral to designing a future-oriented, context-relevant curriculum.

Dr. Amèlie Le Blanc, the curriculum coordinator, requested a meeting of the curriculum committee, made up of representatives from faculty, students, and community health personnel, to discuss contextual factors relevant to a redesigned curriculum. The group decided to schedule a faculty development session to help them with this activity. As a result of this session, several task force groups were formed to determine who would participate, which relevant data to gather, and the sources, methods, and tools needed for this undertaking. The group agreed to meet again when the contextual data-gathering phase was complete.

Questions for Consideration and Analysis of Bellemore University Case

1. Which contextual factors would be most relevant to Bellemore's vision of a future-oriented nursing curriculum?
2. What are the essential data to collect about these contextual factors?
3. Which data-gathering methods and tools might be employed to obtain information about the contextual factors?
4. What would be a suitable time period for collecting and collating these data?
5. Who could best participate in this data-gathering activity? How could they organize to obtain relevant data expeditiously?

Curriculum Development Activities for Consideration in Your Setting

The questions below will assist in determining readiness for data-gathering in your setting.

1. Which are the internal and external contextual factors that we deem important?
2. What are the precise data we need to obtain about each factor?
3. What (or who) are the best sources from which to obtain the data?
4. How should we proceed to obtain the data?
5. Who is available to gather the necessary data?
6. What resources do we have available to prepare data-gathering tools and to analyze data?
7. How do we ensure there is sufficient time for gathering data?
8. What location can we use as a central repository for data?
9. What faculty development activities might best prepare us for data-gathering?

References

Blackburn, S. (Ed.). (1996). *The Oxford Dictionary of Philosophy*. Oxford Reference Online. University of Western Ontario: Oxford University Press. Retrieved November 19, 2007, from http://www.oxfordreference.com/ views/ENTRY.html?subview=Main&entry=t98.e591

Booth, R. G. (2006). Educating the future e-health professional nurse. *International Journal of Nursing Education Scholarship, (3)*1, Article 13, 10. Retrieved November 21, 2007, from http://www.bepress.com/ ijnes/vol3/iss1/art13

Conley, V. C. (1973). *Curriculum and instruction in nursing.* Boston: Little, Brown and Company.

Farrell, M., Wallis, N. C., & Evans, M. T. (2007). A replication study of priorities and attitudes of two nursing programs' communities of interest: An appreciative inquiry. *Journal of Professional Nursing, 23,* 267–277.

Greenfield, S. (2007). Medication error reduction and the use of PDA technology. *Journal of Nursing Education, 46,* 127–131.

Hawkins, J. W., Burke, P. J., & Steinberg, S. (2006). Integrating practice issues in managed care into the curriculum: A Delphi survey. *Journal of the American Academy of Nurse Practitioners, 18,* 582–589.

Keeney, S., Hasson, F., & McKenna, H. (2006). Consulting the oracle: Ten lessons from using the Delphi technique in nursing research. *Journal of Advanced Nursing, 50,* 205–212.

Kenny, A. J. (2005). Interaction in cyberspace: An online focus group. *Journal of Advanced Nursing, 49,* 414–422.

Kreuger, R. A., & Casey, M. A. (2000). *Focus groups: A practical guide for applied research* (3rd ed.). Newbury Park, CA: Sage.

Last, J. M. (Ed.). (2007). *A Dictionary of Public Health.* Oxford Reference Online. Oxford: Oxford University Press. Retrieved November 19, 2007, from http://www.oxfordreference.com/views/ENTRY.html?subview=Main&entry=t235.e1056

Nagle, L. M. (2007). Everything I know about informatics, I didn't learn in nursing school. *Canadian Journal of Nursing Leadership, 20*(3), 22–25. Retrieved Nov 21, 2007, from http://www.longwoods.com/product.php?productid=19285

National League for Nursing. (2005). *The scope of practice for academic nurse educators.* New York: Author.

Nelson, R., Meyers, L., Rizzolo, M. A., Rutar, P., Proto, M. B., & Newbold, S. (2006). The evolution of educational information systems and nurse faculty roles. *Nursing Education Perspectives, 27,* 247–253.

Neuman, L. H. (2006). Creating new futures in nursing education: Envisioning the evolution e-nursing education. *Nursing Education Perspectives, 27,* 12–15.

Ornes, L. L., & Gassert, C. (2007). Computer competencies in a BSN program. *Journal of Nursing Education, 46,* 75–78.

Polit, D. F., & Beck, C. T. (2008). *Nursing research: Generating and assessing evidence for nursing practice* (8th ed.). Philadelphia: Walters Kluwer/Lippincott Williams & Wilkins.

Sitelman, F. G., & Sitelman, R. (2000). Ethics and culture: From the claim that God is dead, it does not follow that everything is permitted. In M. L. Kelley & V. M. Fitzsimons (Eds.), *Understanding cultural diversity: Culture, curriculum and community in nursing* (pp. 11–21). Sudbury, MA: Jones and Bartlett.

Swayne, L. E., Duncan, J. W., & Ginter, P. M. (2006). *Strategic management of health care organization* (5th ed.). Malden, MA: Blackwell.

Whitehead, D. K., Weiss, S. A., & Tappan, R. M. (2007). *Essentials of nursing leadership and management* (4th ed.). Philadelphia: F. A. Davis.

CHAPTER 7

From Contextual Data to Curriculum Nucleus

Chapter Overview

Once data-gathering about the internal and external context is complete, and the data assembled, it is time to integrate the information and determine its meaning for the curriculum. This is the phase when the curriculum possibilities become evident and a context-relevant curriculum begins to take shape.

Following definitions of terms is a description of the cognitive processes involved in the analysis, interpretation, and synthesis of contextual data. These include integrating data, inferring curriculum concepts and professional abilities that a nurse would require, proposing curriculum possibilities, deducing curriculum limitations, and identifying administrative issues that affect curriculum design. Also discussed are syntheses of the ideas generated from the contextual data collectively, and how they lead to the curriculum nucleus. To enhance clarity, the thinking processes that bridge data-gathering and the emerging curriculum nucleus are presented in a procedural fashion. However, the processes are iterative and integrative in nature, with all ideas influencing previous and subsequent thinking.

As in other chapters, some faculty development activities are suggested. After the summary, an extended case is used to illustrate the main ideas. Questions to guide analysis are included, as well as questions to stimulate thinking about developing the curriculum nucleus in individual settings.

Chapter Goals

- Appreciate the multiple cognitive processes inherent in analysis and synthesis of contextual data.
- Understand how the core curriculum concepts and key professional abilities of graduates are derived from the internal and external contextual data.
- Comprehend the nature, formulation, and purposes of the curriculum nucleus.
- Consider faculty development activities related to analysis, interpretation, and synthesis of contextual data, and development of the curriculum nucleus.
- Examine an account of a hypothetical school's development of its curriculum nucleus.

Definition of Terms

A number of terms are introduced that are presented in a conceptually logical order, rather than in a more conventional alphabetical sequence:

Curriculum concepts are abstract ideas that form the substance of the curriculum. The *core curriculum concepts* are essential for graduates to know and use in the context in which they will practice nursing. The core curriculum concepts permeate the curriculum and contribute to the curriculum's uniqueness.

Professional abilities are the capabilities necessary for nursing practice. These include, but are not limited to, cognitive, affective, technical, and interpersonal skills, as well as the integration and judicious use of these skills within the context of nursing. Knowledge is prerequisite to all professional abilities. The *key professional abilities* are essential for nursing practice, emphasized throughout the curriculum, and contribute to the curriculum's uniqueness.

Examples of professional abilities might include:

- Cognitive: Problem solving, critical thinking, clinical reasoning, application of theory
- Affective: Caring, empathy, adherence to professional values and ethics
- Technical: Execution of healthcare procedures, use of health and information technologies
- Interpersonal: Communicating effectively, collaborating, leading, supervising.

Curriculum possibilities are imaginative ideas about potential teaching-learning experiences, curriculum design options, courses, and content areas.

Curriculum limitations are restrictions or constraints on teaching-learning experiences, curriculum design options, or potential content areas.

Administrative issues are those logistical, personnel, and/or budgetary matters that are beyond the authority of faculty members to resolve, but which can significantly affect the curriculum design.

The *curriculum nucleus* simultaneously comprises the foundation and the essence of the curriculum. It is composed of the core curriculum concepts, key professional abilities, principal teaching-learning approaches, and the philosophical approaches (see Chapter 8). It encapsulates the conclusions drawn from an overall synthesis of curriculum concepts, professional abilities, curriculum possibilities and limitations, along with agreed-upon philosophical approaches.

Analysis, Interpretation, and Synthesis of Contextual Data

Analysis (determining essential elements), interpretation (deriving meaning), and synthesis (combining parts to form a whole) of the contextual data to arrive at the curriculum nucleus are iterative and interactive processes that require reflective thought, an open mind, and free communication. Despite the fact that these are clearly non-linear processes, they are deliberately presented separately in this chapter. This should facilitate explanation and understanding of curriculum development processes and make apparent how a context-relevant curriculum is derived.

Analyzing data about contextual factors and deriving meaning to reach conclusions about the curriculum nucleus entail a confluence of examination, integration, interpretation, reflection, and inference-making about curriculum concepts and professional abilities; generation of curriculum possibilities and recognition of contextual limitations; identification of administrative issues; and decision-making. These deliberations occur in collaboration with colleagues whose perspectives, conclusions, and values may be divergent.

The following five processes are described as part of the analysis, interpretation, and synthesis of contextual data:

1. Examining and integrating contextual data; identifying patterns and trends
2. Inferring curriculum concepts and professional abilities
3. Proposing curriculum possibilities
4. Deducing curriculum limitations
5. Identifying administrative issues.

Although presented separately, these processes occur almost in tandem, since ideas about a redesigned curriculum are generated through free-flowing discussion. Ideas relevant to all aspects of the processes arise concurrently, with one thought sparking many others.

Examining and Integrating Contextual Data

Examining and integrating data is an activity for the total faculty group. All those who develop and eventually implement a new curriculum must understand the context in which the curriculum will be operationalized and in which graduates will work. Therefore, individual members should review the data about the contextual factors, determine the influence factors have upon one another, and generate ideas about trends. Individual reviews form the basis for discussion by the total faculty group. Collectively, members discuss the ideas that were generated individually and identify patterns or trends. Data, patterns, and/or trends will reveal the current 'state of affairs' and form the basis of a context-relevant curriculum. Curriculum developers can ask two questions:

- What data are available about this factor?
- What patterns and/or trends emerge from the data about this one factor?

Review and discussion about data and trends for individual factors will make apparent the overlap and connections among contextual data for several factors, and how data and trends about one contextual factor will influence and be influenced by data and trends of other factors. The overall goal of reviewing contextual data and identifying trends is to achieve an integrated view of the data and a shared understanding of the 'big picture' of the context in which the curriculum will be operationalized and graduates will practice nursing. Some of the questions that might be considered include:

- How do data or trends about one particular factor affect trends in other contextual factors? For example, how could the closing of a major industry, that provides healthcare insurance, affect the well-being of families with members employed by that industry?
- If these or any other trends continue, what might that mean for other contextual factors? For instance, what might nursing shortages mean for public health programs?
- What are the dominant features of the context in which graduates will practice nursing?

Predicting possible futures in response to these questions helps curriculum developers anticipate the context for which the curriculum will be developed and in which it will be implemented. In understanding the big picture, curricularists also come to agreement about which contextual factors should be *most important* in determining the curriculum nucleus. *More important* factors may be readily apparent and agreed upon; *less important* ones might require discussion and consensus. There is no need to reach quantitative conclusions about the relative importance of each factor. Instead, faculty members need to reach accord about the comparative weight of all contextual factors so that the *most, more,* and *less important* ones are determined. In this way, the curriculum becomes responsive to the predominant influences of the context.

Inferring Curriculum Concepts and Professional Abilities

Review of contextual data, trends, and patterns will lead to insights about curriculum concepts, which are abstract ideas that form the substance of the curriculum. As well, professional abilities essential for nursing practice can be inferred. The professional abilities, as noted previously, include, but are not limited to, cognitive, affective, technical, and interpersonal skills, as well as integration and judicious use of these skills.

Curriculum concepts and professional abilities are inferred mainly from the external contextual factors, although some may also be evident from internal factors. As well, further ideas are stimulated about these curriculum concepts and professional abilities by those already suggested. The generation of these ideas occurs concurrently, not sequentially. Curriculum developers can ask these questions:

- What inferences about important curriculum concepts that students should know and apply in nursing practice, can be made from the contextual data and from patterns and trends?
- What inferences about professional abilities can be made from the contextual data, from patterns and trends, and from curriculum concepts?
- What additional ideas about relevant curriculum concepts arise from the professional abilities that have been suggested?
- What additional ideas about professional abilities arise from the curriculum concepts that have been suggested?

The intent is to list all the ideas that arise from brainstorming, without censor or concern about the format in which they are expressed.

Proposing Curriculum Possibilities

From ideas about curriculum concepts and professional abilities, thoughts about curriculum possibilities flow spontaneously. Curriculum possibilities (i.e., imaginative ideas about potential teaching-learning experiences, curriculum design options, courses, and content areas) result from creative thinking, unfettered by consideration of logistics. To determine the curriculum possibilities of the contextual data, curriculum concepts, and professional abilities, this question could be posed. What possibilities arise from the contextual data, patterns, trends, curriculum concepts, and professional abilities about:

- Curriculum design options?
- Courses?
- Potential content areas?
- Teaching-learning processes and experiences?

Ideas about curriculum possibilities can be drawn directly from data, trends, curriculum concepts, professional abilities, or from a combination of these. If, for instance, the majority of faculty has educational and experiential credentials in community health, then it will be evident that a community-focused curriculum is possible. If, as another example, the curriculum concept of *professional responsibility* and the professional abilities of *critical thinking* and *political action* are determined, then experience with the political action committee of a professional organization might be proposed as a curriculum possibility.

The intent is to generate many ideas about curriculum possibilities. Some may seem ridiculous or bizarre, and others more conventional. The apparently outlandish possibilities may be appealing, but impractical. However, with subsequent application of pragmatic and logical thinking, these might later be modified into innovative and feasible suggestions.

Inferences about curriculum concepts and professional abilities, and proposals about curriculum possibilities, could lead to considerable discussion and debate, even when only a single contextual factor is being examined. For instance, some faculty may interpret a low fertility rate in the community as signaling the necessity for a curricular emphasis on prenatal assessment and health promotion, while others may conclude that maternal-infant health requires little attention. Some ideas, such as *health promotion*, could be considered a concept, professional ability, and/or a potential content area. It is unnecessary to decide which category it fits best. Rather, it should be recorded in every applicable category. Repeated recording of the same idea in several categories signifies its importance to the curriculum.

It is useful to record all thoughts that occur, and at this stage to avoid debate about suitability, categorization, inclusions, or exclusions. Such decisions will be made in subsequent integrative discussions about the curriculum nucleus, curriculum, and course design. The reason for producing and recording as many ideas as possible is that they naturally arise from an examination of the contextual data, and help curriculum developers move toward the curriculum nucleus. Remember, however, that the ideas being recorded are tentative, should be retained for detailed curriculum and course design, and may be modified as curriculum development proceeds.

Identifying Curriculum Limitations

In contrast to curriculum possibilities, *curriculum limitations* are restrictions or constraints on teaching-learning experiences, curriculum design options, or potential content areas. These are derived from a pragmatic or logical interpretation of the contextual data, trends and patterns, curriculum concepts, professional abilities, and curriculum possibilities. Curriculum builders need to ask:

- How do internal and external contextual data and trends constrain what might be possible in the curriculum?
- What restrictions do curriculum concepts and/or professional abilities place on curriculum possibilities?

Both internal and external contextual data can point to curriculum limitations that warrant serious attention by the curriculum team. For example, a faculty group whose clinical expertise lies mainly in acute care might identify the faculty profile as a limitation, if community-based clinical experiences have been proposed as a curriculum possibility. Another example could be that particular clinical experiences are constrained by limited availability of student placements.

Importantly, some of the curriculum possibilities and limitations can lead to actions that could profoundly change the school and the curriculum. For example, data about the nursing profession would likely include a statement describing the current and projected worldwide shortages of nursing faculty. This fact could limit the likelihood of successfully implementing a small-group, case- or problem-based curriculum, which would require relatively large numbers of faculty. Alternately, it could spur faculty to lobby senior administrators to initiate vigorous faculty recruitment and retention efforts, or to enlist clinicians to lead the small groups.

Deducing Administrative Issues

Invariably, administrative issues that might affect the curriculum will become apparent as contextual data are analyzed and curriculum possibilities and limitations identified. Administrative issues (i.e., those logistical, personnel, and/or budgetary matters that are beyond the authority of faculty members to resolve) can significantly affect the new curriculum. The question to be answered is: What logistical, personnel, and/or budgetary issues should be raised with the dean/director?

It is worthwhile to note administrative issues and bring them to the attention of the dean/director, specifying the effects they could have on the curriculum and the desired resolution. Then, with the dean/director's support and leadership, strategies can be developed to address administrative issues, including securing resources for the future curriculum. Indeed, curriculum design will likely be dependent on the resolution of some of these matters.

Summary of Processes

Several processes have been described to illuminate the thinking that emanates from the contextual data: examining and integrating contextual data, inferring curriculum concepts and professional abilities, proposing curriculum possibilities, identifying curriculum limitations, and deducing administrative issues. Although delineated separately, the processes are interactive and occur almost concurrently, each idea influencing others.

In Table 7-1 is presented an example of the conceptual links that exist between data and curriculum for the external contextual factor of demographics for the Poplarfield case from Chapter 6. Included are an abbreviated set of contextual data, and the patterns and trends arising from the data. Curriculum concepts, professional abilities, curriculum possibilities and limitations, and administrative issues are suggested. The columns in the table provide a convenient and organized method of recording ideas, but are not meant to connote sequential or segmented thinking.

Table 7-1 Example of Conceptual Links Between Contextual Data and Curriculum for Poplarfield University School of Nursing

External Contextual Factor	Data	Patterns and Trends	Curriculum Concepts	Professional Competencies	Curriculum Possibilities (P) and Limitations (L)	Administrative Issues
Demographics	**National**					
	Fertility rate inadequate to sustain population (1.61 children/woman)	Decline in fertility rate Fewer births Reduced proportion of infants and children in the population		Maternal-infant care	**P:** Increased or decreased maternal-infant health **L:** Reduced opportunities for maternal-infant clinical experiences	Preparation of faculty for community-focused care Development of new clinical sites
	Life expectancy = 81.7 years for women; 76.3 for men Largest proportion of population born between 1946–64 (baby boomers)	Increasing numbers and proportion of seniors: seniors will be the largest population group	Nursing care and health promotion of aging population	Care of elderly in homes and community facilities Managing resources	**P:** Clinical experiences in homes; long-term care facilities; inpatient, outpatient, and community settings **P:** Continuum of care from hospital to home	
	Increasing numbers of the very old	Improved health into old age, coupled with increased numbers of those with acute and chronic illness		Health maintenance and promotion throughout the life span	**P:** Nursing in primary, secondary, and tertiary care settings	New clinical practice sites

Population growth through immigration, mainly from mid-East, Eastern Europe, Southeast Asia, Africa, Caribbean	Countries of origin changing from Western Europe to more global pattern	Cultural diversity of recipients of nursing care	Nursing care of those with chronic illness Culturally and ethnically sensitive nursing care Cultural competency Assessment throughout the life span Communication Critical thinking	**P:** Child & adult development **P:** Theoretical or conceptual framework for planning and delivering nursing to individuals of varying cultural beliefs and practices **P:** Approaches to health maintenance and promotion that build on traditions of immigrants

Poplarfield area:

Birth rate = 1.16 children/woman Proportion of 20–40 year olds decreasing, as they migrate to cities	Lower than national rate Numbers of infants and young children will decrease as adults of child-bearing and -rearing age decrease	Pre-conception, prenatal, and perinatal health of both parents Assessment, health promotion		**L:** Pre-, intra-, and post-natal clinical experiences
Retired farmers generally move into the town of Poplarfield	Social and health consequences of lifestyle changes			**P:** Urban and rural clinical experiences Travel difficulties for many students

continues

Table 7-1 Example of Conceptual Links Between Contextual Data and Curriculum for Poplarfield University School of Nursing

External Contextual Factor	Data	Patterns and Trends	Curriculum Concepts	Professional Competencies	Curriculum Possibilities (P) and Limitations (L)	Administrative Issues
	Immigration into town of Poplarfield mainly from Philippines, India	Changing ethnic heritage of Poplarfield residents	Cultural competency	Cultural competency	**P:** Home visiting to expand students' understanding of cultural and ethnic influences on health and illness	
	Seasonal farm workers from Mexico, most of whom do not speak English and do not have health insurance; present from early June to October each year.		Values Culture	Responding to healthcare needs of short-term local residents, for whom cost is a factor Nursing care of marginalized groups Identification of own values, biases	**P:** Rural clinical experiences to address the health needs of migrant workers, urgent care clinics, street nursing	Contracts and insurance for student experience in non-traditional sites
	Large numbers of young adults at local armed forces base		Promotion of life-long health habits during young adult years	Health promotion	**P:** Clinical experiences on armed forces base **P:** Health promotion with members of armed forces	Development of new clinical sites

Determining the Curriculum Nucleus

Descriptions of the *curriculum nucleus* and its components are presented, along with the process to derive it. The curriculum nucleus is both the foundation and essence of the curriculum, and gives clear direction for further curriculum development. Therefore, confirmation of the curriculum nucleus is prerequisite to further curriculum development.

The Curriculum Nucleus

The *curriculum nucleus* simultaneously comprises the foundation and the essence of the curriculum. It has four components:

- Core curriculum concepts
- Key professional abilities
- Principal teaching-learning approaches
- Philosophical approaches (see Chapter 8).

It encapsulates the conclusions drawn from an overall synthesis of curriculum concepts, professional abilities, and curriculum possibilities and limitations, along with agreed-upon philosophical approaches.

The philosophical approaches, which are part of the nucleus, also contribute to the core curriculum concepts. The central ideas in the philosophical approaches will form core concepts in the curriculum, since students must understand them and integrate them into nursing practice. The philosophical approaches also influence the key professional abilities and principal teaching-learning approaches.

The curriculum nucleus can be conceived as being analogous to the gene's of a cell's nucleus which determine its development, growth, and functioning. Similarly, the curriculum nucleus determines the development, direction, and implementation of the curriculum. The constellation of core curriculum concepts, key professional abilities, principal teaching-learning approaches, and philosophical approaches, make the curriculum unique and reflect its relevance for the context in which it is offered.

Figure 7-1 depicts a conceptualization of the curriculum nucleus and its relationship to the total curriculum. The nucleus is surrounded by broken lines to connote that it is not separate from the curriculum. Rather, the influence of the nucleus moves beyond the center into all aspects of the curriculum. The nucleus is omnipresent throughout the curriculum.

Core Curriculum Concepts   *Curriculum concepts* are abstract ideas that form the substance of the curriculum. The *core curriculum concepts* are essential for graduates to know and use in the context in which they will practice nursing, permeate the curriculum, and contribute to the curriculum's uniqueness.

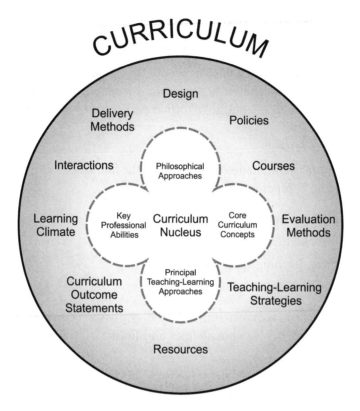

Figure 7-1 Conceptualization of the Relationship between the Curriculum Nucleus and the Curriculum

The process for identifying the core curriculum concepts involves integration and synthesis. First, the curriculum concepts derived from the most important contextual factors are reviewed, and commonalities integrated. Then, the same process is followed separately for the more important and less important contextual factors. The evolving three sets of curriculum concepts that emerge are synthesized, with attention to the factors' relative importance. Concepts not integrated are reexamined to ensure that relevant ones are not omitted. There may be agreement to delete or modify some concepts, or it might seem more suitable to consider that decision later when more detailed curriculum planning occurs.

Simultaneously with analysis of the contextual data, curriculum developers will be identifying the philosophical approaches for the curriculum. The predominant ideas from these philosophical approaches also contribute to the core curriculum concepts.

Synthesis and integration of the curriculum concepts and incorporation of the philo-sophical approaches lead to identification of the core curriculum concepts. The core curriculum concepts:

- are overriding ideas nurses should know
- shape students' views about clients and how nurses think and behave
- permeate and are prominent throughout the curriculum
- are part of the curriculum content and of the structure used to organize content.

Questions to guide synthesis of the core curriculum concepts are suggested in Table 7-2.

Key Professional Abilities *Professional abilities* are the capabilities necessary for nursing practice. These include, but are not limited to, cognitive, affective, technical, and interper-sonal skills, as well as the integration and judicious use of these skills within the context of nursing. The *key professional abilities* are essential for nursing practice, are emphasized throughout the curriculum, and contribute to the curriculum's uniqueness.

To derive the key professional abilities, the professional abilities identified for each fac-tor are synthesized in the same fashion as the curriculum concepts. The synthesized profes-sional abilities lead to identification of the key professional abilities. Similar questions to those proposed in Table 7-2 could be used to determine these. As well, the philosophical approaches influence these key professional abilities.

Table 7-2 Questions to Guide Synthesis of Curriculum Concepts

- What are the commonalities among curriculum concepts inferred from *each* of the *most impor-tant, more important,* and *less important* contextual factors?
- Can curriculum concepts inferred from the *more* and *less important* contextual factors be inte-grated with those of the *most important* contextual factors?
- Of those curriculum concepts that have not been integrated, which should be included in the curriculum?
- Does the synthesis reflect the relative weighting assigned to the contextual factors?
- Are there ideas evident from the combination and inter-relationships of contextual factors that have not been identified?
- Which concepts from the philosophical approaches should also be included?
- Does the synthesis truly encapsulate the important ideas that are essential for graduates to know and use, so they can practice successfully within the present and future societal contexts?

The key professional abilities serve a similar function in the curriculum as the core curriculum concepts. They:

- Are overriding professional abilities that nurses need in all practice contexts
- Shape students' thinking about nursing practice
- Permeate and are emphasized throughout the curriculum
- Are part of the curriculum content and evident in practice experiences

Philosophical Approaches The philosophical approaches to which faculty members subscribe are analogous to the genes of a cell's nucleus, as interpreted previously. They determine the expression of an organism's physical characteristics and functions. Similarly, the philosophical approaches establish the expression and actualization of the curriculum concepts, professional abilities, and teaching-learning approaches.

Principal Teaching-Learning Approaches These are derived from the synthesis of the curriculum possibilities and limitations, according to the same process used for determining the core curriculum concepts and the key professional abilities. The teaching-learning processes that emerge should be assessed within the realities of administrative issues and should reflect the philosophical approaches.

The principal teaching-learning approaches are the predominant processes used to promote student learning throughout the curriculum. They shape students' thinking about knowledge acquisition, development, and creation; and about thinking processes in nursing.

Confirming the Curriculum Nucleus

Finally, the curriculum team must employ its judgment about the curriculum nucleus that has been derived. Members will want to review all the work that has been done and question:

- Is the curriculum nucleus really appropriate for the context?
- Has anything important been missed?
- Are there other core curriculum concepts, key professional abilities, philosophical approaches, and principal teaching-learning approaches that should be discussed?
- Can faculty collectively support the curriculum nucleus that has been determined?

To reach agreement about the curriculum nucleus, considerable discussion could be necessary. Understandably, decisions can be fraught with conflict if aspects of the current curriculum valued by particular faculty members are likely to be excluded or reduced in prominence. It is natural for faculty to use the current curriculum and personal teaching experience as a frame of reference for discussion. If consensus is difficult to reach, it would be wise to review the reasons for curriculum redesign, the data about the most important contextual factors, and values held by faculty. This re-examination could lend objectivity to the discussion.

The total faculty group must achieve resolution about the curriculum nucleus. Confirmation is essential, because a successful curriculum is dependent on total support. Final decisions about the curriculum nucleus should be clearly justifiable by the constellation of contextual data, and responsive to the reasons that led to curriculum development in the first place. Only then can curriculum developers be assured that they are developing a curriculum that will be relevant for its context and the future. Following confirmation of the curriculum nucleus, outcomes are formulated, and curriculum design created.

Once agreement is reached about the curriculum nucleus, a one or two-paragraph description could be written, and used to interpret and promote the curriculum to individuals and groups outside the school of nursing. A document of this type will ensure that all faculty members and students have a similar understanding and provide a consistent explanation of the curriculum.

Faculty Development

The goal of faculty development in relation to analysis, interpretation, and synthesis of contextual data is to expand appreciation and understanding of the processes involved in deriving the curriculum nucleus, and how it gives direction to curriculum development. Participants require knowledge of the process since decisions about the curriculum nucleus will shape the school's teaching-learning activities for a number of years.

Faculty development, in workshop format, can be focused on the processes that will move faculty and other stakeholders from contextual data to the curriculum nucleus. First, participants could discuss the contextual data to gain a common understanding of the environment. Then, they might divide into groups to derive curriculum concepts, professional abilities, curriculum possibilities and limitations, and administrative issues for one contextual factor. In this way, all could have experience in the analysis of the same contextual factor, so that differing perspectives would be evident. Then, the remaining contextual factors could be divided among groups, with each to consider a different factor, thereby expediting the curriculum development process. Practice with the process promotes understanding. Presentation of the subgroups' work could lead to values clarification, and further discussion about the process and purpose of deriving the curriculum nucleus. Faculty development activities can be facilitated by those members with experience in this aspect of curriculum development, or if appropriate, by an outside expert.

Chapter Summary

In this chapter, a further step in the curriculum development process is described, namely the interpretation and synthesis of contextual data to derive the curriculum nucleus. The processes of analyzing, interpreting, and synthesizing the contextual data are emphasized as being iterative and non-linear, although a procedural approach is described for explanatory purposes. Questions are provided to assist in integrating data, inferring curriculum concepts and professional abilities, proposing curriculum possibilities, identifying curriculum limitations, and deducing administrative issues. As well, a description of the curriculum nucleus is provided. Determining and confirming the curriculum nucleus can involve emotions and values. Therefore, open communication, values clarification, and rigorous intellectual discussion are essential to achieve an informed analysis and synthesis of contextual data and the formulation of a future-oriented and contextually relevant curriculum nucleus. Faculty development activities are foundational to prepare participants for this work.

ᴥSynthesis Activities꞉Ꞌꝋ

The Poplarfield University School of Nursing case is continued from Chapter 6 with faculty and other stakeholders now developing the curriculum nucleus. This extended case includes tables to illustrate how contextual data can be analyzed. For purposes of brevity, not all data are presented. The intent is to demonstrate the development of the curriculum nucleus. Questions are provided for analysis of the case.

Because of the length and complexity of the Poplarfield University School of Nursing case, a second case for analysis is not included. The chapter concludes with questions to guide the development of a curriculum nucleus relevant to individual contexts.

Poplarfield University School of Nursing

Members of the Poplarfield University School of Nursing completed their data-gathering about internal and external contextual factors. A curriculum consultant was hired for a 2-day retreat to help the group derive the curriculum nucleus from the data. Dr. Werstiuk, the school director, stated her intention to attend and participate fully. The dean of the faculty of professional schools was also invited, since her support would be needed for any additional resources that might be required for the new curriculum. Faculty believed that the dean's involvement would be an effective way to educate her about the complexity of curriculum planning and the many influences on the nursing curriculum. Additionally, members of the curriculum advisory committee were invited to attend, and two of the 12 members were able to do so.

In preparation for the retreat, data had been organized for each contextual factor on a chart and a hard copy distributed to all faculty members. A copy of the chart was loaded onto laptop computers so that ideas could be immediately recorded and preserved.

The group agreed to derive the curriculum nucleus collectively, starting with a shared understanding of the environment. They were committed to the ideas of inferring curriculum concepts and professional abilities, proposing curriculum possibilities, and deducing curriculum limitations. There was consensus to dismiss identification of administrative issues, because "We already know what the issues are: not enough faculty and not enough money in the budget."

Examining and Integrating Contextual Data

During the course of discussion about contextual data, the faculty tried to focus on the meaning of the data, and the inter-relationships among the contextual factors. They also addressed curriculum concepts, professional abilities, and curriculum possibilities without labeling these ideas as such. They discussed ideas about how:

- The presence of more aged people leads to a greater demand for health care, which increases the requirement for healthcare professionals.
- The growing RN shortage could increase public demand for more seats in nursing programs, and this in turn would necessitate more resources for the school, including human resources.
- RN shortages could lead to more care by nonprofessionals, increasing delegation and supervision by RNs. The RN shortage might result in specialization by all RNs or deprofessionalization of nursing.
- Student skills in information technology could be developed when faculty have limited expertise.
- Professional standards for nursing practice, accreditation standards, and the availability of clinical placements in and near Poplarfield could be reconciled.
- Local health problems might be addressed in a society and healthcare system that are focused on problems of national scope, such as cancer.
- Nursing priorities and mandates must be explicated for a society with a growing proportion of elderly people and a healthcare system where acute care stays are shortened and out-of-hospital care is increased.

The group also talked in detail about some specific data, and how to interpret it. In trying to reach a shared understanding of the context in which the curriculum would be implemented and graduates will practice nursing, several integrated summaries were offered. Each resulted in some disagreement. Finally, at the end of the morning, the group agreed that the environment could be described as one in which:

- There will be less institutionalized health care and growing emphasis on community-based care.
- Independent decision-making and supervision of nonprofessional healthcare providers will become a stronger feature of nursing practice.
- Vulnerable groups in the community may grow in size.
- The proportion of aged people in the community will increase, while young people will likely continue to leave the Poplarfield area.
- Ethnic diversity will become more apparent.
- Agriculture will continue to be a significant contributor to the Poplarfield economy.

In the afternoon, discussion progressed to identification of the factors that should be most influential in shaping the curriculum. Initially, there was a strong sentiment that all contextual factors were of equal weight, apart from the internal factors of *history, philosophy, mission, goals,* and *culture,* all of which seemed less important. The consultant agreed that the factors are highly interconnected and that the division of the data into these factors is somewhat artificial. Yet, she reminded faculty that there must be some basis for identifying the key curriculum influences, and thus for determining the curriculum nucleus.

The group then considered whether it was the recipients of nursing services (*demographics*), the nature of nursing (*professional standards and trends*), or the location and nature of health care (*health care*) that was most important. Faculty phrased this as *who, what, where,* and *how.* Finally, they agreed that most important were the people being served, and therefore, *demographics* and *external culture* would be most significant in determining the curriculum nucleus. *History* was immediately labeled as being of least importance. After further discussion, faculty members concurred about the rank ordering of contextual factors:

1. Demographics, external culture
2. Health care, professional standards and trends; infrastructure
3. Social, political, and economic conditions
4. Technology
5. Environment; philosophy, mission, and goals of the university; and school of nursing, internal culture, history of the school of nursing

Inferring Curriculum Concepts and Professional Abilities, Proposing Curriculum Possibilities, and Deducing Curriculum Limitations

The stakeholders wanted to complete this intellectual work together, in the belief that it was necessary for all to participate in every aspect. Ideas were recorded on the charts, which had previously been loaded onto laptop computers.

It became apparent that one more day would be insufficient to complete this effort, if the group continued in the same way. The consultant suggested that the contextual factors might be divided among smaller faculty groups to complete the formulation of ideas about curriculum concepts, professional abilities, curriculum possibilities, and curriculum limitations. The group agreed to think about this proposal.

The next morning a member of the advisory committee proposed that dividing into small groups would expedite the curriculum work. There was now consensus about this. Three smaller groups were formed, and each took responsibility for some of the internal and external factors.

In reviewing the contextual data, members recognized that curriculum concepts, professional abilities, and curriculum possibilities and limitations did not necessarily arise from each internal factor. However, they noted that the data about some of the factors could ultimately influence decisions about curriculum, either limiting or propelling the curriculum design. For example, when examining the school's infrastructure, they recognized that the existence of computer labs for students meant that computer-mediated learning was a possibility, whereas the school budget and faculty numbers could constrain the curriculum. Accordingly, they reaffirmed their intention to identify the curriculum possibilities and limitations as they examined each contextual factor. As the groups worked, they recognized again that the contextual factors do not operate in isolation and that their ideas reflected the inter-related nature of the internal and external context. The ideas arising from the internal and external contextual data were recorded.

Identifying Administrative Issues

As they continued, faculty quickly recognized that there were administrative issues beyond faculty numbers and budget. Accordingly, the groups considered and recorded the administrative issues. They also recognized that *financial resources* was an important contextual factor.

At the end of their 2 days together, the participants felt proud of their efforts. All were eager to proceed with synthesis of the completed work, and the determination of the curriculum nucleus. See Table 7-1 for analysis of the external contextual factor of *demographics*. Table 7-3 presents the internal factors of *financial resources* and *infrastructure*. Table 7-4 outlines the analysis of the external factors of *culture*, *health care*, and *professional standards and trends*.

Resources were not available for an additional retreat day. Therefore, the group agreed to:

- Distribute hard copies of the analysis of the contextual factors, so all could individually review the work that had been completed by all groups
- Use a regularly scheduled faculty meeting to collectively review the work and add ideas that might have been omitted
- Reorganize individual schedules so they could meet from 3–7 p.m. twice in the next 2 weeks to determine the curriculum nucleus
- Ask Dr. Werstiuk and the dean to discuss the identified administrative issues, and plan further discussion with senior administrators, if necessary.

There was consensus that Professor Rose, chair of the curriculum committee, would lead the discussions. As well, members were enthusiastic about the possibility of adding ideas to the work of other groups. Professor Rose asked that all try to ground their thinking in the work to date and, as much as possible, to look beyond personal beliefs.

The subsequent meetings were lively, and at times, tense. Review of curriculum concepts, professional abilities, curriculum possibilities and limitations, and administrative issues went quickly, with some additional ideas offered. There was a sense of accomplishment at the end of the first meeting, and impatience to get on with the definition of the curriculum nucleus.

Determining Curriculum Nucleus

At the first 4-hour meeting, there was consensus that synthesis of curriculum concepts, professional abilities, and curriculum possibilities should be completed collectively. Some important curriculum concepts were: *aging; health promotion; nursing care of people at home, in the community, and institutions;* and *nurse-client relationships.*

Professor Rose reminded them of the weighting they had assigned to the contextual factors, noting that they had not attended to all the factors they had weighted as second in importance. With this, the group returned to *health care,* agreeing that the curriculum should address local health problems as well as national ones. In considering *professional standards and trends,* faculty confirmed that a strong emphasis on *health promotion* was warranted, and agreed that *illness intervention* must be included. One member noted that *rural health* was an important concept that had been omitted, and there was immediate agreement to include it. Synthesis and further discussion of the curriculum concepts led to the conclusion that the core curriculum concepts would be: *health, aging, health promotion, illness intervention, context (which includes rural),* and *nurse-client relationships.*

In synthesizing curriculum possibilities, the group decided that the principal teaching-learning processes would be *self-direction, collaborative learning,* and *use of information technologies.* Synthesis of the professional abilities led to the conclusion that the key professional abilities would be: *critical thinking, clinical reasoning, independent and collaborative decision-making, cultural competence,* and *life-long learning.*

The group recognized that acceptance of these ideas would require resolution of administrative issues related to human, physical, and financial resources, along with faculty development. Dr. Werstiuk reaffirmed her commitment to work toward resolution of these matters.

The group then turned to a review of the philosophical approaches. These had been proposed by a faculty subgroup and had been tentatively accepted, pending further refinement of the narrative. The philosophical approaches included beliefs about nursing's role in society, social justice, caring, and the nature of the nurse-client relationship, and faculty members' and students' responsibility in the curriculum. They considered the fit between the philosophical beliefs and the concepts, abilities, and teaching-learning approaches that had been identified.

The group confirmed the curriculum nucleus to be comprised of the following:

- Core curriculum concepts: Health, aging, health promotion, illness intervention, context, nurse-client relationships, social justice, and caring (the latter two from the philosophical approaches)
- Key professional abilities: Critical thinking, clinical reasoning, independent and collaborative decision-making, cultural competence, and life-long learning
- Principal teaching-learning approaches: Self-direction, collaborative learning, and use of information technologies
- Philosophical approaches: Social justice, caring, humanism, phenomenology.

The group felt satisfied with the curriculum nucleus and confirmed they could support these ideas as the basis for subsequent curriculum development. Dr. Werstiuk and Professor Rose congratulated the participants for their hard work, creativity in reconciling varying perspectives, and intellectual courage in envisioning a curriculum that would require considerable change and learning by each member. All were proud of themselves individually and collectively, and anxious to begin the intensive planning that would bring their ideas to fruition.

Table 7-3 Conceptual Links Between Internal Contextual Data and Curriculum for Poplarfield University School of Nursing

Internal Contextual Factors	Data	Patterns and Trends	Curriculum Concepts	Professional Competencies	Curriculum Possibilities (P) and Limitations (L)	Administrative Issues
Financial Resources	University budget is dependent on government funding	Prevailing feeling that inadequate budgets constrain activities				Acquisition of additional funding from senior administrators
	School budget meets salary and daily operational costs for current curriculum		Budgeting	Financial management in nursing practice	L: Curriculum design affected by budget	Investigation of new funding sources
	Discretionary funds range from none to "almost none"	Tight budget for many years with no extras			L: Introduction of more expensive teaching approaches	Travel funds necessary to renew, recruit, and retain faculty
	No travel funds for faculty				L: Purchase of learning resources	
	Small budget for annual faculty development day				L: Faculty exposure to nursing education trends through literature only	
	Budget secured from senior administrators for curriculum development				L: Faculty development to support new curriculum	Acquisition of sufficient funds required for ongoing faculty development

Infrastructure a) *Human resources*	*University*			
	Retention of new post-doctoral faculty a concern across campus	Strategies in place in other schools to attract and retain faculty	**P:** Part of curriculum development budget for faculty development	**L:** Recruitment and retention of nursing faculty problematic
	School of Agriculture has highest faculty retention rate among all schools: low teaching loads, extensive research funding, university's sole graduate program			Need for senior administrators to support strategies for nursing faculty recruitment and retention
	All other schools have travel funds to support conference attendance			Learn how School of Agriculture achieved success

continues

Table 7-3 Continued

Internal Contextual Factors	Data	Patterns and Trends	Curriculum Concepts	Professional Competencies	Curriculum Possibilities (P) and Limitations (L)	Administrative Issues
School Faculty:	Director is PhD-prepared				**L:** Few full-time, continuing faculty to develop and implement a high-calibre, rigorous curriculum	Curriculum success dependent on adequate numbers of PhD, full-time, permanent faculty
	8 full-time, masters prepared; 2 to retire within 2 years New full-time faculty receive 2–3 year contract; stay only 2–3 years, leave for larger cities	School has been unable to attract PhD faculty or retain full-time faculty			**L:** Non-researchers may be unable to incorporate research into curriculum **L:** Curriculum developers may not be present for implementation	Need to attract and retain PhD faculty Faculty profile will affect accreditation
	15–22 part-time per term, baccalaureate prepared; approx. $1/2$ work part-time because of family responsibilities; others are	Relatively stable group of part-time faculty			**L:** Many who will implement curriculum are not involved in its development	Need to orient part-time faculty to new curriculum Investigate possibility of converting some

also employed elsewhere			part-time positions to full-time
Students:			
BSN program: 80% from Poplarfield area; remainder from rural areas; 95% directly from secondary school	Rural health	**P:** Eliminate Post-RN program	Possibility of recruiting more students
	Student population is mainly local and rural	**P:** Revitalize Post-RN program with adult learning approaches, accelerated model	Resources to support adult learning approaches
Post-RN students: from Poplarfield and surrounding area	Decreasing interest in Post-RN program		
Staff:			
3 full-time secretaries with roots in the community; all skilled in office computer applications	Stable group of support staff		Retain staff
b) *Physical resources*	School has adequate space for current needs	**L:** Size, number, and configuration of classrooms limit increase in class size or seminar groups	Improved and expanded physical space required
	Nursing building in need of refurbishing; updating		
	Up-to-date computers for faculty and staff	**P:** Increased reliance on computer-based learning	Faculty preparation for alternate
	University ensures that technology is current		

continues

Table 7-3 Continued

Internal Contextual Factors	Data	Patterns and Trends	Curriculum Concepts	Professional Competencies	Curriculum Possibilities (P) and Limitations (L)	Administrative Issues
					P: Computer-based courses	teaching modalities essential
c) *Resources to support teaching and learning*	*Library resources:* Wide range of nursing texts and practice journals					
	Few nursing research journals				**L:** Curriculum devoid of research base for nursing practice and nursing education	Necessary to expand research journals and texts
	Faculty development services:					
	One faculty member appointed full-time to assist with faculty development across campus				**P:** Assistance with alternate teaching and learning approaches	Need for ongoing faculty development
	Nursing faculty have informal mentoring system for new full-time faculty	Continuous mentoring required				Formal mentoring necessary for faculty retention

Orientation program re: clinical teaching and evaluation for all new full- and part-time faculty

Student services:

Computer lab open 18 hrs each day

Academic and personal counseling

Health services

Financial aid services

Resources available to help students be successful

Information technology

Computer literacy

P: Rigorous curriculum

P: Computer-based learning

Faculty development re: new teaching and evaluation approaches

Table 7-4 Conceptual Links Between External Contextual Data and Curriculum for Poplarfield University of Nursing

External Contextual Factors	Data	Patterns and Trends	Curriculum Concepts	Professional Competencies	Curriculum Possibilities (P) and Limitations (L)	Administrative Issues
Culture	Multicultural town No local ethnic radio or TV stations No ethnic restaurants	Dominant culture is North American, with some families retaining elements of culture of origin (e.g., special foods)	Cultural norms, values, safety, traditions	Cultural assessment Cultural competence Family assessment	**P:** Non-nursing course related to culture	Faculty development Negotiation for support course
	Farming community values nature, land, independence, yet always ready to help others	Farm women isolated		Health promotion Assessment of social relationships Provision of support Empathy	**P:** Clinical experiences with farm families	Transportation for students
	Immigrant adults from Philippines and India largely maintain own ethnic traditions and religious practices; children caught between cultures	Over past 5 years, more Filipino and East Indian applicants to nursing program	Intercultural stress	Effective communication with diverse groups	**P:** Health promotion and care of isolated individuals and groups	Access to ethnic groups

Seasonal workers from Mexico do not speak English Military personnel value discipline, order Many younger military personnel socialize in Poplarfield bars on weekends	Seasonal workers are "outsiders" Social distance and distrust between officers and enlisted personnel Increased number of bar brawls in past 2 years	Marginalization	Health care of disadvantaged groups	**P:** Clinical practices with immigrant and community groups	Access for clinical experience
			Health promotion Critical thinking	**P:** Clinical experiences with immigrant and community groups	Access for clinical experience
Drug use considered acceptable by approximately $1/3$ of young adults	Rise in use of "recreational drugs" Change in student culture	Responding appropriately in situations of values conflict Nurses' potential to make a difference	Assessment and intervention re: drug use Self-reflection Critical thinking	**P:** Clinical experiences in schools, drug rehabilitation centers, street clinics	Awareness of policies re: drug use Potential value conflict between faculty and students
Health Care Healthcare insurance available Rising costs of health care	Shorter hospital stays; higher patient acuity; more community- and home-based care to contain costs; greater burden of care on families	Healthcare system Community-based care	Assessment Resource management Independent decision-making Political astuteness	**P:** Home- and community-based care **P:** Analysis of healthcare system	

continues

Table 7-4 continued

External Contextual Factors	Data	Patterns and Trends	Curriculum Concepts	Professional Competencies	Curriculum Possibilities (P) and Limitations (L)	Administrative Issues
	Migrant workers generally do not have health insurance		Marginalization Equity Health care for those uninsured	Cultural competency for care to those who do not have health insurance	**P:** Health care for uninsured	
	Primary health care provided by family physicians, nurse practitioners, and public health units	Less in-hospital care in Poplarfield and surrounding area	Community-based care Health promotion	Health promotion of individuals, families, communities	**P:** Clinical experiences in physicians' offices, walk-in clinics, nurse practitioners	
	Secondary health care provided by Poplarfield Hospital; tertiary care and cancer treatment center 100 miles away	Shorter hospital stays; sicker people at home; home nursing care; increasing burden of care on family			**P:** Emphasis on community-based and outpatient health promotion and acute nursing care	
	Shortened hospital stays		Effective health-care teams			
	Increased in-home nursing care required			Community-based care throughout the life span and health-illness continuum		
	Increased acuity of hospitalized clients					

Many long-term care facilities in and near Poplarfield so residents can be close to home	Increasing numbers of 'old-old' in institutions	Care of permanently institutionalized, with a variety of care needs Psychological, social, and spiritual health, coupled with waning physical (and possibly cognitive) health	Assessment of individuals and families Family health promotion Evidence-based practice Critical thinking Empathy Information search skills	**P:** Clinical experiences in facilities for institutionalized elderly, residential care; mental health, in- and outpatient facilities	Access for practical experience
Major health problems: Local incidence of coronary artery disease and most cancers consistent with national incidence	Expected to continue for the next 20 years until that generation has died	Determinants of health Genetics Lifestyle Heart health Cancer care	Health promotion Screening assessment, intervention	**P:** Clinical experiences related to major health problems in acute, rehabilitation, and outpatient facilities	Negotiation re: practice sites
High incidence of leukemia among older farmers attributed to past unsafe use of fertilizers		Rural health Safety	Health assessment Safety counseling	**P:** Home visits to farms	Logistics of recruiting families for student visits

continues

Table 7-4 continued

External Contextual Factors	Data	Patterns and Trends	Curriculum Concepts	Professional Competencies	Curriculum Possibilities (P) and Limitations (L)	Administrative Issues
	Injury and accidental death of toddlers and young children on farms double the national incidence		Safety in agricultural environments Primary prevention Rural health	Screening assessment, intervention Screening assessment, intervention	**P:** Home visits to farms	
	Family violence recognized as a public health problem	Reporting has increased	Family violence Physical and emotional abuse	Screening assessment, intervention, referral related to family violence and abuse	**P:** Attention to signs of abuse and violence in all clinical settings	
	Nursing workforce: Average age = 48 years Average retirement age = 55 years	Nationwide shortage of registered nurses will worsen markedly	Provision of safe care despite workplace barriers Leadership Supervision of, and delegation to, non-professional care-givers	Maintenance of standards of excellence Leadership, including supervision of, and delegation to, non-professional care-givers Team-building	**P:** Increase enrollment **P:** Leadership experiences, including supervision of non-professionals	Increased resources needed to increase enrollment

	Recruitment and retention of nursing staff of concern		Critical thinking Information search skills Independent decision-making	Creation of empowering workplaces Evidence-based practice Critical thinking	**L:** Fewer mentors and preceptors	Securing, orienting, and rewarding clinical preceptors
Professional Standards and Trends	Professional practice standards	Emphasis on accountability, critical thinking, evidence-based practice, professional development	Professional roles, responsibilities, accountabilities, standards Codes of ethics Critical thinking Evidence-based practice Professional development Interprofessional practice Practice standards	Commitment to ethical standards, life-long learning Competent, ethical practice Interprofessional practice	**P:** Standards could drive curriculum design **P:** Standards and ethics in all courses **P:** Interprofessional courses, practice **P:** Research focus, evidence-based practice guidelines in all courses	Negotiating interprofessional courses
	BSN degree required for all new entrants to nursing profession Competency-based registration examinations that are integrative, not	University preparation for all nursing students	Professionalization of nursing Nursing history Role of professional associations	All competencies of professional nursing	**P:** Increase in applicants to program **P:** Competency-based examinations	Support for program expansion and collaboration with colleges

continues

Table 7-4 continued

External Contextual Factors	Data	Patterns and Trends	Curriculum Concepts	Professional Competencies	Curriculum Possibilities (P) and Limitations (L)	Administrative Issues
	based on medical model Non-university nursing programs closing or forming collaborative degree programs with universities				**P:** Partnering with other educational institutions	Possible loss of some autonomy Need to determine views of senior administrators
	Program accreditation standards include: faculty research, inclusion of research focus in curriculum, link between clinical settings and curriculum			Research focus, evidence-based practice, best practice guidelines in all courses	**L:** Faculty are not researchers **L:** Library holdings scant in area of nursing research	Hiring of PhD faculty and research development support
				Reflective practice Self-directedness	**P:** Research course	Continuous assessment of program
	Feminist, constructivist, phenomenological bases to many nursing curricula	Behaviorist curricula	Nature of relationship with clients, colleagues	Critical thinking Respect Egalitarian relationships	**P:** Concept-based teaching-learning **P:** Practice-driven curriculum **P:** Learner-designed assignments **L:** Faculty preparation and motivation	Time and cost of faculty development Faculty recruitment Supportive environment

Questions for Consideration and Analysis of the Poplarfield Case

1. What strengths and limitations are evident in the processes undertaken by the Poplarfield faculty? How might these processes be applied in other settings?
2. How might the retreat have been organized differently to advance the curriculum work?
3. Review Tables 7-1, 7-3, and 7-4. What gaps and overlaps are present in the contextual data?
4. Examine Tables 7-1, 7-3, and 7-4. Propose other interpretations of the data, concepts, professional abilities, curriculum limitations and possibilities, and administrative issues.
5. Consider the curriculum nucleus identified by the Poplarfield faculty. Does it seem reasonable? What changes could be proposed?
6. If you were the curriculum consultant, how might your actions be similar or different from those of Professor Rose? Why?
7. If you were to assume the role of curriculum consultant for the Poplarfield University School of Nursing, in what way might your actions be similar or different from those of Professor Rose?

Curriculum Development Questions for Consideration in Your Setting

Use the following questions to guide thinking about the development of the curriculum nucleus in your curriculum work.

1. How can the contextual data be organized and displayed in a manner that will be helpful for analysis?
2. What procedures could be used for analyzing, interpreting, and synthesizing the contextual data?
3. How can a common understanding of the contextual data be reached?
4. How can the relative weighting of the contextual factors be determined?
5. How can relevant administrative issues be deduced?
6. What procedures will lead to conclusions about the curriculum nucleus?
7. How can confidence be inspired that the curriculum nucleus is responsive to the reasons that led to curriculum development in the first place, and to the constellation of contextual data?
8. How might divergent viewpoints be addressed constructively?
9. What strategies can be employed to ensure that the identified curriculum nucleus will be supported?

CHAPTER 8

Developing Philosophical Approaches and Formulating Curriculum Outcomes

Chapter Overview

In this chapter, *philosophy* is introduced with definitions and purposes. These are presented from the perspectives of general education and nursing education. Traditional philosophies are considered first, then some of the more current philosophies for nursing curricula, followed by the authors' conceptualization of *philosophical approaches* for curriculum development. It is not the intent of this section to present a detailed description of philosophies. Rather, they are summarized to highlight main ideas, similarities, and differences, and to stimulate pursuit of further understanding.

Subsequent to the section on philosophy, *curriculum outcomes* are described according to definition and purposes. Formulating curriculum outcomes follows. Then, faculty development related to philosophical approaches and curriculum outcomes, and a chapter summary, are presented. Synthesis activities, including two cases, and questions for curriculum developers, conclude the chapter.

Chapter Goals

- Understand definitions and purposes of *philosophical approaches* and *curriculum outcomes* in curriculum development.

- Recognize the value of philosophical approaches and curriculum outcome statements for the nursing curriculum.

- Consider processes for developing philosophical approaches and formulating curriculum outcome statements.

- Reflect on faculty development activities related to developing philosophical approaches and formulating curriculum outcomes.

Curriculum Philosophy

Philosophy is the "love and pursuit of wisdom by intellectual means and moral self-discipline. . . . It comprises statements of enduring values and beliefs held by members of the discipline. . . . Philosophical statements are practical guides for examining issues and clarifying priorities of the discipline" (Haynes, Boese, & Butcher, 2004, p. 77). A curriculum philosophy describes the beliefs held by faculty about the purpose of education, learners, learning, and teaching.

Purposes of a Curriculum Philosophy

General Education   In general education, philosophy statements include assumptions about human nature; the purpose and goals of education, instruction, and learning; and the roles of teachers, students, and programs. John Dewey, one of America's greatest educators, interpreted philosophy as a "general theory of educating", whereas one of his students, Boyd Bode, viewed it as a "source of reflective consideration" (Wiles & Bondi, 1998, p. 35). To Ralph Tyler (1949), a leader in curriculum development throughout much of the 1900s, philosophy defined the purpose of education, clarified objectives and learning activities, specified faculty roles, and guided the selection of learning methods and strategies. More recently, the view of philosophy is that it assists in the following:

- Decision making for the profession (White & Brockett, 1987)
- Professional development (Petress, 2003)
- Curriculum development, such as the determination of overall purpose, objectives, format for instructional delivery, and selection of learning activities and classroom tactics (Wiles & Bondi, 2007)

To Csokasy (2002), "the philosophy provides a framework for discussion of answers to value laden questions related to teaching and learning, and [is] a guide to all activities of the curriculum" (p. 32).

Nursing Education   In the traditional view of philosophy in nursing education, the philosophy provides a value system that grounds the curriculum. It provides a basis for selecting and using curriculum concepts, theories, teaching methods, and learning experiences (Bevis, 1986; Clayton, 1989; Keating, 2006; Yura, 1974), and governs thought and conduct within a nursing program (Lawrence & Lawrence, 1983). Keating further emphasizes that the philosophy should be congruent with that of the parent institution.

Gates (1990) proposes that a philosophy for nursing education should be open rather than hidden, and it should profess the position of the nursing school and curriculum in the wider social context. In a somewhat different vein, Rentschler and Spegman (1996) suggest that the philosophy of the nursing profession is transmitted through a philosophy of education, and that students are socialized into the profession through the lived experience of nursing education.

Traditional views of philosophy prevail, and contain foundational values and beliefs for the nursing curriculum, teaching, and learning (Dillard, Sitkberg, & Laidig, 2005; Csokasy, 2005). These views of philosophy also concentrate on the analysis of thoughts, ideas, and concepts (Clark & Holt, 2001). Philosophies and theories of nursing have been used in nursing curricula to clarify what nursing is, what should be studied, and how nursing differs from other disciplines (Uys & Smit, 1994). Philosophies of nursing include basic premises about the nature and goals of nursing, role of nurses in society and healthcare systems, persons, rights and obligations for health, and environment. It has been suggested that a philosophy could have other major benefits to student learning, such as to:

- help them think, and to think critically
- familiarize them with some philosophical source
- help them evaluate nursing literature, specifically in the areas of nursing knowledge and theory (Clark & Holt, 2001).

Accordingly, megatheories such as Martha Rogers' Unitary Person Model, Newman's Model of Health, and Watson's Theory of Human Caring have been used as theoretical and philosophical bases of curricula. In contrast to these ideas, Bevis (2000a) suggested that a philosophy may not be necessary, and that curriculum developers could substitute assumptions instead.

Although a philosophy for nursing education continues to be supported by curriculum developers, there are some difficulties in how it is used in curricula. For example, statements might be unacceptable to all stakeholders, incongruent with the focus of the curriculum, idealistic rather than real, static, and too general (Torres & Stanton, 1982). As well, philosophy statements may lack meaning and may not be shared with learners, particularly if these statements are viewed merely as a professional or discipline requirement (Kintgen-Andrews, 1988). To ensure that the philosophy reflects faculty beliefs and values, and is relevant to social, cultural, professional, and consumer needs, it should be reviewed and updated periodically (Rentschler & Spegman, 1996). Consistent with this recommendation, in one school the philosophy, vision, and mission were revised 11 times, became a working document, and then was changed three more times in 4 years (King Mixon, Kemp, Towle, & Schrader, 2005).

Traditional Curriculum Philosophies

Although classical philosophies date back some 2500 years to Greek scholars of the 6th century BCE, differences in the philosophical bases of various disciplines began only in the last two centuries (Uys & Smit, 1994). It was not until late into the 1800s that the first well-rounded philosophy about nursing education was developed by Florence Nightingale (Csokasy, 2005). In spite of the development of philosophies specific to disciplines, traditional schools of philosophy (e.g., idealism and realism) emanating from early Greek philosophers, still influence nursing education today.

Idealism According to this philosophy, truth is universal, values are unchanging, and individuals desire to live in a perfect world of high ideals, beauty, and art. The curriculum is built on humanism, liberal arts education, and promotion of intellectual growth. Teachers serve as role models for students, who are encouraged to think and expand their minds by applying knowledge to life.

Realism The main tenet of realism is that natural laws compose the world and regulate all of nature. The curriculum is structured to present and reflect these universal laws, and is organized around content. Teachers provide information sequentially in an efficient, simple-to-complex manner. Students are motivated to learn through positive reinforcement, and they are rewarded for learning basic skills and responding to new experiences with scientific objectivity and analysis.

Learning Theories as Curriculum Philosophies

One or more learning theories could be used as the philosophical base and learning orientation of the nursing curriculum. The theory selected should reflect stakeholder views about learning, teaching, student characteristics, and the educational environment.

An example of a learning theory used as a philosophical base for the curriculum is *behaviorism*. This learning theory is grounded in positivism, the predominant form of scientific reasoning from the latter 1800s to the mid 1900s. With behaviorism, which was the foundation of nursing curricula for much of the 1900s, preeminence is given to behavioral objectives, positive reinforcement, and reward. Curricula are characterized by presentation of real facts and observable phenomena. The responsibility for organizing knowledge lies with the teacher. Students are largely passive learners, and there is limited facilitation of critical analysis, thinking, reasoning, or creativity. Emphases are on learners' ability to master content and transfer formal propositional knowledge into clinical practice, which is generally supervised. Personal development is secondary (Yorks & Sharoff, 2001).

Other learning theories can be conceived as all or part of a philosophical base for a nursing curriculum. Vandeveer and Norton (2005) suggest that cognitive theories, cognitive development, multiple intelligences, some educational frameworks, and interpretive pedagogies could be used as frameworks for a nursing curriculum philosophy.

Current Nursing Curriculum Philosophies

The following nursing curriculum philosophies, albeit merely highlighted, evidence some differences, but also commonalities. As can be detected, there is a blending of philosophy and learning theory, as well as an intermingling of beliefs, values, and teaching and learning applications.

Apprenticeship Hilton (2001) proposed an apprenticeship philosophy based on the epistemology of Michael Polanyi, the Hungarian scientist and philosopher. Polanyi (as cited in Hilton) believes that in an apprenticeship arrangement skills and ways of thinking are learned from experts with intuitive knowledge and by example from authority figures (masters). This is combined with holistic learning that takes place by seeing, doing, touching, experiencing, and by acquiring motor skills first, then building upon them. Using this approach, nursing students would begin with foundation courses (nursing fundamentals), and once they demonstrate mastery of laboratory skills and theoretical knowledge, they would proceed with more difficult material in classrooms, laboratories, and clinical situations. Hilton recommends pairing students as apprentices with experienced nurses throughout the nursing curriculum, in accordance with Polanyi's views.

Similarly, cognitive apprenticeship is a teaching-learning experience in which learners participate with experts in a community of practice to learn expert knowledge, physical skills, procedures, thinking processes, and the culture of the field. Students observe, participate, and discover expert practice through teaching strategies such as modeling, coaching, scaffolding (hints, directions, reminders, physical assistance), and learning strategies such as articulation, reflection, and exploration (Taylor & Care, 1999).

Action-Sensitive Pedagogy This approach "embraces holism, phenomenological human science, and political advocacy" (Averill & Clements, 2007, p. 389) for students, faculty, and the individuals and groups whom nurses serve. Activities are designed to "ignite the curiosity, honor the diversity, and substantially engage . . . students in the enterprise of education" (p. 389). Six patterns of knowing (empirical, ethical, personal, esthetic, socio-political, and unknowing), integration of contexts, holistic thinking, caring, and full engagement of body, mind and spirit, are integral to this pedagogy. It is the "mindful praxis of asking, knowing, mentoring, and acting" (p. 397).

Collaborative Inquiry Collaborative inquiry is a systemic process derived from whole-person epistemology. Learners use experiences to generate new knowledge by action and reflection. Teachers and students share power and responsibility for decision-making. Critical subjectivity in the mutual pursuit of new meaning is practiced, and explicit activity procedures are followed. Collaborative inquiry draws on multiple ways of knowing and legitimizes transformative and holistic learning early in the careers of nursing students.

Constructivism According to this view, knowledge is seen as constructed and all learning as connected. The theory holds that people build knowledge, in contrast to merely acquiring it. With exposure to new perspectives, current understandings are changed, and new knowledge is constructed to make sense of experiences. Reality is perceived as invented. Constructed knowledge is always open to change, as connections are continuously made to previous and new learning and experiences (Belenky, Clinchy, Goldberger, & Tarule, 1986). Meanings resulting from the process of constructing knowledge could vary, depending on the context in which questions are asked and the frame of reference of the questioner. In a curriculum based on this theory, the emphasis is on helping learners interpret and make meaning of knowledge and experiences. As well, their interpretations should be subjected to examination by themselves and others (Haw, 2006).

Post-positivism Recent post-positivist perspectives also center on knowledge and meaning as opposed to prediction and control. Learning and meaning are seen to occur in the context and experience of the evolving co-constructed process between and among nurses, clients, teachers, and students (Walton, 1996). Learning and meaning-making involve connecting the view of others to one's own knowledge, and building a new co-constructed understanding of the shared experience (Surrey, as cited in Walton).

Critical Social Theory This theory is concerned with justice, equality, and freedom. It maintains that knowledge as truth is socially constructed, and facts are relevant only in the lived experiences of persons (Duchscher, 2000). The premise is that all meanings and truths are created and interpreted in the context of social history (Henderson, 1995). Understanding patterns of human behavior involves knowledge of existing social structures and the communication processes that define them. Critical social theory enables students and faculty to share a revisioning and reconstruction of former potentially oppressive and coercive cultural, political, and social ideologies and practices. Nurse educators encourage, listen, express, problem-pose, and philosophize to foster a critical approach to learning. Learners are assisted to take the role of others and develop empathy, confidence, and competence in human relations. These competencies develop through critical self-reflection, self-transformation, discussion, and dialogue (Duchscher). With this action-oriented theory, learners examine health care and other structures (including their own role in oppressive practices), and advocate for changes in the situations that create oppression and influence health (Mohammed, 2006).

Epistemology An epistemological philosophy emphasizes the relationship between persons and knowledge. It is recognized that much significant learning occurs apart from formal educational experiences, and that informal and incidental learning from lived experiences account for most learning. Because learners shape learning through experience, intuition, intellect, and practice (Heron, 1992), value is given to all these ways of knowing.

Feminism Feminism is an ideology originally premised on values and beliefs about women, and relationships of gender, specifically that gender is "a difference that makes a difference" (di Stefano, as cited in Tong, 2007). Although there are many forms of feminism (e.g., liberal, radical, Marxist-socialist, multicultural, global, post-modern, third-wave), they all share the view that women are disadvantaged. Based in feminism, feminist pedagogy serves as a means for educational development and social change to meet educational needs of women. More broadly interpreted, feminism and feminist pedagogy value persons regardless of gender, with the goal of ending previous dehumanizing polarizations. It provides a framework that promotes development of intellectual growth and activism, and incorporates professional nursing values such as self-awareness, independence, empowerment, caring, and nursing's patterns of knowing. Learners question, reflect, and challenge values and assumptions of nursing practice. Together with teachers, they co-construct meaning from life experiences. Students are empowered and test ideas through critical thinking, analysis, synthesis, and self-evaluation.

Humanism A philosophy of humanism is concerned with rights, autonomy, and dignity of human beings and a belief that learning is motivated by a desire for personal growth and fulfillment. In a humanistic-existentialist curriculum, the focus is on personal meaning in human existence (Csokasy, 2005). Teachers question the need for outcome assessment, and rely instead on critical thinking, application of knowledge, and students' interpretation of the learning experience. The role of the teacher is to motivate and encourage experiential learning and facilitate students to establish and attain their own goals.

Interpretive Inquiry and Relational Humanistic Nursing Interpretive inquiry and relational humanistic nursing (relational practice) is a process of intense reflection on events and experiences in which nursing students are part of a relational process of interpreting those events and experiences (Doanne, 2002). Learners are not hampered by the ideas and content of a situation, the interpretation of the content, and what is to be done. Rather, the content becomes whatever arises through the inquiry process. Learners authentically connect with their "self in relation" by inquiring into and interpreting their relational experiences and practices, and move beyond the self through reflection, dialogue, and reenactment.

Life Skills Life skills philosophy is based on the premise that knowledge and facts can be quickly outdated, so students should learn and practice basic skills they will need for a lifetime. These basic skills support acquisition and integration of new knowledge as it is generated, enabling learners to take on new information and adapt to future change. Teaching methods are compatible with producing the workforce of the future, and incorporate a variety of participative learning strategies (Freeman, Voignier, & Scott, 2002).

Phenomenology Phenomenology is an orientation and research method that focuses on lived experience and personal meaning. It emphasizes that people are always situated within a context, that there are multiple realities, and that people's perception of their experiences are valid. In nursing education, consideration is given to the experience of the individual (student, client, teacher), and learning experiences and the curriculum are framed in relation to these experiences.

Narrative pedagogy illustrates an approach to teaching and learning that has a significant basis in interpretative phenomenology, and that also allows for conventional, alternate, and new approaches to converge (Diekelmann, 2001). It relies on the lived experience of faculty, learners, and clinicians as the basis of student learning. The multiple perspectives of those involved in the stories are explored, so that learners gain many views about the meaning of those experiences and about nursing. Public sharing and collective interpretation of the stories enrich learning and make the learning memorable in this student-centered approach. "Thinking is an experience of participative and interpretative practices that attend not only to issues of content (what is known and not known), but also to multi-perspectival issues of significance" (Ironside, 2005, p. 447).

Pragmatism Central to pragmatism is the testing of ideas, a combination of idealism and realism. Pragmatism in education is based on progressive and reconstructive theories, whereby learners are actively engaged in learning and exploring, in laboratory work, simulations, field trips, and social and community activities. Learners are encouraged to take in new information, interpret, and apply it to previous learning and current client experiences (Csokasy, 2002). Learning outcomes are assessed through examinations and observation of students interacting with clients.

The preceding is merely an overview, as it is beyond the scope of this book to provide a comprehensive description of philosophies. The philosophies, singly or in combination, give rise to implications for nursing education. Implications of some are summarized in Table 8-1.

Philosophical Approaches

The curriculum should be built on a philosophical base that is then embodied throughout the curriculum. Since most, if not all, nursing education curricula are based on blended ideas drawn from several philosophies, the term *philosophical approach(es)* seems more fitting than *philosophy*. This conceptualization implies a liberal interpretation of the term *philosophy* and can encompass eclecticism, pluralism, assumptions, beliefs, and values. Latitude

Table 8-1 Implications of Philosophical Approaches for Nursing Education

Philosophical Approaches	Key Ideas for Curriculum	Implications for Learners
Action-sensitive pedagogy	Holistic thinking, caring, phenomenological human science, political advocacy	Engage in learning (body, mind, spirit) through patterns of knowing, curiosity, diversity, mentoring, asking and acting
Apprenticeship; Cognitive apprenticeship	Master-apprentice relationship; learning by example and from intuition of experts	Learn by example from experienced clinicians early in the curriculum and throughout the curriculum
Behaviorism/positivism	Positive reinforcement and reward; simple-to-complex curriculum; scientific objectivity; achievement of behavioral objectives	Learn by positive reinforcement and reward; learn content and transfer knowledge to clinical experience; able to practice as graduates if prescribed curriculum objectives and standards are met
Collaborative inquiry	Generation of new knowledge from reflection, shared power, active learning, and decision-making; four ways of knowing	Use all four ways of knowing; use experiences to generate new knowledge
Constructivism; Post-positivism	Meaning and knowledge are constructed; learning is connected; new understandings occur between and among students, teachers, and clients	Construct knowledge by taking own and others' views to build new knowledge and a co-constructed understanding; learning and meaning-making arise from connecting others' views to own knowledge
Critical social theory	Meanings and truth are interpreted in context of history; critical self-reflection develops capacity to examine experience in different ways; involves autonomy, social responsibility, emancipation, empowerment, and understanding	Share in revisioning and reconstructing formerly oppressive or coercive ideologies and practices

continues

Table 8-1   continued

Philosophical Approaches	Key Ideas for Curriculum	Implications for Learners
Epistemology	Relationship between learner and knowledge; informal, incidental, lived experience learning	Comprehend that a relationship exists between self and knowledge, and informal, incidental, and lived experiences form most of learning
Feminism	Lived experiences; creative and critical thinking; empowerment	Become empowered to question, reflect, challenge values and assumptions of nursing practice; incorporate life experience in learning
Humanism-existentialism	Critical thinking; application of knowledge; "being" in nursing; experiential learning	Be motivated towards experiential learning; establishing and meeting own goals

and some diversity in thoughts, views, values, assumptions, principles, and beliefs are thus possible. There must, however, be logical consistency in the espoused philosophical approaches. As well, they must be congruent with the values of faculty and the educational institution. Philosophical approaches can be expressed through philosophical or value statements, or through assumptions.

Developing Philosophical Approaches

A sound beginning for a philosophical approaches subcommittee is to conduct a literature search about nursing, curriculum, and nursing education philosophies. Then the committee should review the philosophical statements of other schools of nursing. This will assist the subcommittee members to:

- Appreciate the range of philosophical ideas that could influence nursing curricula.
- Identify ideas that resonate for them.
- Assess the style in which statements of philosophical beliefs are expressed in other schools of nursing.

From this review of literature and other schools' statements, members can make a decision about whether to use a formal philosophy (or more than one), philosophical approaches, value statements, or assumptions.

The subcommittee should strive to understand the beliefs and values of colleagues, as all faculty implement the curriculum. One strategy could be to summarize the main precepts of several philosophies gleaned from the literature and request that stakeholders indicate those that best fit their ideas. Alternately, a template could be given to faculty and other stakeholders, with a request that they write their beliefs about matters such as teaching and learning, the nature and purpose of student-faculty and nurse-client relationships, health, and so forth. Common ideas within the responses could be the basis of the curriculum's philosophical approaches. A third activity might be to delineate the teaching and learning implications of several philosophical approaches, and seek information about stakeholders' preferences.

Once information is obtained from stakeholders, philosophical approaches for the curriculum can be drafted and distributed with a request for feedback. This requires considerable discussion since it is likely that differing beliefs will have to be reconciled (Oliva, 2005). Several drafts are generally required before agreement is reached about the philosophical approaches.

The following questions could be considered when developing the philosophical approaches for the nursing curriculum:

- How can we become more knowledgeable about philosophical approaches in general education and nursing education?
- Should value statements, assumptions, or a single, pluralistic, or eclectic approach be used for the curriculum? What are the advantages and disadvantages of each?
- How can stakeholders' views be determined in a reasonable time period?
- Which philosophical approaches seem most consistent with the beliefs and values of stakeholders and the educational institution?
- What are the curriculum implications of the philosophical approaches we prefer?

Confirming Philosophical Approaches

The importance of consensus among the total faculty group about the philosophical approaches cannot be overemphasized. The philosophical approaches are the basis of the entire curriculum. There must be agreement and a common understanding about philosophical approaches when the curriculum nucleus is defined, and before subsequent curriculum work is undertaken. The philosophical approaches are part of the curriculum nucleus, and thus are foundational to further curriculum development. Time spent on reaching a shared understanding and agreement by the total faculty group is time well spent. Once this is achieved, the philosophical approaches subcommittee can attend to perfecting the written statements.

Curriculum Outcomes

The educational destination that students are supposed to achieve at the end of the nursing program must be specified, since this description becomes the basis for subsequent curriculum decisions. In this book, the term *outcomes* is used, although in some curricula the terms *objectives, goals,* or *ends-in-view* label the anticipated professional abilities of graduating students. Each term connotes a different idea from the others, although all are written to be meaningful to several audiences. The formulation of statements to describe the educational destination is, like other aspects of curriculum development, a group activity requiring confirmation by the total faculty group.

Clarification of Terms

Curriculum outcomes are statements of the professional abilities learners are projected to attain as the result of an educational program. They are practice-oriented statements, integrating several domains of knowledge so that higher-level functions, such as nursing care, can be performed. The focus is on a pattern and complexity of knowledge domains pertinent to, and evident in, professional practice. Outcomes are assessable (Glennon, 2006). In the Model of Context-Relevant Curriculum Development, the outcome statements incorporate the philosophical approaches, indicate the core curriculum concepts, and describe the key professional abilities in a comprehensive, holistic fashion.

In nursing education literature, the term *outcomes* has been used with two connotations. First, the term is employed to explain the *intended or expected* cognitive processes and practice behaviors that learners will exhibit at program completion. Although generally termed *outcomes,* it is really the *outcome statements* that embody the anticipated professional abilities of graduates and to which curriculum writers give attention. Secondly, the word has been used to describe the *actual* cognitive processes and practice behaviors of graduates. These actual outcomes can be known only through follow-up studies of graduates and employers. Therefore, the curriculum outcome statements should be written in a manner that will provide direction to these studies.

Terminal objectives, based on the work of Ralph Tyler (1949), are generally associated with a behaviorist philosophy, and are a method to describe the learning achieved in a nursing curriculum. However, behavioral objectives each describe only one behavior in the cognitive (Bloom, Englehart, Furst, Hill, & Krathwohl, 1956; Anderson et al., 2001; Krathwohl, 2002), affective (Krathwohl, Bloom, & Masia, as cited in Oermann & Gaberson, 2006), or psychomotor (Dave, as cited in Oermann & Gaberson, 2006) domain, and therefore, they are too specific to describe the end point of a program of learning. Accordingly, although the phrase *terminal objectives* may be used, these statements may resemble *goals.*

Curriculum goals are broad statements that describe the educational destination to be reached by graduating students. The goals reflect the philosophical approaches, core curriculum concepts, and multiple objectives. Goals incorporate cognitive, interpersonal, and psychomotor aspects of professional practice. Because goals encompass many objectives, they have been described as "multidimensional" (Bastable & Doody, 2008).

Finally, *ends-in-view* are intended to "... point directions and to provide subjects or topics that become the rubric under which a wide range of content can fall" (Bevis, 2000b, p. 139). The open form of ends-in-view statements reflect the idea that cognitive understandings cannot be prescribed in the same manner as behaviors associated with skills learning. Ends-in-view are not as specific as outcomes, objectives, or goals. As such, benchmarking and evaluation may be less straightforward. The term, *ends-in-view*, is used less frequently than the others, possibly because it is difficult to align ideas about accountability in education with such open-ended descriptions of learning. Examples of outcome statements, terminal objectives, goals, and ends-in-view are provided in Table 8-2.

If the outcome statements are written, then the level and course expectations are generally referred to as *competencies*. When *goals, objectives*, or *ends-in-view* are used to describe the expectation of students at graduation, the same term is typically used consistently throughout the curriculum. In this book, the terms *outcomes* or *outcome statements* are used to refer to the description of learners at program completion.

Table 8-2   Examples of Statements Describing Learner Abilities at Program Completion

Statement Type	Example
Ends-in-view	• Consider the leadership dimensions inherent in planning, providing, and evaluating nursing care in all settings. • Work toward advancement of the nursing profession.
Goals	• Employ leadership skills in planning, providing, managing, and evaluating care in institutional and community settings. • Promote justifiable positions to advance professional nursing practice and healthcare policies that are responsive to societal needs.
Outcomes	• Integrate theory from nursing, biological, and psycho-social sciences when collaboratively planning, providing, and evaluating care. • Incorporate knowledge of political action, health, and social justice to prepare justifiable position statements about the nursing profession and health policy.
Terminal objectives	• Provide nursing care to diverse clients in accordance with standards of practice. • Advocate for healthy work environments for nurses.

Purpose of Curriculum Outcome Statements for Various Audiences

The outcome statements, which appear in published descriptions of the curriculum, have several audiences; each reads them for a different purpose. All have a legitimate interest in curriculum outcome statements.

Curriculum Developers This group uses the outcome statements as a source of direction for all subsequent aspects of curriculum planning, implementation, and evaluation. This implies that the curriculum design, level and course competencies, learning activities and assignments, and evaluation of learning, all derive their focus and intent from the curriculum outcome statements. Curriculum developers are obligated to create and sequence learning experiences that will allow motivated and capable learners to achieve the intended curriculum outcomes.

Faculty Faculty designing individual courses turn to curriculum outcomes (from which more specific level and course competencies emanate) as their reference point for course planning, teaching-learning strategies, and assessments of student learning. The curriculum outcomes are the standards for students to achieve and against which faculty members assess the suitability of learning experiences.

Current Students Students enrolled in a school of nursing look to curriculum outcome statements as the target they should reach by graduation, and to course competencies as targets for smaller units of learning. To make outcome statements meaningful to learners, faculty should refer to them frequently, identifying how particular learning activities contribute to achievement of the outcomes. In this way, the outcome statements have an educational value to learners, and are not merely rhetoric that seems unrelated to courses. Additionally, frequent and explicit reference to curriculum outcome statements helps learners articulate their professional abilities and achievements.

Prospective Students Potential applicants can review the outcome statements to determine if the curriculum will match their view of nursing, personal expectations, and philosophical orientation. Outcome statements can attract applicants whose interests are aligned with the curriculum purposes and processes. A curriculum based on feminist approaches, for example, may be of great interest to some, and unappealing to others. Similarly, outcome statements that incorporate an emphasis on community health could attract those interested in working in non-institutional settings, while prospective students interested in critical care would be unlikely to apply to that program.

Clinicians and Potential Employers These groups can use the published outcome statements to understand, in general terms, what learners are expected to accomplish and what professional abilities they will have at graduation. Reference to outcome statements by faculty can be effective in helping clinicians appreciate why the nursing curriculum may not prepare learners in the manner some clinicians might prefer. Similarly, outcome statements that indicate curriculum concepts and competencies such as critical thinking, reflective and collaborative practice, or leadership, could assist employers to recognize the value graduates can bring to organizations, following a suitable period of orientation.

Other Members of the Educational Institution Faculty teaching non-nursing courses, chairs of institution-wide committees concerned with curricula and standards, and administrators are interested in whether the nursing curriculum outcome statements are congruent with the mission and values of the parent institution. If institution-wide outcomes have been delineated for programs, these should be apparent in the nursing outcome statements, although presented within the context of nursing practice. However, nursing curriculum outcomes might exceed the institutional expectations.

Representatives of Accrediting Organizations, State Boards of Nursing, and Provincial Licensing Bodies Representatives of organizations concerned with nursing education and nursing practice standards also have a legitimate interest in the curriculum outcome statements. They want to be assured that the intended outcomes match the expectations for the program level (practical nursing, associate degree, diploma, baccalaureate, or graduate) and are congruent with practice standards. Additionally, curriculum outcome statements, among other information, are evaluated when graduates seek licensure in jurisdictions other than where they were originally licensed.

Members of Professional Nursing Organizations These persons review nursing curriculum outcome statements to keep abreast of educational expectations and professional abilities of new graduates. As well, the outcome statements could signal the type of placement experiences that might be requested for students within the professional organization. The outcome statements might contribute to the rationale used to substantiate recommendations to legislators about nursing practice and healthcare policy.

Members of the Public Healthcare recipients generally read curriculum outcome statements only when they encounter a problem in nursing practice. In those instances, if a complaint to a licensing body or a lawsuit is considered, members of the public and/or their legal representatives may want to determine the curriculum outcomes graduates should have achieved.

Formulating Curriculum Outcome Statements

As previously stated, curriculum outcome statements are developed from the agreed-upon philosophical approaches, core curriculum concepts, and key professional abilities. These should be evident in the final outcome statements. The outcome statements must be congruent with the mission, vision, and goals of the school of nursing and educational institution. There could be considerable similarity in the curriculum outcome statements of many schools of nursing because curriculum developers are guided by similar contextual influences, such as nursing practice or performance standards; codes of ethics; licensure and accreditation requirements; provincial, state, or national positions on higher education; and prevailing educational philosophies. Yet, as much as possible, the outcome statements should give an indication of the uniqueness and context-relevance of each school's curriculum.

The language and format of the curriculum outcome statements must be consistent with the philosophical approaches and incorporate the key professional abilities and core curriculum concepts. When writing these statements, curriculum developers should be mindful of the intended audiences and ensure that the terminology is understandable. The statements are to be comprehensive, yet concrete enough to be meaningful, and sufficiently broad to allow for ongoing curriculum refinement.

Synthetic thinking, artful writing, and ongoing discussion among faculty are required for outcome statements that reflect the intent of the curriculum. The subcommittee preparing the outcome statements should be immersed in the philosophical approaches, core curriculum concepts, key professional abilities, nursing education and practice standards, and other relevant information assembled as part of the contextual data. Goal or outcome statements from other schools can also provide useful ideas.

When developing outcome statements for the nursing curriculum, the outcomes subcommittee might consider:

- What format is compatible with the philosophical approaches? Should outcome statements, terminal objectives, goals, or ends-in-view be used? Why?
- What are the most relevant nursing education and practice standards that must be evident (or exceeded) in the statements?
- How can graduating students' professional abilities, and the context in which these will be evident, be meaningfully described?
- What is necessary to ensure that the curriculum outcomes are appropriate for the program level?
- How can the curriculum outcomes be grounded in the curriculum nucleus?
- How can feedback from stakeholders be obtained expeditiously?

Formulating outcome statements can be laborious and controversial. Because the statements encapsulate graduates' professional abilities, the use of unambiguous language is essential. Faculty members are rightfully concerned about accuracy, reasonableness, and comprehensiveness in the outcome statements and, therefore, discussion about both the substance and phraseology can be anticipated before approval by the total faculty group is achieved.

Faculty Development

Faculty development can focus on the purpose of philosophical approaches in the curriculum. Values and beliefs about nursing, education, persons, learning, and so forth should be discussed. Examples of standard philosophies could be circulated to help those in attendance see what others have developed. Beginning belief and value statements could be drafted, and the purpose and formulation of outcome statements could be addressed. Some practice with writing these statements would be valuable, particularly if the format of the statements is changing from the existing one. Members experienced in curriculum development can facilitate these sessions.

Chapter Summary

The philosophical approaches of the nursing curriculum reflect the beliefs, values, and convictions of stakeholders. These approaches should be evident throughout the entire curriculum. The curriculum outcome statements describe the characteristics and professional abilities of graduates. Together, the philosophical approaches and outcome statements form the basis of the nursing curriculum, and must be congruent with those of the educational institution.

In this chapter, the definition and purposes of a curriculum philosophy are presented. Some traditional and current curriculum philosophies are briefly described. The authors' view of philosophical approaches and how to develop these approaches for the curriculum are suggested. Similarly, the definition, purposes, and formulation of curriculum outcome statements are described, along with possible faculty development activities.

Synthesis Activities

As in other chapters, two cases are presented for review and discussion. The first case is critiqued; the second is for analysis. Following the cases, questions are offered about developing curriculum philosophies and outcome statements, to guide curriculum development in individual settings.

Southwestern University School of Nursing

Southwestern University School of Nursing has been offering a baccalaureate nursing curriculum that was originally developed 10 years ago. Many faculty members who developed the curriculum have left the university and new ones have been hired. These newer faculty have placed their preferred emphases into their courses and have introduced ideas such as social justice and phenomenology, at times altering course competencies to match these ideas. Consequently, the integrity and unity of the intended curriculum has been reduced, and this became apparent to all faculty when they undertook an extensive curriculum evaluation.

The faculty members agree that it is time to reconsider the curriculum. They are uncertain about whether they should revise the current curriculum or begin anew with a completely reconceptualized curriculum. They decide to gather contextual data, and they agree that the analysis of the data will help them with this decision.

Concurrently with the data collection, a group of four faculty members, the philosophical approaches task force, are beginning the work of formulating a draft statement of philosophical approaches for the curriculum. They review the literature and the Web sites of prominent nursing schools in North America. Then, they prepare a chart indicating possible curriculum implications of the various philosophical stances. They also survey faculty members, asking about their beliefs and values related to person, health, nursing, nurse, nursing education, and learning. The predominant ideas from the faculty are incorporated into the chart, which is circulated to all with a request for feedback about which ideas resonate best with individuals' beliefs.

The ideas with the highest frequency of agreement are to be the basis of a draft statement of philosophical approaches. Unfortunately, some ideas that might seem conflicting have received an almost equal amount of support. For example, some faculty support the idea that they should facilitate students' capacity to be active resource-seekers in nursing practice, while others believe they should ensure students are "thoroughly prepared" to function effectively during clinical practice. The task force arranges a meeting of faculty to discuss the results, instead of proceeding with the preparation of a statement. They believe that members' fuller explanation will lead to resolution of the apparent conflicts and that ultimately, faster resolution of the philosophical approaches will be reached.

Critique

The curriculum evaluation revealed the necessity for curriculum reconceptualization, and faculty have undertaken this task. It is commendable that they are willing to do this in a thorough fashion in order to have a context-relevant curriculum. The early appointment of a task force to develop a statement of philosophical approaches will make the definition of the curriculum nucleus possible, once the contextual data are analyzed.

The philosophical approaches task force has been thorough in obtaining published information about philosophical approaches. However, the literature includes relatively few accounts of concerns that might arise with implementation of the various philosophical approaches in the curriculum. Therefore, the task force might also contact appropriate members of other schools using varying philosophical approaches to learn more about implementation of the approaches. Such information could enrich discussion among faculty members and be significant in the final selection of philo-sophical approaches.

The decision to have a meeting with faculty members is sound. Discussion about in-dividuals' beliefs, preferences about philosophical approaches for the curriculum, and the consequences of these approaches for Southwestern University School of Nursing will en-hance faculty members' understanding and facilitate resolution. Once there is informal agreement about which philosophical approaches will be adopted, the statement can be written, refined, and then formally approved. Resolution about the philosophical ap-proaches will enable faculty to proceed with other decisions about the curriculum nucleus and subsequent curriculum development.

Michaelson County Community College

Michaelson County Community College is one of two post-secondary institutions lo-cated in a small city with a largely working-class population of 39,000. One 150-bed gen-eral hospital, a 98-bed residential care facility, and two health clinics provide services to the community. The college offers 1- and 2-year certificate and associate-degree programs during day, evening, and weekend hours. Approximately 6400 full- and part-time students are enrolled in technology and health-related programs.

The associate-degree nursing (ADN) program is open to applicants who qualify after completing a high school diploma. It was introduced in 1976 and has since graduated over 1600 nurses. A 78% success rate on first-time attempts at NCLEX in the early years has increased to 92%.

The ADN curriculum has undergone several changes in keeping with new approaches in nursing education and practice. Mildred Spenser, MSN, RN, present chair of the nurs-ing department, has been meeting for several months with the nursing faculty and the cur-riculum committee to discuss changes to the curriculum. They have been reviewing environmental, socio-economic, cultural, professional, and institutional factors related to the college, community, and the ADN program. As well, they have been working at dif-ferentiating *curriculum outcomes* from *curriculum goals*, since they want to change their statements to be congruent with more recent thinking in nursing education. Current cur-riculum development activity is focused on the philosophical approaches and curriculum outcome statements.

Guided by the curriculum coordinator, the committee (composed of faculty, students, and agency representatives) has already determined that apprenticeship or cognitive ap-prenticeship philosophical approaches would be suitable. They have drafted an updated, all-encompassing purpose for the program: to prepare students to provide safe, ethical, culturally-sensitive nursing practice, in collaboration with other healthcare providers, to individuals, families, and communities. The intent now is to articulate more specifically curriculum outcomes. A schedule of future meetings has been posted.

Questions for Consideration and Analysis of Michaelson County Community College Case

1. What philosophical assumptions or statements can be derived from the apprenticeship or cognitive apprenticeship approaches?

2. How will these assumptions or statements guide the curriculum?

3. What effect will the philosophical approaches have on the curriculum outcome statements?

4. What must the curriculum committee do to formalize the curriculum outcome statements?

5. Describe the process of developing curriculum outcome statements from the curriculum nucleus.

6. How can the following be formulated:

   • A description of the apprenticeship or cognitive apprenticeship philosophical approaches for the ADN curriculum.

   • ADN curriculum outcomes based on apprenticeship or cognitive apprenticeship philosophical approaches.

Curriculum Development Activities for Consideration in Your Setting

The questions below are intended to stimulate thinking about developing philosophical approaches and formulating curriculum outcome statements in your setting.

1. How will contextual data influence the philosophical approaches and curriculum outcome statements?

2. Who should be involved in the development of the philosophical approaches and curriculum outcome statements?

3. How should the development of philosophical approaches and outcome statements for the curriculum proceed?

4. Which philosophical approaches would be consistent with our ideas, beliefs, convictions, and values, and those of our faculty colleagues?

5. If faculty members ascribe to more than one philosophical approach, would an eclectic or a pluralistic approach more clearly express our views?

6. How can we assure that our philosophical approaches are congruent with those of the educational institution?

7. How can we articulate our philosophical approaches and curriculum outcomes?

8. How can we resolve the manner in which we will describe graduating students' professional abilities? Will we construct outcome statements, goals, terminal objectives, or ends-in-view? What criteria will guide our choice?

9. How can we ensure that the curriculum outcome statements reflect the curriculum nucleus?

10. What resources will be required to complete the work of developing philosophical approaches and curriculum outcome statements?

11. What is a reasonable time period for completion of these curriculum elements?

12. What faculty development activities could help us develop the philosophical approaches and curriculum outcome statements?

References

Anderson, L. W., Krathwohl, D. R., Airasian, P. W., Cruikshank, K. A., Mayer, R. E., et al. (Eds.). (2001). *A taxonomy for learning, teaching, and assessing.* New York: Longman.

Averill, J. B., & Clements, P. T. (2007). Patterns of knowing as a foundation for action-sensitive pedagogy. *Qualitative Health Research, 17*(3), 386–399.

Bastable, S. B., & Doody, J. A. (2008). Behavioral objectives. In S. B. Bastable (Ed.), *Nurse as educator. Principles of teaching and learning for nursing practice* (3rd ed., pp. 319–354). Sudbury, MA: Jones and Bartlett.

Belenky, M. F., Clinchy, B. M., Goldberger, N. R., & Tarule, J. M. (1986). *Women's ways of knowing.* New York: Basic Books.

Bevis, E. O. (1986). *Curriculum building in nursing: A process* (3rd ed.). St. Louis, MO: C.V. Mosby.

Bevis, E. O. (2000a). Illuminating the issues. In E. O. Bevis & J. Watson (Eds.), *Toward a caring curriculum. A new pedagogy for nursing* (pp. 13–35). Boston: Jones and Bartlett.

Bevis, E. O. (2000b). Practical decision making about curriculum. In E. O. Bevis & J. Watson (Eds.), *Toward a caring curriculum. A new pedagogy for nursing* (pp. 107–152). Boston: Jones and Bartlett.

Bloom, B. S., Englehart, M. D., Furst, E. J., Hill, W. H., & Krathwohl, D. R. (1956). *Taxonomy of educational objectives. The classification of educational goals: Handbook 1: Cognitive domain.* New York: David McKay.

Clark, D., & Holt, J. (2001). Philosophy: A key to open the door to critical thinking. *Nurse Education Today, 21*(1), 71–78.

Clayton, G. M. (1989). Curriculum revolution: Defining the concepts. *Journal of Professional Nursing, 5*(1), 6, 55.

Csokasy, J. (2002). A congruent curriculum philosophical integrity from philosophy to outcomes. *Journal of Nursing Education, 41*(1), 32–33.

Csokasy, J. (2005). Philosophical foundations of the curriculum. In D. Billings & J. Halstead (Eds.), *Teaching in nursing: A guide for faculty* (2nd ed., pp. 125–143). St. Louis, MO: Elsevier Saunders.

Diekelmann, N. (2001). Heideggerian hermeneutical analyses of lived experiences of students, teachers, and clinicians. *ANS, Advances in Nursing Science, 23*(3), 53–71.

Dillard, N., Sitkberg, L., & Laidig, J. (2005). Curriculum development. An overview. In D. M. Billings & J. Halstead (Eds.), *Teaching in nursing: A guide for faculty* (2nd ed., pp. 87–107). St. Louis, MO: Elsevier Saunders.

Duchscher, J. E. B. (2000). Bending a habit: Critical social theory as a framework for humanistic nursing education. *Nurse Education Today, 20*(6), 453–462.

Doanne, G. A. H. (2002). Beyond behavioral skills to human-involved processes. Relational nursing practice and interpretive pedagogy. *Journal of Nursing Education, 41*(8), 400–404.

Freeman, L. H., Voignier, R. R., & Scott, D. L. (2002). New curriculum for a new century: Beyond repackaging. *Journal of Nursing Education, 41*(1), 36–40.

Gates, R. (1990). From educational philosophy to educational practice: Fidelity and the curriculum in context. *Nurse Education Today, 10*(6), 420–427.

Glennon, C. D. (2006). Reconceptualizing program outcomes. *Journal of Nursing Education, 45*(2), 55–58.

Haw, M. A. (2006). Learning theories applied to nursing curriculum development. In S. B. Keating (Ed.), *Curriculum development and evaluation in nursing* (pp. 49–60). Philadelphia: Lippincott Williams & Wilkins.

Haynes, L., Boese, T., & Butcher, H. (2004). *Nursing in contemporary society. Issues, trends, and transition to practice.* Upper Saddle River, NJ: Pearson Prentice Hall.

Henderson, D. J. (1995). Consciousness-raising in participatory research: Method and methodology for emancipatory inquiry. *Advances in Nursing Science, 17*, 58–69.

Heron, J. (1992). *Feeling and personhood. Psychology in another key.* Newbury Park, CA: Sage.

Hilton, J. J. (2001). Polanyi's philosophy. A new look at a theoretical framework. *Nurse Educator, 27*(6), 249–250.

Ironside, P. (2005). Teaching thinking and reaching the limits of memorization: Enacting new pedagogies. *Journal of Nursing Education, 44*(10), 441–449.

Keating, S. B. (2006). Components of the curriculum. In S. B. Keating (Ed.), *Curriculum development and evaluation in nursing* (pp. 163–208). Philadelphia: Lippincott Williams & Wilkins.

King Mixon, D., Kemp, M. A., Towle, M. A., & Schrader, V. C. (2005). Negotiating the merger of three nursing programs into one: Turning mission impossible into mission possible. *Annual Review of Nursing Education, 3,* 187–203.

Kintgen-Andrews, J. (1988). Philosophy statements: Challenging beliefs and values. *Nursing and Health Care, 9*(8), 436–438.

Krathwohl, D. R. (2002). A revision of Bloom's taxonomy: An overview. *Theory into Practice, 41*(4), 212–218.

Lawrence, S. A., & Lawrence, R. M. (1983). Curriculum development: Philosophy, objectives, and conceptual framework. *Nursing Outlook, 3*(3), 160–163.

Mohammed, S. A. (2006). (Re)Examining health disparities: Critical social theory in pediatric nursing. *Journal for Specialists in Pediatric Nursing, 11,* 68–71.

Oermann, M. H., & Gaberson, K. B. (2006). *Evaluation and testing in nursing education* (2nd ed.). New York: Springer.

Oliva, P. F. (2005). *Developing the curriculum* (6th ed.). Boston: Pearson Education.

Petress, K. (2003). An educational philosophy guides the pedagogical process. *College Student Journal, 37*(1), 128–135.

Rentschler, D. D., & Spegman, A. M. (1996). Curriculum revolution. Realities of change. *Journal of Nursing Education, 35*(9), 389–393.

Taylor, K. L., & Care, D. W. (1999). Nursing education as cognitive apprenticeship. *Nurse Educator, 24*(4), 31–36.

Tong, R. (2007). Feminist thought in transition: Never a dull moment. *Social Science Journal, 44*(1), 23–39.

Torres, G., & Stanton, M. (1982). *Curriculum process in nursing.* Englewood Cliffs, NJ: Prentice-Hall.

Tyler, R. W. (1949). *Basic principles of curriculum and instruction.* Chicago: University of Chicago Press.

Uys, L. R., & Smit, J. H. (1994). Writing a philosophy of nursing. *Journal of Advanced Nursing, 20*(2), 239–244.

Vandeveer, M., & Norton, B. (2005). From teaching to learning. Theoretical foundations. In D. Billings & J. Halstead (Eds.), *Teaching in nursing: A guide for faculty* (2nd ed., pp. 231–281). St. Louis, MO: Elsevier Saunders.

Walton, J. C. (1996). The changing environment. New challenges for nursing education. *Journal of Nursing Education, 35*(9), 400–405.

White, B., & Brockett, R. (1987). Putting philosophy into practice. *Journal of Extension, 25*(2). Retrieved August 4, 2008, from http://joe.org/joe/1987summer/a3.html

Wiles, J., & Bondi, J. (1998). *Curriculum development. A guide to practice* (5th ed.). Upper Saddle River, NJ: Pearson Merrill Prentice Hall.

Wiles, J., & Bondi, J. (2007). *Curriculum development. A guide to practice* (7th ed.). Upper Saddle River, NJ: Pearson Merrill Prentice Hall.

Yorks, L., & Sharoff, L. (2001). An extended epistemology for fostering transformative learning in holistic nursing education. *Holistic Nursing Practice, 16*(1), 21–29.

Yura, H. (1974). Curriculum development process. In *Faculty curriculum development: Part 1: The process of curriculum development.* New York: National League for Nursing.

CHAPTER 9

Curriculum Design

Chapter Overview

In this chapter, information about curriculum design is presented first. Included are terminology, program type, structure, delivery, and models. General and health professional education designs, organizing strategies for nursing curricula, and patterns for nursing course sequencing follow. Then, the design process is described. Although presented in a linear fashion, curriculum design does not occur through a prescribed sequence, but rather through iterative discussion, generation of design ideas, and critique. Following a brief discussion of faculty development related to curriculum design and a chapter summary, two cases are presented. The first case is critiqued; the second is for analysis. Questions to determine curriculum design activities in individual settings conclude the chapter.

Chapter Goals

- Understand the process of curriculum design.
- Identify factors important in curriculum design decisions.
- Appreciate variations in curriculum design.

- Consider human and financial implications of curriculum design.
- Reflect on faculty development activities pertinent to curriculum design.

Curriculum Design

The term *curriculum design*, when used as a noun, refers to the configuration of the program of studies. It includes the courses selected, their sequencing, the relationships between and among courses, and associated curriculum policies.

The process of designing the curriculum, or the *curriculum design process*, refers to the discussions and decision making that lead to the configuration of the program of studies. This process can feel like the heart of curriculum development, and its outcome is the written curriculum plan. The completed design makes the future curriculum tangible. Curriculum developers experience a strong sense of accomplishment, ownership, and satisfaction when they are able to say, "This is our curriculum."

It may be helpful to clarify some of the terminology used when undertaking the design phase of curriculum development. Terms such as *design*, *structure*, and *model* are often used interchangeably in the nursing education literature. To add to the confusion, descriptors such as *block*, *integrated*, *2 + 2*, *accelerated*, and *collaborative* have been referred to as *designs*, *programs*, *structures*, *models*, or *patterns*. For conceptual clarity, the following interpretations are used in this book and are more fully described in subsequent sections.

A *program* can be described according to the following characteristics:

- Type: Educational level (i.e., doctoral, masters, baccalaureate, associate degree, diploma, or practical nurse)
- Structure: Arrangement as to program length and semester or quarter divisions
- Delivery: Means by which faculty offer the curriculum
- Model: Overall organization of the curriculum that typically describes the arrangement of nursing and nonnursing courses (e.g., articulated, generic, or upper-division nursing program).

These design elements affect the configuration of courses.

Program Type and Structure

The *program type*, or educational level, has a significant influence on the curriculum design, since the nature and number of courses will be linked to the expected outcomes for graduating students. The program type is evident in the curriculum outcome statements, which should be internalized by curriculum planners.

Program structure refers to the duration of the program and the arrangement of divisions within the academic year. The duration is usually a function of program type, although alternative program lengths can be considered, such as an accelerated baccalaureate program which can be 11 to 24 months in length (Ouellet & MacIntosh, 2007; Supplee & Glasgow, 2008). Once established, the program length is a boundary within which the curriculum must be designed. The division of the academic year into quarters, semesters, or terms is established by the educational institution. These divisions are the temporal units in which year (or level), semester, and course competencies must be achievable.

Program Delivery

Program delivery, another design element, refers to the method that the curriculum is offered to students. Traditionally, this has been through provision of courses at the educational institution that awards the academic credential. Now, however, programs are extended through flexible delivery and partnerships.

Traditional Delivery

The traditional approach for delivering nursing curricula has been face-to-face instruction, in which the teacher and students are physically present in the same classroom, lab, or clinical learning environment, at the same time, for a designated time period. This time- and place-dependent approach has evolved to include more flexible scheduling and delivery. For example, nursing classes can be scheduled on one day of the week, in the evenings, or on weekends to accommodate learners' work and family schedules. As well, faculty can travel to distant locations to offer classes for those unable to attend the credential-granting educational institution. Availability of faculty and suitable locations, as well as costs associated with time and travel, are some issues related to flexible, traditional delivery.

Distance Delivery

Distance delivery is a means to provide an educational offering when the education is physically separate from learners. Terms often used interchangeably to describe the educational process whereby learners and educators are physically separated or in different off-campus locations include *distance education, distance teaching, distance learning, open learning, distributed learning, asynchronous learning, telelearning,* and *flexible learning* (Picciano, 2001). The word *distance* is somewhat misleading as it implies a disconnection, albeit physical, among participants engaged in the educational endeavor. Yet, physical distance should not automatically evoke images of students and instructors who are detached from one another. Although course participants may be sprinkled around the globe, contemporary technology makes it possible for them to feel psychologically connected while actively and collectively sharing the learning experience.

Flexibility should be a core element of distance delivery and uptake of courses. Many variations are possible in the execution of distance courses, although they normally include the use of technology to connect learners with faculty and each other. Courses can be conceptualized and offered using a single technology, or several, to accommodate students' learning styles, life roles, and inability to be traditional on-campus learners. As well, courses can be paced or not paced. A paced course, typical in undergraduate and degree completion programs, is completed in a specified time period. Alternatively, if the course is not paced, students have more flexibility in timing. Course materials can be print based, computer based, video and audio recordings, or a combination of these and/or other technologies. The following are some examples of the commonly used flexible delivery methods.

Correspondence Courses Correspondence courses are offered and completed through the postal mail. Printed and/or audio course materials and assignments are mailed to learners, who then send completed assignments back to the course instructor for grading. Thus, these courses are independent of place: learners can be anywhere the postal mail can reach them. Hence, they can complete course work wherever they choose, indoors or outdoors. This approach has been popular for many years, and although students usually have regular contact with faculty by mail, phone, fax, or e-mail, they often lack the benefit of dialogue and ongoing interaction with faculty and peers.

Although correspondence courses as a sole method of delivery have become less prominent in North America, they continue to be important internationally. In Kenya, for instance, where technology is lacking or very costly, correspondence courses are important to upgrade nurses' credentials. Rural nurses generally lack computers and cannot leave their families and communities to enroll in programs offered through traditional delivery. As well, the universities cannot send faculty to small towns to provide courses on-site. Therefore, correspondence courses are the only way for nurses to continue their education (C. Mureithi, personal communication, December 1, 2006).

Broadcast Television Through satellite or local television networks, broadcast television provides synchronous (same time) delivery to learners in different locations. Transmission of course information flows primarily in one direction, from instructor to students. Learners can communicate with the instructor by mail, phone, fax, or e-mail. Although normally in their own homes, students could be at designated sites with others taking the same course. If physically together, they have the added benefit of interaction, perhaps with the help of a tutor.

In some Canadian provinces, credit courses are delivered through publicly funded television stations. The broadcasts are available to all television viewers, although only those who are formally enrolled and who complete course requirements, receive course credit.

Video Technologies Video technologies allow for the provision or transmission of visual images and sound. Both synchronous and asynchronous delivery is possible, depending on the technology being used. Asynchronous video technologies include video tapes and interactive video disks (Curran, 2006). If the necessary technology is available, there can be synchronous interaction between the originating site and one or more sites, or among several sites. The method requires all participants to be present at the same time at locations with video-conferencing facilities.

Audio Technologies Audio technologies involve voice transmission, and like video technologies, can be used for either synchronous or asynchronous learning. Teleconferencing, also referred to as *audio conferencing,* is a synchronous delivery method that engages participants in real time interaction. Many-to-many communication is possible (Curran, 2006); however, for this to occur, participants must be able to phone into the teleconferencing system at the same time. Place independence is possible in that participants can be anywhere there is a telephone. Audiotapes are used for asynchronous learning, typically in correspondence courses.

Web-Based Learning Platforms Learning platforms, such as Blackboard or WebCT provide a system for online teaching and learning, usually asynchronously. Students and teachers are connected in a shared learning space via the Internet. These platforms allow posting of course materials with links to other Web sites, creation of discussion groups, threaded discussion, assignment submission, e-mailing, tutorial sessions, posting and writing of examinations, grade management, and so forth. Written or verbal interactions constructed during discussions are stored on the host computer, and these can be reviewed by participants as needed. Other features can be added, such as a real-time virtual classroom where live lectures and demonstrations can occur (Cornelius & Smith Glasgow, 2007).

Voice tools make it possible to insert voice announcements, voice e-mail, real-time discussions, threaded voice discussions, and so forth into the learning platform. The use of a voice tool reduces the need for typing, and may make the learning process more comfortable for some. Voice discussion can be either synchronous or asynchronous. If synchronous, only one person can speak at one time, and participants' opportunities to speak are managed by a moderator. Built-in audio recording makes asynchronous discussion possible and allows preservation of synchronous dialogue. Elluminate and Skype are two examples of Web-based conferencing platforms that integrate multiple methods of communication such as two-way audio, text messaging, and a shared whiteboard.

Learning platforms allow for the range of activities and interactions that occur in a classroom. As such, they are used for both undergraduate and graduate courses, as well as for entire programs. The sophistication of the platforms, and the ease with which most students learn to navigate them, has transformed much of nursing education. RN-BSN, master's (Cornelius & Smith Glasgow, 2007), and doctoral nursing programs (Woodward Leners, Wilson, & Sitzman, 2007) are offered completely online.

Podcasts "A podcast is a media file that is distributed over the Internet for playback on personal computers . . . and portable media players" (Copley, 2007, p. 387). New files are automatically downloaded to subscribers. Lectures and supplementary materials can be delivered through audio and video podcasts to learners on and off campus. For on-campus students who attend regular lectures, a podcast is an example of e-learning (Guri-Rosenbitt, as cited in Copley). For off-campus learners, the podcast is a flexible delivery method.

Streaming Media   *Streaming video* is a sequence of moving images sent in compressed form over the Internet and displayed by the viewer as they arrive. *Streaming media* is both video and sound. Recipients do not have to wait to download the file before seeing the video or hearing the sound. Instead, the media is sent in a continuous stream and is played as it arrives. The user requires a media player, which is a special program that uncompresses and sends video data to the display and audio data to speakers (SearchUnifiedCommunications.com, 2005). Typically, the player is available from a software provider or downloaded from a Web site. The transmission and viewing can be synchronous, or the media file can be available on a server for learners to access when convenient.

Hybrid or Blended Approaches

Combining two or more delivery approaches is also possible in a curriculum or within individual courses. For example, podcasts can be used along with traditional courses (Copley, 2007). As well, computer-based discussions through a learning platform could be used to complement classroom and clinical courses, when additional interaction among participants is desired. This approach was used during a final 3-month integrative practicum when BScN students were located in healthcare agencies throughout a region. Through the computer-based conferencing, learners felt connected with one another, shared their experiences, supported one another, and learned (Babenko-Mould, Andrusyszyn, & Goldenberg, 2004).

Another example of an effective use of a hybrid approach to course offerings was in a graduate nursing leadership course. In addition to traditional classes in each of their countries, students and faculty from Canada and Norway connected to jointly address nursing leadership content through asynchronous computer conferencing and synchronous video conferencing (Iwasiw et al., 2000).

Delivery Through Partnerships

Partnerships are formal arrangements that exist between and among institutions. In the nursing education literature, the terms *partnership, collaboration, collaborative partnership,* and *consortia* are often used without sufficient definition or differentiation. They do, however, refer to formal or informal affiliations or alliances developed by educational institutions with service agencies for clinical or service-learning experiences, or to arrangements that exist between and among educational institutions for the purpose of providing nursing education.

Educational institution partnerships are formed when more than one institution offers all or part of the same program. These agreements require a high level of trust and cooperation. In collaborative partnerships and consortia with a common curriculum, negotiations and a willingness to let go of treasured aspects of individual programs are necessary to achieve the larger purpose of the partnership. Contractual arrangements typically specify the responsibilities of all parties in developing, approving, implementing, and evaluating the curriculum, as well as administrative arrangements, including financial provisions. Additionally, details about the curriculum design can be specified.

The nature of contractual arrangements can have a profound effect on curriculum design. Clauses about design (such as where, how, and which courses will be offered), as well as resource sharing and requirements about faculty credentials, could be written to ensure curriculum quality. Details such as course sequencing, or the provision of particular courses at specified sites, are sometimes seen as desirable to guarantee the role of partners. Yet, the more specific the curriculum detail in the signed agreements and the greater the number of institutions involved, the more difficult it can be to modify the curriculum as time passes. Curriculum revision or complete reconceptualization of the curriculum will require approval from all partners, and possibly new contracts. It is wise to minimize references to specific design details when agreements are first developed.

Three principal forms of partnerships exist between and among educational institutions. These are *fee-for-service*, *collaborative partnerships*, and *consortium* arrangements. There are no precise conceptual, functional, or quantitative demarcations between partnerships and consortia, so groupings of nursing programs use the term deemed most appropriate.

Fee-for-Service Partnership   In this arrangement, one institution purchases the courses of another. This is the least complex of the partnership agreements. Elements of the contract could include the nature of the course, number of students, delivery mode(s), and the fee, which may be based on enrollment numbers. The provider is unlikely to participate in the purchaser's curriculum development.

Collaborative Partnership   A collaborative partnership denotes a higher degree of involvement between (or among) educational institutions. The collaborating partners share in curriculum development, implementation, and evaluation. Each partnership determines matters such as:

- Admissions policies and procedures
- Flexibility within the agreed-upon curriculum in response to the local context
- Sharing of human and physical resources
- Decision making and approval processes
- Delivery modes.

A simple partnership could involve two partners that support the same goal. The more partners, the more intricate can be the contractual agreements between and among them.

In the Canadian province of Ontario, the universities and colleges of applied arts and technology (which had previously offered diploma, not degree, nursing programs) are collaboratively offering 4-year collaborative baccalaureate programs. Universities, which confer the degree, have one or more college partner(s), with each partnership having one common curriculum. The formal arrangements, in which nursing courses are offered in all 4 years, include the following:

- Two years at a college for all students, followed by 2 years at the university
- Enrollment in either the college or university for the first 2 years of the program, with all students enrolled at the university for the final 2 years
- Simultaneous enrollment in both the college and university, with all students taking courses at both sites throughout the 4 years
- Simultaneous delivery of the entire program at each of the university and college sites, with students being enrolled in only one site.

Consortium A consortium is a cooperative association of many partners formed to achieve common goals. It is an extended collaborative partnership. One example is the Collaboration for Academic Education in Nursing (CAEN), comprising nine partner schools of nursing in British Columbia and one in the Northwest Territories. Four of them grant degrees, six offer the entire curriculum, with the remaining three offering part of the curriculum (M. Chapman, personal communication, January 29, 2008). The original partnerships were formed in response to the baccalaureate entry-to-practice position of the Canadian Nurses Association, government initiatives to increase university accessibility, and healthcare reform. Over time, the number of partners and interinstitutional relationships have changed (Molzahn & Purkis, 2004). Each CAEN partner has an equal voice in administrative and curriculum decisions, with each institution's curriculum-approval processes being followed. Flexibility within the shared curriculum is possible so that each school can respond to local conditions (M. Chapman, personal communication, January 29, 2008).

Another example is the Oregon Consortium for Nursing Education (OCNE), a statewide consortium of nursing programs created to double the number of nursing graduates. This is "a voluntary coalition of associate degree (ADN) and public and private baccalaureate degree (BSN) programs" (Gubrud-Howe et al., 2003, p. 166). The common curriculum culminates in a BSN degree, although community college students will be able to receive an ADN credential and take the NCLEX-RN before BSN studies. The intent is to share faculty, laboratories, classrooms, and learning resources across nursing programs. There are common admission standards, a shared application process, and student transferability between schools (OCNE, 2006).

Advantages of Collaborative Partnerships and Consortia The advantages of collaborative partnerships and consortia lie in the optimal use of resources to develop and share curricula and resources across institutions (Molzahn & Purkis, 2004). In Canada, these partnerships and consortia increase access to baccalaureate degrees, mandatory for entry to practice (except the provinces of Quebec and Manitoba), and maintain a supply of new entrants to the profession. In the United States, they also increase access to baccalaureate degrees, expanding the capacity of students to gain this professional credential and advance the practice and profession of nursing. Faculty development about teaching and scholarship are possible across the partnership. Collaboration can lead to cohesion among nursing educators, who collectively, can influence government funding, educational policy, and nursing organizations.

Program Models

The program model is the overall organization of the curriculum. This organization can vary according to the arrangement and numbers of required nursing courses, required non-nursing (commonly called *support courses*), elective courses, and program length. All models are designed to facilitate students' achievement of the intended program outcomes. In essence, the model determines where particular courses (including clinical courses) can be placed in the curriculum. The name given to the model may include a reference to the program length. It is important not to confuse program model with *conceptual model* or *paradigm*.

One example of a model is a 4-year baccalaureate program, with an exit option to take licensure examinations after 3 years. In this model, courses deemed essential for RN practice must be included in the first 3 years. The fourth year includes courses necessary to meet institutional requirements for the nursing degree. In a 4-year generic, or basic program, nursing and non-nursing courses are given throughout the entire program, whereas in an upper-division program, nursing courses are offered after foundation courses in other disciplines. Integrated programs combine or blend concepts so that courses are connected in a meaningful way (Pennington, 1986). Articulated programs have a planned progression from a lower to a higher level of learning, for example, LPN to ADN, ADN to BSN or MSN. External degree models, for ADN or BSN study, are not centered on traditional patterns of institutional-based study. Rather, the focus is on the concept of providing credit on the basis of what one knows, not on how one has achieved it.

The program model is an important element of design. If a nursing program is being created in an institution where nursing did not formerly exist, then there is freedom to choose the program model. However, if there is a desire to change an existing model, considerable negotiation may be required, as there can be scheduling, faculty, and budgetary implications for the school of nursing and other departments.

Curriculum Designs in General and Health Professional Education

Curriculum design, as noted at the beginning of this chapter, refers to the configuration of the program of studies, including the courses selected, sequencing, the relationships between and among courses, and associated curriculum policies. Two typologies of curriculum design in general education are described, and designs for health professional curricula are presented.

Curriculum Designs in General Education

Selection and Organization of Content Five types of curriculum designs, all based on the selection and organization of content have been identified (Armstrong, 2003). Some can be recognized in nursing curricula. Most nursing curricula do not use only one design, but rather a combination of these approaches.

In an *academic subject design,* particular subjects are included in each or most years of the curriculum. This design pattern is represented by nursing courses such as Professional Nursing, which is often included more than once in a curriculum, with increasing complexity in competencies in subsequent courses.

Subjects are combined to form new content areas in a *fusion design.* Again, a Professional Nursing course would be an example. Knowledge from sociology, management, psychology, and gender studies is combined in a way that the originating disciplines are not readily identifiable.

Broad-fields designs seek a new unity that cuts across an entire branch of knowledge. An example in the school system is Social Studies, which combines economics, sociology, psychology, and history.

A *special topic design* is flexible. Content is drawn from several subjects to address important issues, problems, or areas of interest. As issues emerge, courses are developed, and then discontinued once they are no longer timely. In nursing curricula, courses about *international nursing* or *global health* were often introduced as elective offerings, and then altered to become a formal part of the curriculum once it became apparent that they were an enduring, rather than a special topic.

In *student-centered designs,* courses are provided in response to student interests. In nursing, giving choice about clinical placement sites is an example of student centeredness, as is the provision of electives in the curriculum.

Ordering or Construction of Knowledge Wiles and Bondi (2007) describe five patterns of constructing or ordering knowledge in a curriculum. All can be identified within nursing curricula.

In a *building blocks design,* a clearly defined body of knowledge or skills is organized into a pyramid arrangement. The base is made up of foundational knowledge, and the middle portion of the pyramid is composed of increasingly specialized material. The pinnacle contains in-depth, specialized knowledge. The sequence is prescribed and deviation is not allowed.

A *branching design* is a variation of the building blocks design. The endpoints of learning are known in advance. The curriculum starts with foundational knowledge and then there is some choice within prescribed areas beyond the common experiences.

In a *spiral design*, the same content area is repeatedly revisited at higher levels of complexity. There can be some flexibility, but this is likely limited.

With a *specific tasks or skills design*, content and experiences are intended to assist students to achieve specified competencies. There can be flexibility in the content and the ordering of content.

In a *process* design, there is a fluid organization of knowledge. The emphasis is on the process to be learned, and content is the medium through which specified processes are addressed.

Nursing curricula typically employ all five means of organizing or constructing knowledge. A *building blocks* approach is evident in a curriculum where students first encounter clients experiencing limited psychological stress and physiological alterations, then those with moderate levels of psychological and/or psychological problems, and finally, clients with complex health and social problems. Curricula with course choices (i.e., *branching*), would reflect a belief that there is more than one path to reach the outcomes. Many programs have a final practicum, and this experience provides an example of both *branching* and *spiraling*. A variety of placements for a practicum represents a *branching* design. Students who repeat a placement they have previously experienced are in a spiral situation: they are returning to the same practice area with more knowledge and experience. Plans for psychomotor skills learning in many curricula are reflective of a *specific tasks or skills* design.

Curriculum Designs in Health Professional Education

Traditionally, health professional courses have been unidisciplinary. Curricula were planned by members of one health professional discipline for students in that discipline. However, there is growing recognition that if learners are educated in isolation from one another, they likely will have difficulty collaborating in meaningful ways once they are practicing professionals. Therefore, there is increasing interest in the development of shared learning experiences during health professional education. Within higher education, interdisciplinary courses can be categorized according to the disciplinary focus of the content, or the members of the planning and teaching team. Moving beyond interdisciplinary courses are interprofessional courses.

Disciplinary Focus Lattuca (as cited in Lattuca, Voight, & Fath, 2004) has defined four types of interdisciplinary courses (*discipline* meaning academic discipline), according to the questions or issues that motivate the teaching:

- Informed disciplinarity: Instructors focus on one discipline and call on information from other disciplines to illustrate or illuminate course content.

- Synthetic disciplinarity: Instructors combine theories and concepts from different disciplines, with the contributing disciplines remaining identifiable.
- Transdisciplinarity: Instructors apply and test theories from several disciplines across disciplines so that they are no longer associated with the originating disciplines.
- Conceptual interdisciplinarity: Instructors include disciplinary perspectives, but the course has no compelling disciplinary focus.

Members of the Planning and Teaching Team   Courses that include students from more than one health professional program can be *multidisciplinary, interdisciplinary,* or *transdisciplinary.* The type of course depends on the extent to which faculty members from two or more health professions:

- Are committed to a shared vision that includes fostering collaborative interprofessional relationships
- Believe that some healthcare knowledge is not the domain of only one discipline
- Recognize and value the contributions of members from other health professions to health care
- Are involved in shared course development, delivery, and evaluation.

Dyer (2003) has summarized multi-, inter-, and transdisciplinary models.

A *multidisciplinary* model is one in which a single discipline-specific faculty member determines which additional disciplines should be involved in providing resources relevant for student learning. In this model, a specific course is taught by a faculty member from one discipline, while recognizing and helping all participating students achieve outcomes critical to their specific disciplines.

The *interdisciplinary* model requires greater collaboration and interdependence among team members from relevant disciplines. Members from the collaborating disciplines take responsibility for jointly planning, developing, and teaching portions of the course for which they are expert, to students from the participating disciplines.

A *transdisciplinary* model requires a greater degree of team sharing and collaboration. In course development and delivery, expertise from different disciplines is shared across these disciplines. Concepts and processes are integrated. Some boundary blurring occurs, as well as mutual trust and respect for discipline-specific expertise.

Interprofessional Education   Building on the ideas of conceptual interdisciplinarity and transdisciplinary education is *interprofessional education* (IPE). IPE is the provision of "occasions when members (or students) of two or more professions associated with health or social care engage in learning with, from, and about each other" (Freeth et al., as cited in Reeves, Goldman, & Oandasan, 2007, p. 231). The goal is to facilitate learners' development of attitudes, knowledge, skills, and behaviors that are expected to lead to successful collaboration and thus, increased patient safety, when they are practicing professionals. Effective strategies include learners from two or more disciplines engaging in problem-based learning, patient-focused case studies, or acquisition of clinical skills (Barnsteiner, Disch, Hall, Mayer, & Moore, 2007). As well, reflection on interactions and learning is an essential element of IPE. Although growing in popularity and intuitively appealing, the theoretical bases or frameworks for IPE have not been explicated and tested (Clark, 2006), and the evidence linking IPE to successful professional collaboration is not yet compelling.

Barnsteiner et al. (2007) propose six criteria for full engagement of IPE in an organization:

- Explicit and widely known organizational philosophy of IPE
- Shared development of learning experiences by faculty members from different professions
- Embedding of IPE as a required part of curricula
- Inclusion of integrated and experiential opportunities to learn teamwork and collaboration, and how these group skills relate to safe care delivery
- Requirement that all learners demonstrate competence in a single set of interprofessional competencies
- Presence of organizational infrastructure that fosters IPE.

Organizing Strategies for Nursing Curriculum Design

A *curriculum organizing strategy* is the structure or scaffolding upon which courses are built. It gives direction to the nature, choice, and placement of courses and learning experiences.

Nursing has always used an organizing strategy for curriculum design, beginning with Nightingale's statements about the environment. Since then, numerous organizing strategies have been developed. The one selected should:

- Correspond with the curriculum nucleus.
- Respond to the context of the program.
- Ensure opportunities for students to meet expected outcomes.
- Be logical and justifiable.
- Provide optimal usefulness and consistency.

Additionally, Boland (2005) emphasizes that the organizing strategy "must reflect the domain of nursing practice, the phenomena of concern to nurses, and how nurses relate to others who are dealing with health concerns" (p.168). Moreover, one criterion for the quality standard of curriculum and instruction used by the National League for Nursing Accrediting Commission (NLNAC) (2005) is that, "Curriculum developed by nursing faculty flows from the nursing education unit philosophy/mission through an organizing framework into a logical progression of course outcomes and learning activities to achieve desired program objectives/outcomes" (p. 15). Thus, the organizing framework must be explicitly attended to during curriculum development.

Traditional Organizing Strategies

Medical Model In the medical model of organizing nursing curricula, popular for more than half of the 1900s, content was organized according to the following components: disease (teaching by body system), knowledge (learning by parts and adding on), terms or vocabulary (precise definitions), concept of nurse (whose function is incidental and who "does things" to the patient and environment), and concept of patient (as a repository of disease and recipient of nursing care). In this organizing strategy, courses are ordered in specific sequences. The content to be learned and how it is to be learned are identified. Nursing courses and nursing skills are delineated first, then the required non-nursing courses, critical learning experiences, and evaluation methods to assess what students have learned.

The traditional hospital clinical areas (maternity, medicine, pediatrics, psychiatry, surgery) are the focus of learning, with the addition of a community experience. Advantages of this organizing strategy include the wide availability of nursing textbooks written according to the medical model, a good fit with hospital organization and faculty members' areas of expertise, and a match with popular perceptions of nursing. However, a risk is that nursing knowledge may not be given prominence in the curriculum.

The decline of the medical model as an organizing framework for nursing programs is evident in the results of a national US survey. Only 25% of diploma, associate degree, and baccalaureate nursing programs indicated use of the medical model, and this was the smallest percentage of all organizing or conceptual frameworks reported (McEwan & Brown, 2002).

Simple-to-Complex In a simple-to-complex organizing strategy, another traditional approach, knowledge is organized so that learning occurs sequentially. Students learn progressively more about a specific concept or process over time. For example, the curriculum might first address nursing care of individuals, then families, then aggregate groups. The advantage rests with the innate logic of incremental learning: students are expected to be responsive first to one person, then to a small group, and then to a community. However, this organization does not reflect the reality of nursing practice, since nurses typically respond to families along with individuals, to individuals within families and groups, and to both individuals and small groups within aggregates.

Stages of Illness Health and its meaning are considered first when employing stages of illness as the organizing strategy. Content addressing acute-care nursing is followed by content about rehabilitative, and then chronic-care nursing. Normal life processes such as pregnancy and aging do not fit easily into this approach, nor does health promotion of families and groups. Nonetheless, this strategy can encompass both institutional and community-based practice.

Contemporary Organizing Strategies

Nursing Conceptual Framework, Model, or Theory The curriculum can be organized according to one nursing conceptual framework, model, or theory, for example Orem's theory of self-care, Leininger's cultural care, or Watson's human science, human care. These can be employed individually. Each conceptual framework, model, or theory offers a somewhat different perspective of nursing with its own accompanying vocabulary. With this organizing strategy, the concepts and components of the selected theory or practice framework are predominant in all courses and experiences. The nursing focus is foremost in the curriculum and directs learners to view theory and practice with a specific perspective. However, a single nursing conceptual framework, model, or theory may not reflect the views of all faculty and students, and may not easily fit all nursing practice contexts. Also, the language and critical concepts may be too abstract for some learners. Finally, textbooks and other references are not likely to be organized according to the chosen perspective.

Multiple or eclectic nursing conceptual (or theoretical) frameworks can also be adopted. Curriculum designers select concepts and definitions that best fit their values and beliefs about nursing. Several conceptual frameworks, models, or theories within the curriculum (pluralism), might be used, with different ones being given prominence in different courses. Combining parts of two or more theories (eclecticism) is also possible. This would combine what is best understood from several nursing frameworks, models or theories. Adaptation of elements from multiple perspectives could generate creative curriculum designs. Pluralism or eclecticism might be less constraining than reliance on only one. Nevertheless, a multiple approach could jeopardize the body of knowledge from one model, or take away from that which is uniquely nursing. Distortion of original concepts, definitions, characteristics, and attributes of one or more of the original models or theories might result.

Outcomes An outcomes approach is another organizing strategy. These outcomes, which could form components of the design, could include critical thinking, collaborative skills, shared decision making, analyses, and interventions at individual, family, aggregate, and systems levels (Boland, 2005). Candela and Benzel-Lindley (2006) view the outcomes as the basis for designing the curriculum, as does Glennon (2006).

If curriculum developers are concerned with outcomes or end-stages, this might suggest that the curriculum design proceed from this point first. In this way, curriculum designers would initially identify the outcomes students should demonstrate, and accordingly shape the concepts embedded in the outcomes and competencies. For example, if health promotion, critical thinking, collaborative skills, and shared decision making are necessary outcomes, these concepts or competencies will form components of the curriculum. Curriculum developers would first identify essential qualities of graduates, then identify competencies or competency statements for each year or level of the program necessary to attain the outcomes (which also become the evaluation criteria). Curriculum developers would then determine the antecedents or factors necessary for achieving the competencies, the learning experiences, teaching methods, learning resources, and assessment strategies (Boland, 1998; 2005).

Dalley, Candela, and Benzel-Lindley (2008) have also proposed developing curriculum outcomes as the starting point of curriculum design. They then suggest that faculty list all the possible content, concepts, and abilities pertinent to their teaching area, and then categorize items from that list:

- Foundational content, concepts, and abilities that should be mastered in early nursing courses and be evident in all subsequent courses
- Specialty concepts and abilities associated with specialized areas of nursing practice
- Content that learners can discover for themselves.

Once this is completed, all faculty make decisions about leveling and placement of content based on the outcomes.

Other Theories, Concepts, and Philosophies   Theories, concepts, and philosophies, which influence the development of the curriculum philosophical approaches, could also be the basis of the curriculum design. For example, views related to theories of knowledge development, domains of practice, feminism, or existentialism, singly or in combination, can be used to organize the curriculum or parts of the curriculum.

Giddens and Brady (2007) advocate the use of concepts to organize the nursing curriculum and to be the foci of courses. Among concepts suggested for inclusion throughout the curriculum are *family strengths* (Sittner, Hudson, & Defrain, 2007), *holistic comfort* (Goodwin, Sener, & Steiner, 2007), and *global health* (Hodson Carlton, Ryan, Nagia, & Kelsy, 2007). An example of an organizing concept suggested for a particular course is *social justice* for a professional nursing course (Boutain, 2005).

The many ideas about concepts to incorporate into a curriculum, or the use of different concepts to be the focus of different courses, highlights that one conceptual framework is probably not suitable for all situations. The abundance of these concepts and course frameworks indicates that nurse educators accept pluralism as a sound basis for curriculum development, and that curricula are evolving as new ideas are proposed within nursing and other disciplines. If pluralism is the basis of curriculum design, the frameworks must be consistent with the philosophical approaches and with each other.

In the Model of Context-Relevant Curriculum Development in nursing education, illustrated in Chapter 1, the core curriculum concepts are derived from the contextual data and the philosophical approaches. Therefore, these concepts are relevant to the context, aligned with curriculum developers' beliefs, and logically consistent.

The core concepts provide the organizing framework of the curriculum. These core concepts and subconcepts must be carefully defined so there is a common understanding by curriculum developers, and subsequently by students.

Course Sequencing Patterns

Within the organizing strategy used to design the curriculum, courses can be sequenced in block, concurrent, mixed, or immersion-residency patterns. A block pattern specifies theory and clinical courses in sequence, each separate from the other and becoming the foundation for those that follow. In a concurrent pattern, theory and clinical courses are scheduled simultaneously throughout the curriculum.

A mixed pattern is also possible, with different parts of the curriculum having different patterns. A program with concurrent theory and practice, followed by a concentrated clinical practicum without formal classes, is an example of a mixed pattern for course sequencing.

A new pattern is the *immersion-residency* pattern, developed by the University of Delaware School of Nursing. Students have nursing theory courses in the first 3 years of the curriculum, with clinical experiences reserved for a full-year immersion residency in the final year of the program (Diefenbeck, Plowfield, & Herman, 2006).

Curriculum Design Process: Creating a Context-Relevant Nursing Curriculum

Creating a curriculum design involves many processes. These include confirming the goal of the design process; defining curriculum parameters; deliberating about delivery approaches, program models, organizing strategies, and course sequencing; identifying courses; and attending to program policies and resources. Iterative discussions lead to the generation of design proposals, critique, and decision making. There is no formula for curriculum design, such that a particular model and organizing strategy results in a predetermined design. Each design team establishes procedures, and through use of creative and logical thinking, produces a design relevant for its own context. Invariably, the design group's work will be characterized by ongoing deliberation and negotiation.

Concurrent with the curriculum design process is creation of a plan for curriculum evaluation. This important and often overlooked aspect of curriculum development is described fully in Chapter 12.

Confirming the Goal of the Curriculum Design Process

Nurse educators strive to develop curricula that will build students' professional knowledge and skills so that graduates will practice nursing competently in a changing healthcare environment, thereby contributing to the health and quality of life of those they serve. It is valuable to clarify the goal of the curriculum design process, since members of the development team may have varying expectations. The goal is to design a curriculum that is:

- Context-relevant
- Congruent with the philosophical approaches and principal teaching-learning approaches chosen for the curriculum
- Allows for the continuous and evident presence of the core curriculum concepts and key professional abilities
- Provides opportunities for learners to achieve the curriculum outcomes
- Feasible within the context in which the curriculum will be offered
- Meets requirements for approval and accreditation
- Supported by stakeholders and the educational institution

Defining Curriculum Parameters

Attention to curriculum design (i.e., the configuration of the program of studies) cannot occur in isolation from the context in which the curriculum will be offered. The context and previous curriculum decisions determine the *curriculum parameters,* that is, *the limits within which the curriculum must be designed and operationalized.*

Many curriculum parameters will have been identified during collection and analysis of the contextual data, although they might not have been labeled in this way. A review of contextual data can highlight relevant information that curriculum designers must keep in mind. Internal contextual data include information about faculty numbers, infrastructure, institutional policies, partnerships, as well as the ability of other departments to mount new courses. Critical data from the external context includes the types of health services available in the community, and standards for state or provincial approval and national accreditation.

In addition to contextual limitations, the design is affected by all curriculum decisions made to date. These decisions give direction to the design, while also requiring curriculum developers to limit themselves to ideas that are congruent with the curriculum nucleus, that is, philosophical approaches, core curriculum concepts, key professional abilities, and principal teaching-learning approaches. The curriculum nucleus makes some designs possible, while ruling out others.

A review of contextual data and analysis of the data can highlight relevant information that curriculum designers must keep in mind. As well, a return to the nucleus will refresh developers about the essence of the curriculum. It is important for curriculum designers to be clear about the parameters that affect the design, so that a realistic, feasible, and logical curriculum can be created.

Facilitating the Design Process

Designing the curriculum, which requires time and considerable intellectual effort, can be facilitated by reviewing current literature, visiting other schools, consulting with colleagues regionally and nationally, and attending nursing education conferences. Surveys of catalogues of highly rated schools (particularly those using similar philosophical approaches), with attention to program designs, could prove beneficial and move the process forward.

To solicit input, the design team could develop a template and ask stakeholders to respond to the designated elements. Following formulation of statements about the philosophical approaches, core curriculum concepts, and curriculum outcomes, the template could include space for year outcomes, semester outcomes, possible courses, credit allocations, sequencing, clinical experiences, and other items deemed relevant. The collation of this information can provide a basis for curriculum design. As well, assistance from an expert in curriculum design could be profitable to provide ideas about possible designs.

A two-dimensional grid or matrix is another way to facilitate the design process (Heinrich, Karner, Gaglione, & Lambert, 2002). The grid, with pertinent horizontal and vertical headings, can be useful to illustrate the emerging curriculum. The matrix would indicate such items as:

- Development of concepts across the curriculum
- Interrelationships among concepts
- Outcome and content links between and among courses
- Gaps and redundancies in the knowledge base, experiences, or skills.

The matrix serves as a visual depiction of the developing curriculum, indicating the plan for continuity and increasing depth of concepts. It is a recording of prominent ideas for each nursing course and the basis for detailed course and evaluation planning. Once finalized, the matrix becomes a blueprint against which the operationalized curriculum can be compared and assessed. See Table 9-1 for a simplified example of a matrix.

Table 9-1 Example of Matrix Showing Core Curriculum Concepts in Courses

Nursing Courses	Core Curriculum Concepts				
	Health Promotion	Empowerment	Interpersonal Relationships	Caring	Social Justice
Theoretical Foundations of Professional Nursing	Introduction of concept in health and illness	Introduction of concept and its value in nursing practice	Professional boundaries; self-awareness and reflection; active listening; responding to requests	Caring in social and family relationships vs caring in professional relationships	Introduction of concept; application to client situations
Personal Empowerment for Professional Nursing		Strategies for self, colleagues, and the profession	Assertiveness; conflict resolution, advocacy	For self and colleagues	Power relationships in nursing practice
Empowering Individuals through Health Promotion	Health and health promotion in illness situations	Supporting client decision-making	Collaboration with clients, nurses, and other health professionals; advocacy with/for clients	Evidence-based nursing interventions; client choice vs system demands	Social (in)justices in institution-based care
Knowledge Development: Empowerment of the Profession	Purposes of nursing research; relation to health	Knowledge & power; types of knowledge and evidence; creation, critique, and dissemination	Researcher-participant interaction	Research ethics	Types of studies funded
Health Promotion of Expanding Families	Knowledge related to health in pregnancy, labor and delivery, fetal and infant development; family relationships; nursing interventions in response to family needs	Empowerment of clients through provision of information, referral to resources; support of decision-making	Helping relationships during normal life events and during stressful periods	As expressed through health promotion and the provision of appropriate interventions during labor, delivery, post-partal period; care for partner and other family members	Examination of disparities in services for various groups

Deliberating about Curriculum Design

It can be worthwhile to review the curriculum work done to date to rekindle agreed-upon perspectives. As in all aspects of curriculum development, similarities should be capitalized upon, previous decisions recalled, and differences negotiated. A review of the analysis of the contextual data will refresh members about previously proposed design ideas.

Deliberations about curriculum design encompass integrative discussion about all aspects of design as well as focused discussion about the specific components of design. If diagrammed, discussion would resemble many overlapping and repeated zig-zags among the design components, not a segmented, linear progression of ideas. The dialogue could address the following questions:

- How can the philosophical approaches be operationalized?
- How can the core curriculum concepts be addressed throughout the curriculum?
- How can the curriculum be designed so students will have opportunities to achieve the key professional abilities and the curriculum outcomes?
- What design ideas stem from the principal teaching-learning approaches to which we have agreed?
- Which ideas from our analysis of the contextual data do we want to discuss in detail?
- Will flexible delivery, on-campus classes, or a combination be used?
- If we have a choice about the program model, what is our preference? Why?
- What could be the overall organizing strategy for the design?
- Which pattern for sequencing learning experiences matches our beliefs about learning?
- What are the learning experiences (theory and practice) that students require to achieve curriculum outcomes?
- Which are the necessary nursing and non-nursing courses?
- If we support the idea of shared education for health professional students, do we prefer multidisciplinary, interdisciplinary, or transdisciplinary, or interprofessional experiences?
- Which courses could be optional for students?
- What configurations of courses are possible to maximize learning?
- What is the rationale for the delivery approach, model, organizing strategy, and configuration chosen?
- What academic policies should be considered as part of the design?

Some design components are addressed in detail below. Notably, these include selecting delivery approaches, a program model, an organizing strategy, and course-sequencing pattern.

Selecting a Delivery Approach   Decisions about delivery (traditional or flexible) form an important part of the overall discussion, if this has not already been defined as a parameter. Referring to contextual data about faculty, institutional support for flexible delivery, and available infrastructure, designers might question:

- Is the use of only one delivery approach congruent with philosophical approaches and curriculum outcomes, or should a combination be used?
- Which modalities would best suit the nature of the curriculum?
- What resources would faculty require?
- What resources will learners require for flexible delivery (e.g., personal computers, access to video-conferencing facilities)?
- How might delivery approaches affect the configuration of courses?

Selecting a Program Model   When curriculum designers have the option of creating a new program model, their deliberations are strongly guided by beliefs about learning. They can ask themselves:

- Which arrangement of nursing and non-nursing courses best match the philosophical approaches, curriculum outcomes, and principal teaching-learning approaches?
- Which arrangements can be ruled out?
- Which model will be feasible and acceptable to students, faculty, and the educational institution?

Selecting an Organizing Strategy and a Course-Sequencing Pattern   The choice of an organizing strategy will depend on the philosophical approaches previously determined for the curriculum and the core curriculum concepts identified from the analysis of the contextual data. Stakeholders working on design might ask themselves questions such as:

- What are appropriate criteria for choosing an organizing strategy and sequencing pattern?
- Which organizing strategies can be ruled out?
- Which organizing strategies might fit with the philosophical approaches and beliefs about teaching and learning?
- Do faculty support one theory of nursing, pluralism, or eclecticism?
- Is there a natural fit with core curriculum concepts and one of the organizing strategies?
- Can some of the organizing strategies be combined in a meaningful way?
- Should a block, concurrent, mixed, or immersion-residency pattern of course sequencing be used?

These, and other points of discussion, will occur in a recursive fashion, leading to a conclusion about an organizing strategy and sequencing pattern. Like other aspects of curriculum development, ideas are proposed and, following exploration, debate, and review of previous decisions, modifications are made and new ideas added.

Identifying Courses

Discussion about courses to include in the curriculum requires attention to many ideas concurrently. The scope and depth (i.e., what is to be learned), the sequence (order of the units), and continuity (logical relationship or progression from one unit to another) are significant concerns for curriculum designers. The balance between process and content can be a source of much deliberation, possibly reflecting differing values in the group.

Identifying appropriate courses begins with an examination of the curriculum outcomes, followed by discussion about prerequisite knowledge and experiences (Boland, 2005; Friesner, 1978; Gagné, Briggs, & Wager, 1992; Taba, 1962). Recognition of courses that are not suitable occurs as part of the discussion and helps to define which ideas are relevant. The prerequisite knowledge and experiences form the basis of nursing and non-nursing courses.

Typically, the curriculum outcomes are those for the graduating year or final semester of the program. Working backward from these, level (year) or semester competencies are identified and then analyzed to derive competencies for the nursing courses. In this way, the link between individual units of learning (courses) and the curriculum outcomes are evident. An example of leveling of one curriculum outcome statement for a 4-year, baccalaureate-nursing program is given in Table 9-2. Further refinement is required for individual courses.

Table 9-2 Example of Leveling One Curriculum Outcome in a Four-Year Baccalaureate Curriculum

Curriculum and Year 4 Outcome	Incorporate best evidence; respect for the diversity and culture of individuals, families, and communities; and nursing practice standards in written reports of nursing care
Year 3 Competencies	1. Synthesize evidence for one aspect of nursing practice in a scholarly paper
	2. Integrate concepts of cultural sensitivity and nursing standards in weekly reflective journal entries about own nursing practice
Year 2 Competencies	1. Incorporate clients' cultural perspectives in written summaries of health promotion activities
	2. Integrate evidence for nursing interventions in clinical presentations
Year 1 Competencies	1. Integrate evidence for nursing interventions in written care plans
	2. Incorporate theory about interpersonal communication in clinical presentations about clients and nursing care

This approach forms part of the Model of Context-Relevant Curriculum Development in nursing education. The curriculum outcomes encompass the key professional abilities and the core curriculum concepts. Therefore, during the delineation of prerequisite professional abilities and subconcepts, the interrelationships among the professional abilities, and among the concepts, is revealed. Ultimately, this process results in a logical progression from the learning expectations and experiences in the first courses to those in subsequent courses, and to the expected curriculum outcomes.

Nursing Courses Nursing courses are typically defined first. The interface between level and semester competencies and the organization of identified concepts gives rise to decisions about the nature, number, and configuration of nursing courses. These decisions rest upon the program model, structure, organizing strategy, course sequencing pattern, and all previous decisions about the curriculum.

A review of the curriculum nucleus provides a strong basis for planning. As well, this is the time to examine all the curriculum possibilities that were proposed when contextual data were analyzed (see Chapter 7). Among the possibilities may be ideas for courses, or several possibilities might be combined to form a course. The value of the time spent in analyzing the contextual data and brainstorming about curriculum possibilities becomes readily apparent when nursing courses are being defined.

When thinking about nursing courses, curriculum designers should consider whether courses in other disciplines or with other health science disciplines, would be suitable instead of developing their own course. The following questions could shape the discussion:

- Which of the curriculum possibilities that were proposed during the analysis of the contextual data fit best with the curriculum nucleus?
- Are there curriculum possibilities that logically combine to form meaningful courses?
- Which ideas about curriculum possibilities should be further developed?
- How can core curriculum concepts be integrated with increasing depth throughout the curriculum?
- How could concepts be grouped into courses?
- How many nursing courses are possible within the program structure?
- Which nursing courses could be included?
- How will the overall focus of each course contribute to curriculum outcomes?
- What could be the competencies for the proposed courses?
- What is a reasonable sequence for these courses?

In defining the general substance of each course, curriculum designers may struggle with the tension between essential knowledge for nursing and adherence to the curriculum nucleus and curriculum outcomes. If committed to a teaching-learning approach that includes interpretative pedagogies, "The challenge for nurse educators is to ... overcome the focus on covering content at the expense of engaging students in thinking" (Ironside, 2004, p. 6), and to recognize that lectures are not the best way to introduce learners to content (Ironside, 2005). This challenge exists when first describing each course and later when planning and implementing courses.

Although course details will be defined later, at this time it is important to be clear about the general focus of each course. Brief course descriptions and possible competencies should be drafted. These will give members of the curriculum development team an understanding of the intent of all nursing courses.

The titles of nursing courses merit attention. Generic titles, such as Nursing Care of Adults or Clinical Practicum, do not provide information about the important ideas or professional abilities that will be addressed. Rather, nursing course titles should match the curriculum nucleus. This nomenclature conveys the intellectual dimension of nursing, and gives both conceptual and visual unity to the curriculum.

Non-nursing Courses   Consideration is given to non-nursing courses that contribute to students' knowledge and understanding of nursing. Formerly called *support courses*, the term preferred in this book is *non-nursing courses* because they are an integral part of the nursing curriculum. They do not merely support the curriculum; they are a significant part of the curriculum.

Substantive knowledge from liberal arts and psychosocial and health sciences is essential to the development of open-minded, educated, and informed practitioners. Students' interaction with an array of concepts, processes, and worldviews expands the depth and scope of their learning, and helps them to think critically from a broader, more comprehensive knowledge base.

Consideration is given to which required non-nursing courses to include, prerequisites, and the number of electives. Modification of existing non-nursing courses, or development of new ones, could be discussed. These ideas would require negotiation with the departments offering the courses. Conclusions about non-nursing courses are reached through discussion about their nature, contribution to students' achievement of curriculum outcomes, and fit in the curriculum.

Multidisciplinary, Interdisciplinary, Transdisciplinary, and Interprofessional Courses
Courses shared across health science disciplines can form part of the curriculum as elective or required classroom or clinical courses. Because it is important for nursing students to respect the goals and perspectives of other disciplines, and to learn to work collaboratively with members of many health disciplines, they should be provided with opportunities to learn and interact in varied disciplinary teams and practice settings. Faculty committed to interdisciplinary and interprofessional education and practice should design and schedule courses in concert

with faculty from other disciplines, bearing in mind each discipline's curriculum outcomes, philosophies, and roles. Intellectual cross-pollination among students should be a constant feature of courses through discussion, projects, and shared clinical learning.

A decision to include interprofessional experiences in the curriculum requires attention to operational and logistical matters such as:

- Identifying faculty from other disciplines committed to interprofessional education, or at least willing to learn about and test such courses
- Developing a shared vision and philosophy (Barnsteiner et al., 2007)
- Agreeing when interprofessional education best belongs in the curricula of all disciplines: before or after learners' socialization to their own professions
- Agreeing about the nature, goals, and processes of the courses
- Interpreting shared clinical experiences to agencies
- Developing expert facilitators
- Ensuring ongoing facilitator development and support (Reeves et al., 2007)
- Scheduling
- Building enthusiasm for the endeavor in the organization and among students and clinicians.

Elective Courses   Elective or optional courses, both within and outside of nursing, can be a valuable component of the curriculum design. The purpose of elective courses is to provide students opportunities to meet personal learning outcomes and freedom to explore interests in nursing and other disciplines. The design team may require electives at a specific academic level or from particular disciplines. Conversely, faculty may believe that learners should choose elective courses freely, without constraint. These decisions will hinge on the institutional mission, as well as the philosophical approaches and intended outcomes of the nursing curriculum.

Determining Policies and Guidelines

Developing new policies, or modifying existing ones, is part of the curriculum design process. A policy is a firm course of action that must be adhered to in every situation (e.g., appeals policy). The function of policies is to support and guide the achievement of the program and institutional mission and outcomes (Applegate, 1998). When devising policies, curriculum designers should differentiate between policies and less formal guidelines for action. Guidelines, or guiding principles, present an appropriate course of action for a specific situation, although there may be some context-dependent flexibility (e.g., dress code).

Some policies will be in place within the educational institution and apply to all academic constituencies, while others will be discipline-specific. The latter must be consistent with those of the larger institution, as well as with philosophical approaches of the curriculum. Policies must be readily available to all members of the academic community so that the 'rules' are known. The number and nature of policies will vary among nursing programs. Nevertheless, there are some fundamental matters about which policies will be evident in all programs. The following are examples:

- Admissions and progressions: Admissions policies state the criteria used to determine whether an applicant meets admission standards. Progressions policies address advancement in the program, specifically the requirements to progress to subsequent semesters or levels. These normally include statements about passing grades for classroom and clinical courses, required grade point average, and whether failing courses can be repeated.
- Academic rights and responsibilities: Academic rights and responsibilities include, among others, an appeals policy and a code of student conduct. An appeal is a formal request by a student to have an academic decision about a grade or adherence to a policy reviewed and changed. Normally, the institution will have a formal process for students and faculty to follow. A code of student conduct outlines what is viewed as acceptable behavior in the institution and may be an example of a policy with more flexibility than an admission policy.

Other policies and guidelines can be formulated specifically for the nursing program, such as attendance (clinical, laboratories, and/or class), definition and consequences of unsafe clinical practice, immunization, language proficiency standards, and dress code. Additional institutional policies can include those related to transfer from other institutions (Purcell, 2006), student involvement in institutional governance, scholastic discipline, student support, enrollment status, graduation requirements, non-discrimination, and human rights.

Considering Human and Financial Implications

Each curriculum has human and financial implications, and therefore, the curriculum leader should keep the dean/director informed of the emerging design. A successful design depends on the availability of adequate resources for implementation, and the dean/director is in the best position to know if those resources will be present.

If, for example, the new curriculum includes more nursing courses than previously, or more clinical practice time, there will be increased teaching costs. If financial resources in the school cannot support the proposed design, then the dean/director knows how and with whom to negotiate for additional funding. Modifications to the design will be necessary if adequate financial resources are not forthcoming.

Alternately, a curriculum redesign may mean that some faculty will no longer be required. A change from supervised clinical experience to more independent practice, for example, could result in reduced numbers of clinical faculty. The dean/director may need to inform long-standing, part-time clinical faculty that their employment will be decreased in amount or cease entirely. Concomitant with decreased faculty costs could be a decreased budget for the school. If so, strategic planning will be necessary to at least retain the school's budget.

A reconceptualized curriculum design might mean significantly changed teaching assignments for some faculty. Again, the dean/director should be fully apprised of the emerging design so that teaching assignments and faculty development can be planned.

Possible financial implications for students should be taken into account when designing a curriculum. An increased reliance on flexible delivery could make it possible for geographically dispersed learners to enroll in the nursing program. Yet, if those students must then travel a considerable distance for dispersed clinical experience, the associated costs could preclude their enrollment. Similarly, on-campus students may find travel to new practice sites difficult. It is important that the anticipated costs to learners be considered and that accurate information be provided to prospective applicants.

Deciding on the Design

When deciding on a curriculum design, developers should probably construct several designs, with different configurations of courses, and judge the advantages and disadvantages of each. Ultimately, one design will be proposed and this should be optimally useful, responsive to current and future social contexts, flexible enough to allow for ongoing refinement, and congruent with the curriculum nucleus.

Like other aspects of curriculum development, the design subcommittee's work must be reviewed and approved by the total faculty group. The subcommittee presents the level or semester competencies, configuration of courses, draft course competencies, and brief course descriptions to the total faculty group. Inclusion of the matrix or template can facilitate the group's understanding. Ultimately, the total faculty group should ask:

- Does the design represent a context-relevant curriculum?
- Is the design congruent with the philosophical approaches and principal teaching-learning approaches?
- Will the design allow for the continuous and evident presence of the core curriculum concepts and key professional abilities?

- Are there opportunities for students to achieve the intended curriculum outcomes?
- Is the design supported by stakeholders?
- Is the design feasible within our school of nursing and the external context?
- Does the design support the institutional mission?
- Is anything missing?
- Can faculty and other stakeholders commit to this curriculum?

Summary of Curriculum Design Process

The complex process of curriculum design cannot be accurately described in a formulaic manner. Faculty must be cognizant of the parameters in which the curriculum will be operationalized so their efforts are directed toward the creation of a curriculum that will be supported by the school, educational institution, and the community. The curriculum nucleus and curriculum outcomes, as well as other parameters (such as the program structure, partnership, commitments about delivery approaches) affect all deliberations and decisions. Determinations about the organizing strategy, program model, courses and their sequencing, and so forth, must be philosophically and logically consistent with the curriculum nucleus and outcomes. Discussion is iterative and integrative, with ideas about curriculum design emerging for critique, negotiation, development, and action.

Faculty Development

The overall goal of faculty development in relation to curriculum design is to expand members' knowledge and appreciation of curriculum design. As with all aspects of faculty development, the precise activities will be dependent on faculty needs.

Faculty development can include a brief review of the goal of the curriculum design process and the parameters that constrain it. Then, attention can be given to the process of curriculum design, and possible configurations of courses that could be congruent with the philosophical approaches and curriculum outcomes. In a workshop setting, a template might be introduced for small groups to complete. The completed templates could be given to the design team for consideration. In this way, the faculty development activity contributes directly to the design process.

An additional activity would be to introduce a curriculum matrix, with course names and concepts identified. Workshop participants could complete the matrix, which would help them understand the interrelatedness of concepts and design possibilities. Those members with expertise in curriculum development can readily facilitate these activities.

Chapter Summary

The curriculum design is the configuration of the program of studies. The design must be congruent with the institution and school's mission and purpose, and with the faculty's values and beliefs. It should be directed and oriented to student learning, and it should reflect the curriculum nucleus, outcomes, and context of nursing. Curriculum developers should have a clear sense of purpose and commitment to completing the task of design. Because of human and financial implications, the dean/director must be apprised of the emerging design.

The chapter includes descriptions of elements important in curriculum design such as partnerships, delivery approaches, curriculum models, organizing strategies, and patterns for course sequencing. The process of designing curricula is detailed, beginning with confirming the goal; identifying curriculum parameters; selecting delivery approaches, program model, and organizing strategies; and identifying courses. Policy development is addressed, as are human and financial implications of curriculum design.

✦Synthesis
Activities

Below are two case studies. First is Eastern Harbor University followed by a critique. Discuss the case and its analysis, considering additional ideas that arise. The second is McLanahan University with questions to guide examination. Questions to assist the curriculum design process in individual settings conclude the chapter.

Eastern Harbor University

Eastern Harbor is a large public university on the Atlantic Coast. The school of nursing has a history of research collaboration with the schools of medicine and social work. More recently, research collaborations have developed with the school of occupational therapy. The school of nursing is undergoing curriculum redesign, and during the data-gathering phase, faculty members took note of interprofessional courses in some nursing curricula. They investigated interprofessional education and the reasons for its development more thoroughly.

The total faculty group agreed that interprofessional collaboration should be one of the key professional abilities in the curriculum nucleus, in response to concerns about patient safety. They asked the chair of the curriculum committee, Dr. Adhiambo Kalume, to initiate discussions about interprofessional education with members of the other health professional schools. The faculty group agreed that they should first know if there is a willingness among the other disciplines to develop interprofessional education before they proceed with curriculum design. The champions of interprofessional education began to discuss where these courses would best be placed in the nursing curriculum.

The representatives of the other professional schools agreed that planning interprofessional education could be a valuable initiative and that short courses, possibly for credit as electives, could be developed over time. The idea of required interprofessional education in the curricula of all the health professional schools was seen as premature without first piloting a course and garnering widespread support. The school representatives agreed to convene a meeting of faculty members interested in learning more about interprofessional education, with the expectation that possible course foci could emerge. Dr. Kalume believed that if the first course was a success, the initiative would grow.

Dr. Kalume reported back to the nursing faculty, and they realized that they cannot include required interprofessional courses in the nursing curriculum. However, they agreed that as they proceeded with curriculum design, they would make provision for elective courses, which could include an interprofessional course once it is developed.

Critique

The nursing faculty has agreed that interprofessional collaboration is a key professional ability. This professional ability responds directly to concerns about patient safety and is aligned with current trends in health professional education. As such, this aspect of the curriculum nucleus is context-relevant.

Although the enthusiasm may be understandable, discussion about the placement of interprofessional courses in the nursing curriculum does not take into account an important parameter of curriculum design, the availability of desired courses. As well, consideration of the placement of particular courses before further deliberations about the complete design is an indication that there may not be full understanding of the requirement for the total curriculum to "hang together" in a unified, logical manner. It is not wise to make decisions about the placement of particular courses in isolation.

A decision to include electives is appropriate if electives reflect a belief that some branching in the curriculum is appropriate. Presumably, this is consistent with the philosophical approaches. The idea that interprofessional courses might one day be viewed as optional courses will give flexibility to the curriculum, since limited or no formal curriculum revision will be necessary when these courses are developed. If the organizational culture of the health professional schools changes to such an extent that interprofessional courses become mandatory, some curriculum redesign will be necessary.

Until interprofessional courses are available, the design team should ensure that students have opportunities to achieve the key professional ability of interprofessional collaboration. They could consider, for example, students' attendance at interdisciplinary, client-centered conferences in clinical areas. Or, as a beginning, those keen about interprofessional education might be able to develop a short-term, shared student clinical experience with an interested faculty member from another discipline.

McLanahan University

McLanahan University is an accredited university of approximately 28,000 full-time and 12,000 part-time students, offering baccalaureate, masters, and doctoral programs. It is located in a multicultural city of 1,200,000 inhabitants. There are five acute care hospitals, one of which is a 375-bed magnet hospital. Other healthcare facilities in the city include three chronic and long-term care agencies, numerous nursing homes, eight home healthcare agencies, a public health unit, physicians' and nurse practitioners' offices, and walk-in clinics.

Dr. Seranous Koupouyro is the director of the McLanahan School of Nursing, which comprises 10 masters-prepared and 11 doctorally-prepared full-time nursing faculty. Faculty have been meeting for 4 months to redesign the BSN curriculum. Part-time faculty have been regularly invited to join the curriculum work, but their involvement has been slight. The goal is to implement the revised curriculum in 18 months for a class of 125 students.

The total faculty group endorsed the existing humanistic-caring, feminist philosophical approaches. Core curriculum concepts, key professional abilities, and principal teaching-learning approaches were identified and the curriculum nucleus endorsed.

The curriculum committee has developed the outcome statements, and after these were approved, they formulated the level competencies. The outcome statements address the provision of evidence-based nursing care in accordance with regulatory standards, effective communication and management, ethical and cultural competence, and advocacy to enhance social justice. The faculty are now ready to consider the curriculum design.

Questions for Consideration and Analysis of the McLanahan University Case

1. How should the curriculum committee proceed with the work yet to be done?
2. What should the curriculum committee consider next?
3. What resources would assist the committee in its curriculum design process?
4. What should be included in the curriculum design?
5. How will the curriculum nucleus influence the curriculum design?
6. How could nursing and non-nursing courses be determined?
7. What policies should be taken into account for the curriculum design?

Curriculum Development Activities for Consideration in Your Setting

Use the following questions to guide thinking about designing your curriculum:

1. Which program structure is most appropriate for the type of program we are developing and for our educational institution?
2. Which program model most clearly reflects our beliefs about learning?
3. How do our partnerships and delivery methods influence the design?
4. What organizing strategy might we select to assure a logical progression to, and achievement of, curriculum outcomes?
5. What should we include in the curriculum matrix?
6. What nursing, non-nursing, and elective courses will best facilitate achievement of curriculum outcomes? Should there be interdisciplinary, multidisciplinary, transdisciplinary, or interprofessional courses? What steps do we need to take to develop these courses?
7. What configuration of courses should be considered?
8. How can courses be titled to ensure conceptual and visual unity?
9. What negotiations should take place with other academic units to operationalize the envisioned curriculum?
10. Which existing institutional policies influence our design?
11. Which specific policies need to be developed?
12. What are the resource implications of our curriculum design?
13. What approaches might be considered to enhance faculty understanding about, and commitment to, the curriculum design process?

References

Applegate, M. A. (1998). Educational program evaluation. In D. M. Billings & J. A. Halstead (Eds.), *Teaching in nursing. A guide for faculty* (pp. 423–457). Philadelphia: W. B. Saunders Co.

Armstrong, D. G. (2003). *Curriculum today.* Upper Saddle River, NJ: Merrill Prentice Hall.

Babenko-Mould, Y., Andrusyszyn, M. A., & Goldenberg, D. (2004). Effects of computer-based clinical conferencing on nursing students' self-efficacy. *Journal of Nursing Education, 43*(4), 149–155.

Barnsteiner, J. H., Disch, J. M., Hall, L., Mayer, D., & Moore, S. M. (2007). Promoting interprofessional education. *Nursing Outlook, 55*(3), 144–150.

Boland, D. L. (1998). Developing curriculum frameworks, outcomes and competencies. In D. M. Billings & J. A. Halstead (Eds.), *Teaching in nursing. A guide for faculty* (pp. 135–150). Philadelphia: W. B. Saunders Co.

Boland, D. L. (2005). Developing curriculum frameworks, outcomes and competencies. In D. M. Billings & J. A. Halstead (Eds.), *Teaching in nursing. A guide for faculty* (2nd ed., pp. 167–185). St. Louis, MO: Elsevier Saunders.

Boutain, D. M. (2005). Social justice as a framework for professional nursing. *Journal of Nursing Education, 44*(9), 404–408.

Candela, L., & Benzel-Lindley, J. (2006). A case for learner-centered curricula. *Journal of Nursing Education, 45*(2), 59–66.

Clark, P. G. (2006). What would a theory of interprofessional education look like? Some suggestions for developing a theoretical framework for teamwork training. *Journal of Interprofessional Care, 20*(6), 577–589.

Copley, J. (2007). Audio and video podcasts of lectures for campus-based students: Production and evaluation of student use. *Innovations in Education and Teaching International, 44*(4), 387–389.

Cornelius, F., & Smith Glasgow, M. E. (2007). The development and infrastructure needs required for success—one college's model: Online nursing education at Drexel University. *Techtrends, 51*(6), 32–35.

Curran, V. R. (2006). Tele-education. *Journal of Telemedicine and Telecare, 12*(2), 57–63.

Dalley, K., Candela, L., & Benzel-Lindley, J. (2008). Learning to let go: The challenge of de-crowding the curriculum. *Nursing Education Today, 28*(1), 62–69.

Diefenbeck, C. A., Plowfield, L. A., & Herman, J. W. (2006). Clinical immersion: A residency model for nursing education. *Nursing Education Perspectives, 27*(2), 72–79.

Dyer, J. (2003). Multidisciplinary, interdisciplinary, and transdisciplinary educational models and nursing education. *Nursing Education Perspectives, 24*(4), 186–188.

Friesner, A. (1978). Curriculum process for developing or revising a baccalaureate nursing program. In *NLN. Curriculum process for developing or revising a baccalaureate nursing program* (pp. 13–22). New York: Author.

Gagné, R. M., Briggs, L. J., & Wager, W. W. (1992). Principles of instructional design (4th ed.). Fort Worth, TX: Harcourt Brace Jovanovich.

Giddens, J. F., & Brady, D. P. (2007). Rescuing nursing education from content saturation: The case for a concept-based curriculum. *Journal of Nursing Education, 46*(2), 65–69.

Glennon, C. D. (2006). Reconceptualizing program outcomes. *Journal of Nursing Education, 45*(2), 55–58.

Goodwin, M., Sener, I., & Steiner, S. H. (2007). A novel theory for nursing education: Holistic comfort. *Journal of Holistic Nursing, 25*(4), 278–284.

Gubrud-Howe, P., Shaver, K. S., Tanner, C. A., Bennett-Stillmaker, J., Davidson, S. B., Flaherty-Robb, M., et al. (2003). A challenge to meet the future: Nursing education in Oregon, 2010. *Journal of Nursing Education, 42*(4), 163–167.

Heinrich, C. R., Karner, K. J., Gaglione, B. H., & Lambert, L. J. (2002). Order out of chaos. The use of a matrix to validate curriculum integrity. *Nurse Educator, 27*(3), 136–140.

Hodson Carlton, K., Ryan, M., Nagia, S. A., & Kelsy, B. (2007). Integration of global health concepts in nursing curricula: A national study. *Nursing Education Perspectives, 28*(3), 124–129.

Ironside, P. M. (2004). "Covering content" and teaching thinking: Deconstructing the additive curriculum. *Journal of Nursing Education, 43*(1), 5–12.

Ironside, P. M. (2005). Teaching thinking and reaching the limits of memorization: Enacting new pedagogies. *Journal of Nursing Education, 44*(10), 441–449.

Iwasiw, C., Andrusyszyn, A., Moen, A., Østbye, T., Davie, L., Stovring, T., et al. (2000). Canada-Norway graduate education in nursing leadership through distance technologies. *Journal of Nursing Education, 39*(2), 81–86.

King Mixon, D., Kemp, M. A., Towle, M. A., & Schrader, V. C. (2005). Negotiating the merger of three nursing programs into one: Turning mission impossible into mission possible. *Annual Review of Nursing Education, 3*, 187–203.

Lattuca, L. R., Voight, L. J., & Fath, K. Q. (2004). Does interdisciplinarity promote learning? Theoretical support and researchable questions. *Review of Higher Education, 28*, 23–48.

McEwan, M., & Brown, S. C. (2002). Conceptual frameworks in undergraduate nursing curricula: Report of a national survey. *Journal of Nursing Education, 41*(1), 5–14.

Molzahn, A. E., & Purkis, M. E. (2004). Collaborative nursing education programs: Challenges and issues. *Nursing Leadership(CJNL), 17*(4), 41–53.

NLNAC. (2005). *Accreditation manual with interpretative guidelines by program type for post-secondary and higher degree programs in nursing.* Accessed January 27, 2008, from http://www.nlnac.org/manuals/NLNACManual2005.pdf

Oregon Consortium for Nursing Education (OCNE). (2006). Update on progress. Accessed January 26, 2008, from http://www.ocne.org/update.php

Ouellet, L. L., & MacIntosh, J. (2007). The rise of accelerated baccalaureate programs. *Canadian Nurse, 103*(7), 28–31.

Pennington, E. A. (1986). The integrated curriculum: A 15-year perspective. In E. A. Pennington (Ed.), *Curriculum revisited: An update of curriculum design* (pp. 37–48). New York: National League for Nursing.

Picciano, A. G. (2001). *Distance learning: Making connection across virtual space and time.* Upper Saddle River, NJ: Prentice-Hall.

Purcell, F. B. (2006). Smooth transfer: A once mundane administrative issue re-emerges as a key tool for equity. *Connection. New England's Journal of Higher Education, 21*(1), 20–21.

Reeves, S., Goldman, J., & Oandasan, I. (2007). Key factors in planning and implementing interprofessional education in health care settings. *Journal of Allied Health, 36*(4), 231–235.

SearchUnifiedCommunications.com (2005). *Definitions.* Retrieved February 7, 2008, from http://searchunifiedcommunications.techtarget.com/sDefinition/0,,sid186_gci213055, 00.html

Sittner, B. J., Hudson, D. B., & Defrain, J. (2007). Using the concept of FAMILY STRENGTHS to enhance nursing care. *MCN, the American Journal of Maternal Child Nursing, 32*(6), 353–357.

Supplee, P. D., & Glasgow, M. E. (2008). Curriculum innovation in an accelerated BSN program: The ACE model. *International Journal of Nursing Education Scholarship, 5*, Article 1, Retrieved February 6, 2008, from http://www.bepress.com/ ijnes/vol5/iss1/art1

Taba, H. (1962). *Curriculum development: Theory and practice.* New York: Harcourt Brace Jovanovich.

Wiles, J., & Bondi, J. (2007). *Curriculum development: A guide to practice* (7th ed.). Upper Saddle River, NJ: Merrill.

Woodward Leners, D., Wilson, V. W., & Sitzman, K. L. (2007). Twenty-first century doctoral education: Online with a focus on nursing education. *Nursing Education Perspectives, 28*(6), 332–336.

CHAPTER 10

Course Design

Chapter Overview

Following completion of the curriculum design, attention turns to the design of individual courses. In this chapter, descriptions of course components and design parameters are followed by approaches to course design. A brief overview of teaching-learning strategies is presented. The process of course design is detailed, followed by ideas about designing individual classes and possible activities for faculty development. The chapter concludes with a summary and synthesis activities.

Chapter Goals

- Identify course components.
- Consider parameters influencing course design.
- Examine approaches to course design.
- Understand the process of course design.
- Reflect on faculty development activities to facilitate course design.

Course Design

An academic course is a recognized unit of learning within an overall curriculum. It is designed with components that outline the purpose of the course, what students are to achieve, and what they are to do. The intent of course design is to achieve unity and coherence within each course and among courses. Course design begins as soon as a curriculum design has been approved, and truly never ends, since courses are refined throughout the life of the curriculum. It is a cyclical process: after implementation, courses are evaluated and designs modified.

The term *course design*, when used as a noun, refers to the configuration of a course. The design encompasses all components (title, purpose, and description; outcomes, teaching-learning strategies, content; classes; opportunities for students to demonstrate learning and faculty evaluation of student achievement), and the relationships between and among them. The process of designing courses, or the *course design process*, refers to discussions and decision-making that lead to the configuration of a course. The course design process personalizes the impending curriculum since faculty members feel a sense of ownership about the courses they create and teach.

Course design proceeds once the curriculum design is approved. The level, year, or semester competencies; brief course descriptions; and draft course competencies developed during curriculum design become the starting point for designing courses. The philosophical approaches and outcomes approved for the curriculum are realized within courses.

The terminology used to describe course components varies among nursing programs. Nonetheless, they are present in all academic courses, whether they are theory, practice, or laboratory, or offered through traditional or distance delivery.

Course Title, Purpose, and Description

The course title should convey the main conceptual, process, or content focus of the course in accordance with the overall curriculum design. Collectively, course titles should present a picture of a unified curriculum.

All courses have a purpose in a nursing curriculum. A statement of purpose makes evident why the course is part of the curriculum and how it contributes to students' achievement of curriculum outcomes. Although the purpose may be readily apparent to curriculum designers, the reason for the existence of the course in the curriculum might not be obvious to learners. Therefore, explicit statements about the purpose and how it contributes to their development as professional nurses, can orient learners to the value of the course in their progress toward career goals.

Each course requires a brief description that is published in the institutional catalogue or calendar. This description is expanded in course materials to provide more detail for learners enrolled in the course. It provides information about the scope of the course, preparation required for classes, the nature of class meetings, participation expected of learners, and other information that faculty consider important to explain the intent and character of the course. This can be written in the second person to personalize the ideas so they will have more impact for each learner. Class or practice hours and course credits are generally stated. Table 10-1 is an example of a course purpose and expanded description.

Table 10-1 Course Purpose and Expanded Description

Nursing 376 Teaching and Learning in Nursing Practice

Description

In this course, students will explore the role of the nurse as teacher and learner in a variety of contexts. Educational theories for teaching, learning, and motivation for health behavior change will be addressed. Concepts and processes involved in teaching and learning will be included. Workshops, group presentations and projects, and dialogue about clinical practice will provide opportunities to integrate theory and practice. Preparation and active participation is integral to all classes. 3 hours per week, 13 weeks. 3 credits.

Purpose of the course

The purpose of this course is to assist you to expand your:

- Skill in assessing health learning needs, providing health information that is meaningful to clients, and evaluating learning
- Ability to integrate knowledge of the processes of teaching and learning into peer presentations and nursing practice
- Capacity to assess your own leaning needs and plan how to meet them.

How this course will contribute to your development as a professional nurse

Nurses teach clients formally or informally in all their interactions. For example, when saying that it will take 20 minutes before the effects of an analgesic will be felt, a nurse is teaching. When explaining that health-promoting actions can have a lifelong influence on a person's health, a nurse is teaching. Nurses teach in all settings with clients of all ages. However, teaching is more than simply telling. To be effective, nurses must assess the client and tailor the information and style of providing the information to individuals, families, or community groups. As well, nurses should be able to work successfully in teams and make presentations to peers. Therefore, the learning you gain in this course will contribute to your nursing practice throughout your career.

Successful completion of this course moves you toward achievement of the following curriculum outcomes:

- Incorporate best evidence; respect for the diversity and culture of individuals, families, and communities; and nursing practice standards in written teaching plans.
- Integrate self-assessment, knowledge of professional standards and competencies, and aspirations of the profession into a written plan for ongoing professional development.

continues

Table 10-1 continued

Nursing 376 Teaching and Learning in Nursing Practice

How we will work together

Classes will be interactive and include both large and small group discussion. Therefore, you will learn from your colleagues and contribute to their learning. To gain the most from each class, and to contribute meaningfully to your colleagues' understandings, it is important that you bring to class your insights and questions about the weekly readings. Sharing of insights and experiences will make the learning experience as rich as possible.

There are two workshops planned so you can practice learning needs assessment and provide a small teaching intervention with 3 or 4 colleagues. As well, you will plan and provide a short presentation for the class, with 5–6 colleagues. These sessions will allow you to apply what you are learning in a collegial environment.

Together we will discuss and critique the readings; consider their application to nursing practice through case studies and personal experience; and provide support as we incorporate principles of teaching and learning into our repertoire of professional behaviors.

Course Competencies

Competency statements are another component of courses. They describe the abilities or competencies expected of students at the end of the course and are written in the same format as overall curriculum outcomes. Learning, a process that leads to the acquisition or development of new knowledge, understandings, and abilities, is the ultimate purpose for which courses are designed. The nature of the desired learning is expressed in the course competency statements. Preliminary course competencies, derived from curriculum outcomes and level or semester competencies, are formulated when courses are identified and configured as part of curriculum design. These must be refined to make them specific for each course.

Course competency statements delineate the achievements expected of students within the context of the course experiences. Important course concepts should be evident in the statements. Typically, the number of course competencies exceeds the number written for each semester because the expectations for courses are more specific. The course competencies should collectively 'add up' to the semester outcomes, although each course does not typically address all the semester outcomes.

Teaching-Learning Strategies

Teaching-learning strategies are specific actions planned by an instructor to facilitate students' learning. These can include lectures, discussions, seminars, demonstrations, role-playing, gaming, and so forth. They are termed *teaching-learning strategies*, and not merely *teaching strate-*

gies to emphasize that the intent of the activities is that learning occurs. Moreover, through teaching, faculty members expand their own as well as students' understanding and insights. As Joseph Joubert, the 19th century French philosopher said, "To teach is to learn twice" (Great Quotes.com, n.d.).

The strategies selected should, of course, be congruent with faculty members' beliefs about learning, as expressed in the philosophical approaches and evident in the principal teaching-learning approaches delineated in the curriculum nucleus. These principal teaching-learning approaches will predominate in the nursing courses, although others may be used as well. The specific strategies selected should assist learners in their progression toward achievement of the course competencies.

Direct teaching strategies, such as a lecture or small group discussion, require face-to-face interaction with learners. The lecture may be complemented by indirect strategies such as readings from books and journals, or watching video-clips. When direct and indirect strategies are combined, they serve to stimulate learning through multiple sensory channels (Van Hoozer et al., 1987).

Traditional Teaching-Learning Strategies Traditional teaching-learning strategies are those that have been relied upon for decades, perhaps chosen by the instructor for convenience, comfort, and efficiency. The lecture, for example, often selected as a primary classroom teaching strategy due to large class size, actively engages the instructor in the act of teaching. Students, however, may be more passively involved in the learning process unless active learning strategies are incorporated into lectures (Bowles, 2006; Oermann, 2004). Other examples of traditional strategies include discussions, seminars, questioning, and use of audiovisual presentations of course content (DeYoung, 2003).

Contemporary Teaching-Learning Strategies Contemporary teaching-learning strategies promote more active learner engagement than do traditional strategies. Students take an active role in learning experiences individually and/or with their colleagues through cooperative and collaborative projects, in computer-assisted instruction or other multimedia applications, in simulated clinical situations, in virtual reality laboratories, and in creation and synthesis of knowledge in the classroom.

Clinical Teaching-Learning Strategies Teaching-learning strategies for clinical courses are influenced by the size and level of the student group and the learning opportunities available in the setting. Pre- and post-conferences, on-the-spot consultations, and questioning are commonly employed, as are direct client care and observational experiences, peer teaching, and preceptoring.

Much has been written about teaching-learning strategies, but it is beyond the scope of this text to examine each strategy in detail. Table 10-2 outlines characteristics that a novice nurse educator might find helpful when making decisions about using specific strategies. In this table, group size indicates the class size for which the strategy is suitable. Cost and infrastructure are the extent of financial and other organizational resources necessary to implement the strategy.

Instructor preparation time refers to the amount of time required by an instructor to prepare a unit of learning. *Learning curve* is a term adapted from industry that refers to the rate at which learning takes place to yield the desired outcome. If the learning curve associated with use of a specific teaching-learning strategy is steep, then an alternative one may be considered. *Learner engagement* is the extent to which students participate in the learning process when a particular strategy is used. *Intent* refers to the abilities expected of students.

Table 10-2   Characteristics of Commonly Used Teaching-Learning Strategies

Teaching-Learning Strategy	Group Size	Cost/Infrastructure	Instructor Preparation Time/Learning Curve	Learner Engagement/Learning Curve	Intent
Algorithms	Both	Low/Low	High/Steep	Active/Minimal	Analysis, CT*
Audio-conferencing	Small	High/High	High/Moderate	Passive/Minimal	Understanding
Buzz groups	Both	Low/Low	Low/Minimal	Active/Minimal	Application
Clinical observation	Small	Low/Low	Medium/Minimal	Active/Moderate	Understanding
Computer-assisted instruction	Large	High/High	High/Steep	Active/Moderate	CT, Application, Synthesis
Computer-conferencing	Small	High/High	High/Moderate	Active/Steep	CT, Synthesis, Evaluation
Concept mapping	Small	Low/Low	High/Moderate	Active/Moderate	Analysis, CT, Synthesis
Debate	Both	Low/Low	High/Steep	Active/Minimal	Analysis, CT
Direct client care	Small	Low/High	High/Steep	Active/Steep	CT, Synthesis, Evaluation
High-fidelity simulations	Small	High/High	High/Steep	Active/Steep	Application, CT, Synthesis, Evaluation
Gaming	Both	Low/Low	High/Moderate	Active/Minimal	Application, CT, Synthesis
Laboratory practice	Small	High/High	High/Moderate	Active/Moderate	Application, CT, Synthesis
Lecture	Large	Low/Low	High/Moderate	Passive/Minimal	Understanding
Lecture-discussion	Large	Low/Low	High/Moderate	Active/Minimal	Understanding
Live patient simulations	Small	High/High	High/Steep	Active/Moderate	Application, CT, Synthesis, Evaluation

Table 10-2   continued

Teaching-Learning Strategy	Characteristics				
	Group Size	Cost/ Infrastructure	Instructor Preparation Time/Learning Curve	Learner Engagement/ Learning Curve	Intent
Metaphor	Both	Low/Low	High/Moderate	Active/Moderate	CT, Critical Reflection, Synthesis
Multimedia	Large	High/High	High/Steep	Active/Steep	Application
Narrative dialogue	Small	Low/Low	Medium/Moderate	Active/Minimal	Critical Reflection, CT, Synthesis
One-minute paper	Both	Low/Low	Low/Minimal	Active/Minimal	Understanding
Oral examinations	Small	Low/Low	High/Steep	Active/Steep	CT, Evaluation
Peer teaching	Small	Low/Low	Medium/Moderate	Active/Steep	Understanding
Preceptorships	Small	Low/High	Medium/Low	Active/Minimal	Application, CT, Synthesis, Evaluation
Pre- and post-conferences	Small	Low/Low	High/Steep	Active/Minimal	Understanding, CT, Synthesis, Evaluation
Questioning	Both	Low/Low	High/Moderate	Active/Minimal	Understanding, CT, Synthesis, Evaluation
Reflective journaling	Small	Low/Low	High/Moderate	Active/Steep	Critical Reflection, CT, Synthesis
Role play	Small	Low/Low	High/Moderate	Active/Moderate	Application, CT
Student presentation	Both	Low/Low	High/Moderate	Active/Steep	CT, Synthesis
Think-pair-share	Large	Low/Low	High/Minimal	Active/Minimal	Application, CT
Video-conferencing	Small	High/High	High/Steep	Active/Steep	Understanding, Synthesis
Videotape	Small	High/Low	High/Steep	Passive/Minimal	Understanding
Virtual reality	Small	High/High	High/Steep	Active/Steep	Application, CT, Synthesis
Written assignments	Both	Low/Low	High/Steep	Active/ Moderate	CT, Synthesis, Evaluation

*CT = Critical Thinking

Course Content

The course content is the component that can be of most interest to students who want to know what they need to learn. The scope of content is specified for each course, and this typically is conveyed to learners in the form of titles or topics for each session, along with a list of required readings.

Courses contain substantive knowledge (facts, concepts, hypotheses, and methods, to name a few) through which the thinking processes for nursing practice are developed. No matter how the information is addressed, each course has content. The content must be judiciously selected, with only the most pertinent chosen.

In courses where faculty are most concerned with learners' engagement with content, that is, creating meaning and discerning its significance to practice (Ironside, 2004, 2005), the content continues to be important. Even though processing of information is primary, learners must acquire content as one of the building blocks of their thinking. Therefore, the basic issue of identifying and organizing suitable content remains.

Content in clinical courses is the knowledge and skills to practice in designated clinical situations, the clinical situations themselves, and the insights and understandings developed during the experience. Being in the situation, applying previously held and new knowledge and abilities, seeking learning opportunities, and formulating new understandings are the intent of clinical courses. Therefore, a weekly topical schedule is not applicable, although faculty can identify particular concepts or professional abilities as the focus of clinical sessions.

Classes

Each course has a specified number and duration of formal sessions when faculty and students interact. These sessions can be conducted in classrooms, clinical settings, labs, or through cyberspace. In classroom courses, a topic is typically identified for each session. Although the structure of courses offered through flexible delivery may vary, they generally retain the idea of a 'class' in which a conceptually meaningful unit of content is addressed weekly. For clinical or laboratory courses, the "class" is each practice session.

Student learning activities can be planned for each class, and if so, they become part of the course syllabus. These describe the preparatory, in-class, and follow-up activities that learners are expected to complete. The preparatory activities can include reading, interviews with clients, visits to community agencies, writing a vignette from clinical practice, and so forth. The intent is that learners arrive at class ready to engage with the content and not merely to receive it. The in-class activities typically include opportunities to process information and experiences, and work toward achievement of course competencies through interaction with course content, faculty, peers, clinicians, and/or clients. The follow-up activities provide suggestions for reflection, application, and development of deeper understandings.

The key feature of student learning activities is that they require active engagement of learners, and thus reflect a belief that learning is optimized when students are responsible for acquiring basic knowledge, and participating in the development of understandings, analysis, and synthesis of that knowledge. Although results of studies of the outcomes of active and traditional teaching methods are not consistent (Ridley, 2007), there is a widespread movement in nursing education toward interactive teaching-learning approaches, based on a constructivist model of education.

Opportunities for Students to Demonstrate Learning and Faculty Evaluation of Student Achievement

Students must demonstrate achievement of course competencies so faculty can be assured that they are ready to progress in the program and ultimately, to graduate. Therefore, *opportunities for students to demonstrate learning and faculty evaluation of student achievement,* are viewed as a course component. This view is taken since the student activity of demonstrating learning and the faculty activity of evaluating the products of learning are inextricably linked. They are therefore viewed as one component.

Opportunities to demonstrate learning is the term used in this book for what are typically called *assignments, course requirements,* or simply *evaluation of student work.* This connotes a more positive perspective and conveys the idea that learners have a responsibility to provide evidence that they are achieving the course competencies.

The opportunities for students to demonstrate learning can include a host of activities, including:

- True-false, multiple-choice, multiple-response exams
- Completion and essay exams (Oermann & Gaberson)
- Term papers and other written assignments, such as journal writing
- Class presentations and other oral reports
- Objective structured clinical examinations
- Verbal questioning
- Checklists, rating scales, anecdotal reports, observations, simulations, concept or mind mapping
- Process recordings, care plans, case studies, teaching plans, clinical documentation, portfolios, group projects, self-evaluation (Oermann & Gaberson)
- Reports of self-evaluation.

Activities included in the course design must be consistent with the philosophical and principal teaching-learning approaches. They must, of course, allow learners to demonstrate their level of success in achieving course competencies. Completion of the work is inherently a learning activity, and hence a dual purpose is achieved; students learn and they demonstrate their achievement.

In some courses, learners have choices among several assignments, can propose their own ideas about how to demonstrate achievement, or can assign the weighting for several assignments. In this way, they are given options within the course structure.

Once students fulfill their responsibility and present their evidence of learning, the faculty member's reciprocal obligation is to evaluate the completed work fairly. The purposes of evaluation are to "measure learning and other outcomes, judge performance, determine competence to practice, and arrive at other decisions about students. . . ." (Oermann & Gaberson, 2006, p. 1). Evaluation can be *formative,* intended to provide feedback to learners about their progress, or *summative,* an assessment of achievement at the conclusion of a course. Information from the evaluation tells learners how well they are doing in the course.

Opportunities for students to demonstrate learning and faculty evaluation of student learning, a component of course design, requires thoughtful attention. Decisions about this component will be influenced by many factors, including: philosophical approaches, course outcomes, purpose of the evaluation (formative/summative), content, course level, learning domain, class size, educational delivery medium, reliability, validity, utility, evaluation frequency, and availability of resources.

Approaches to Course Design

The approach to course design is strongly influenced by faculty members' abilities, interests, and comfort level, as well as the background knowledge, life experiences, and capabilities of students. Often, faculty use a familiar approach without giving careful thought to what is consistent with the philosophical approaches and intended curriculum outcomes. Indeed, many faculty teach as they were taught 15–20 years ago (Chipas, as cited by Moore Schaefer & Zygmont, 2003). If it seems that some courses are not being designed in accordance with the philosophical and principal teaching-learning approaches specified in the curriculum nucleus, then wider faculty discussion may be needed about the amount of flexibility in course design that is acceptable within the overall curriculum.

Irrespective of the approach to course design, attention should be given to learner diversity. Accordingly, course designers strive to ensure that:

• Written course materials and oral expression are clear and unambiguous.
• Important ideas receive prominence in course materials.
• Web sites are readily understandable and intuitive.

- Opportunities exist for alternate evaluation methods.
- Physical facilities are accessible and comfortable, with good sight lines (Bowe, 2000).

Extending from the idea of making courses intellectually and physically accessible, is the belief that courses should be culturally comfortable for learners of differing heritages. Therefore, deliberate effort is made to avoid ethnocentric and gender-limited language, texts, readings, and learning experiences. Additionally, authors with varied backgrounds should be represented in course readings (Saunders & Kardia, 2004). The intent is to make the course as inclusive as possible so all students feel welcome and accepted in an environment conducive to learning.

Traditional Approaches

In traditional approaches to course design, planning proceeds in a logical, step-wise fashion, starting with objectives. The intent is to design a course and lessons that will lead students to achieve specific objectives and learn specific content in a readily identified and prescribed way. The traditional, behaviorist course design is structured, supports knowledge as being absolute, and is teacher-centered. Faculty have responsibility for identifying the nature, purpose, and objectives of the course, as well as content, teaching-learning strategies, and evaluation methods. Students are the recipients of knowledge and decisions.

With this approach, a course description is written first. Then, course objectives are formulated according to taxonomies that address cognitive, psychomotor, and affective learning domains. The course objectives state what the learner will be able to do, think, or feel. They are drawn from program and level objectives, the course description, and content necessary for desired behaviors to occur. As well, unit or module objectives are specified, with the units being defined by content groupings. "Courses are constructed around the content deemed necessary to produce the desired target behaviors" (Bevis, 1982, p. 195). Teaching strategies, media, and evaluation methods are then selected.

Gagné, Briggs, and Wager (1992) propose a more detailed approach, whereby following the specification of program outcomes, an instructional analysis is completed to identify the skills involved in reaching those outcomes. This entails a task analysis to delineate the steps or skills in the behavior and an information-processing analysis to identify the mental processes required to enact each outcome. From these, objectives are prepared. Next, criterion-referenced evaluation procedures are created and instructional strategies and media selected.

Lesson planning is an important element of traditional approaches. For each lesson, objectives are delineated and appropriate instructional events defined. Written lesson plans specify activities that the teacher will carry out. See Table 10-3 for a sample of a traditional lesson plan.

The following criteria for judging the quality of a lesson plan have been suggested:

- Coherence is evident in the link between what students should know, understand, and be able to do.

Table 10-3 Lesson Plan for a 2-Hour Class

Purpose: Provide students with information necessary for health education and promotion

Objectives	Content	Teaching Strategies	Time	Resources	Evaluation Methods
Identify 3 goals of health promotion	Health promotion goals	Lecture-discussion	10 min	Chalk board Overhead or PowerPoint slides	Pre-testing
Describe how the Health Belief Model can be used to influence behavior	Health Belief Model	Lecture-discussion	25 min	PowerPoint slides	Question and answer
Assess concerns of families seeking health promotion interventions	Family health	Case study or role play Discussion	35 min	Guests Discussion questions on overheads or slides	Question and answer
Recall guidelines for health promotion	Guidelines for health promotion	Brainstorming Large group discussion	20 min	Flip-charts	Question and answer
Examine health promotion measures	Review of course goals	Lecture-discussion	30 min	Questionnaire	Post-testing

- Activities are motivating and designed to meet the learning needs of different types of learners.
- The lesson supports the intent of the curriculum and is worthy of the time given to it (Erikson, 2007).

These criteria are applicable for all class plans, whether traditional lesson plans are used or not.

Contemporary Approaches

With a more contemporary or conceptual approach to course design, courses are planned so the focus of learning is on inquiry and the active pursuit of experiences that contribute to learning. These learning-centered course designs incorporate recognition and acceptance of the values, beliefs, knowledge, and experience that learners bring. Courses are designed in accordance with the premises that learning and contextual knowledge:

- Evolve from processes such as discussion, dialogue, debate, and other heuristics that promote active engagement and sharing of knowledge.
- Occur in an environment that advances trust and critique among all participants.

This approach to course design is based on adherence to values of human freedom and self-reflection, and an epistemology of transactional constructivism. Therefore, course procedures are designed to emphasize learners' information-processing and construction of understandings and meanings through transactions with others (Sutinen, 2008). Process-oriented courses further integrative learning, de-emphasize specific content, and reduce reliance on the lecture method. Attention is given to how students, faculty, and clients, together, bring life experiences to knowledge and learning. Understanding develops through thoughtful deliberation and critical analysis of information, dialogue about its meaning, and reflection on its fit with personal beliefs and values.

Faculty and students share course design, jointly creating the climate and cultural reality in which collaboration flourishes. Together, they determine course competencies, establish appropriate methods for learners to achieve them, and agree on the evaluation procedures. In this way, students gain a sense of ownership for the course and learning process. They become active constructors of knowledge and meaning (Seaton-Sykes, 2003), and shape their learning through participation in course design and activities. The instructor is an expert learner, metastrategist, and facilitator (Bevis, 2000a), who empowers, fosters creativity, stimulates intellectual inquiry, and maintains rigor.

Central to contemporary course design is conceptualizing learning activities. As stated previously, these enable learners to process information and work toward achievement of course competencies through interaction with course content, peers, and faculty. They are activities that students undertake with the intent that learning occurs, and can be developed collaboratively, as a part of course design. Learning activities replace didactic instruction; require active involvement and participation; encourage self-responsibility for learning; foster synthesis and analysis; and lead to critical thinking, autonomy, personal and professional integrity, and competency (Bevis, 2000b).

The success of this approach is highly dependent on the interpersonal dynamics between and among instructors and students. For student engagement to grow, instructors ought to "offer a welcome, warmth, a sense of sharing and respect, . . . and [create] a setting where a sense of belonging and mutuality can flourish" (Bryson & Hand, 2007, p. 360). Moreover, learners must engage in authentic communication with the instructor and each other, while involved in activities "focused on constructing, comprehending, reflecting, and communicating meanings, as well as creative and critical thinking" (Ridley, 2007, p. 205).

The instructional responsibilities are to nurture the creation of a psychologically safe environment, design the structure in which purposeful learning can occur, and provide formative feedback about students' progress (McAlpine, 2004). Fulfilling these instructional obligations requires focused attention during the design of courses and individual classes.

Blended Approaches

In a blended approach, there is a mix of contemporary and traditional approaches. In small classes, a contemporary approach may be possible since faculty and student collaboration could occur in all aspects of course design. In large undergraduate courses, however, some predetermined structure is required because of class size, agreements with clinical agencies, and policies of the educational institution. Faculty who support constructivism might rely upon an approach to course design that blends both traditional and contemporary perspectives.

For the most part, faculty members design the course structure (i.e., define the description, competencies, general scope of content, and opportunities to demonstrate learning) in a way that appears to mirror traditional approaches. Nonetheless, there could be opportunities for student choice within specified limits (Iwasiw, 1987). For example, learners may choose from a number of broadly defined essays or projects or collectively determine assignment due dates.

While courses are designed with a predetermined structure, their intent is to support process learning. A contemporary approach becomes apparent in the teaching-learning strategies and planned learning activities that occur. For example, planned student activities in lectures (Oermann, 2004), peer teaching (Goldenberg & Iwasiw, 1992; Iwasiw & Goldenberg, 1993), narrative pedagogy (Diekelmann, 2001; Ironside, 2003), and problem-based learning, among others, require students to be active participants in learning and knowledge construction. Additionally, faculty can develop guidelines that emphasize process learning in course sessions and make these available to students. The guidelines are learning-centered, specify class preparation activities, make evident the information processing skills expected, and allow fluidity in the conduct of classes. Readings are typically included as part of preparatory activities. See Table 10-4 for an example of class guidelines.

Table 10-4 Class Guidelines

Nursing 376 Teaching and Learning in Nursing Practice

Class Title: **Course Synthesis**

Overview:

In this course you were invited to engage in several learning activities to build on and expand your knowledge in, and expertise with, teaching and learning interactions. We addressed many foundational principles important in providing health education to clients and families and in our own learning. Now that the course is ending, it is important to reflect upon the growth achieved individually and collectively; recognize how this learning has influenced your repertoire of professional behaviors; and critically evaluate the way(s) in which the knowledge and experiences in this course have influenced you as a learner and as a teacher.

Class Outcomes:

1. Synthesize your knowledge about teaching and learning in nursing practice, and your own learning, in group discussion.
2. Integrate your understanding of evaluation of learning, and a self-assessment of your learning in this course, in group discussion.
3. Incorporate your understandings of teaching and learning, and appreciative inquiry, in a verbal synopsis of a group discussion about the course.

In Preparation:

1. Examine the course as a whole and identify:
   a. Insights that were new to you and made an impact upon you as a learner and as a professional
   b. Areas in which you would like to pursue further professional development
2. Review the expected course outcomes, the course processes, and the processes of appreciative inquiry.

In Class:

1. In small groups, discuss your:
   • Gains in understanding and how these have influenced your professional behaviors
   • Ideas about continued development related to teaching and learning in nursing
   • Evaluation of the course according to the stages of appreciative inquiry. Share key points with the class.
2. Complete the formal university teaching and course evaluations.

On Further Reflection

Reflect upon the insights you gained from your colleagues, readings, and experiences in this course. How will you continue to integrate your learning into your nursing practice?

Course Design Process

Designing a course is an iterative process with decisions about each course component affecting deliberations about other components. The process involves writing, modifying, critiquing, and revising before plans are finalized. The intent is to devise a course that adheres to curriculum philosophical and principal teaching-learning approaches, facilitates students' achievement of curriculum outcomes, and is effective within the school's context. There should be unity within the course, such that the relationships among the course components are apparent.

Course titles, brief descriptions, placement in the program, draft competencies, major curriculum concepts, principal teaching-learning approaches, and so forth, are determined as part of the curriculum design process. These, along with ideas about curriculum possibilities (content and learning experiences) generated during the analysis of contextual data, are reviewed as intensive course design begins.

Typically, courses are designed in the order in which they are to be implemented. During the design process, courses should be compared to the curriculum matrix to maintain adherence to the original curriculum intent. Reasons for deviations should be explained and agreement reached about their acceptability. Variations from the curriculum matrix might necessitate changes in subsequent courses (Heinrich, Karner, Gaglione, & Lambert, 2002).

Course design is not an activity undertaken in isolation. Ongoing consultation is required among course designers to ensure that:

- The curriculum intent and integrity are maintained.
- Concurrent courses are complementary.
- Sequenced courses build in depth and complexity without redundancy.
- Curriculum outcomes can be achieved.
- Student and faculty workloads are reasonable.

The design process begins with a review of parameters that influence the design, selection of a course design approach, and then proceeds to creation of the course components. Although attention is given to the components individually, ideas arise about all of them simultaneously. This concurrent thinking leads to course unity. The process concludes with a critique of the course design and preparation of information for learners.

Reviewing Course Parameters

Course parameters are boundaries that limit the range faculty have in creating courses, yet compel them to exercise creativity and ingenuity in designing courses that are motivating and promote positive learning experiences. Reviewing these parameters and how they will affect the course design is a necessary beginning.

Curriculum Nucleus and Curriculum Outcomes The overriding parameters for all courses are the school's curriculum nucleus (philosophical approaches, core curriculum concepts, key professional abilities, and principal teaching-learning approaches), and curriculum outcomes. Courses must be congruent with these. If the curriculum is being organized according to specified theories, conceptual models, or frameworks, these must be evident in the course components. Importantly, the philosophical approaches influence all learning experiences and evaluation procedures. They also define the desired learning climate.

Course Level, Structure, and Delivery The course level, that is, the semester and year in the curriculum gives course designers information about students' prior learning, which determines the depth and scope possible in the course to be designed. Course structure (i.e., length and frequency, duration, and length of sessions) also has a direct bearing on the competencies to be achieved, the extent of the subject matter, and evaluation. Course delivery approaches establish how learners access and engage in the course.

Learner Characteristics Learner numbers, and their attitudes toward learning, technology, participation, and evaluation, are important to know. These characteristics, as well as students' cultural and generational diversity, maturity, motivation, interests, and other commitments, have a bearing on course design.

Physical Environment Desk arrangements, temperature, windows, ventilation, and lighting affect attention, fatigue, and interactions, and must be considered in course design. This cannot always be known in advance of designing a course, and indeed, the finalized design will influence the classroom space that is required. As well, for clinical courses, the physical setting, such as the availability of a room for clinical conferences, influences learning opportunities.

Human and Material Resources The numbers of faculty and graduate teaching assistants, and their experience, have a bearing on the decisions made about individual courses. As well, clients and personnel in health care and community agencies influence clinical courses. Library and computer resources, and technical equipment in classrooms, among other material resources, must also be considered.

Policies and Contractual Agreements Finally, educational institutions have policies or regulations that must be respected in course design. For example, there may be requirements about the timing of evaluation and examinations. For clinical courses, contractual arrangements with clinical or community agencies regulate learning experiences.

To reinforce the parameters in the minds of those designing courses, they might ask:

- What are the institutional requirements related to course design?
- Which of the core curriculum concepts and major professional abilities will be addressed in this course?
- What are the implications of the philosophical approaches for course design?

- What are the principal teaching-learning approaches for the curriculum?
- What is the learning climate we wish to achieve in the course?
- Which delivery method(s) will be employed? Could multiple methods be used? Is the infrastructure sufficient to support the preferred method(s)?
- What resources will be available for the course?
- What are the knowledge and experiences that learners bring to this course?
- How many students are likely to be enrolled? What are their characteristics?
- Will the students be:
  - Direct from secondary institutions?
  - Those with previous diplomas, degrees, or some postsecondary education?
  - Adults with strong values about lifelong learning and continuing their education?
  - Individuals who, in addition to academic responsibilities, juggle multiple life roles?
  - Learners with special needs for whom certain accommodations need to be made?
  - Diverse or homogenous?

Choosing an Approach for Course Design

The choice of an approach for course design could be guided by the alignment between a traditional, contemporary, or blended approach with:

- Philosophical and principal teaching-learning approaches of the curriculum
- Faculty and student preferences
- Feasibility
- Institutional requirements

Identifying the Course Title, Purpose, and Description

Identifying the course title and purpose sets the stage for subsequent discussion. Course designers should question:

- What is the focus of this course?
- What is the reason for having this course in the curriculum?
- What is the main intent of this course? How can this be expressed in the title?
- Does our proposed title reflect the course intent and purpose?
- Does the course title convey that it is a part of a unified curriculum?
- How will this course move learners toward semester competencies and curriculum outcomes?

- How will this course assist learners in their development as professional nurses, and how can that be expressed?

Once a title is decided upon, a preliminary course description is written, and this undergoes many revisions during course design. The initial description represents the ideas that faculty first discuss as possibilities for the course. The course description is not finalized until all other design components are completed. In general, the following questions are raised as the description is discussed and written:

- Which curriculum possibilities, identified during the analysis of the contextual data, should be considered? What other learning experiences could be suitable?
- What would be the nature of interactions in these learning experiences?
- What could be the scope of the content, or the nature of practice experiences?
- How should learners participate in this course?
- If there is choice about delivery modes, which one(s) would be most fitting?
- If face-to-face delivery, what is suitable scheduling?

Formulating Course Competencies

The draft course competencies developed during the curriculum design process are refined, and perhaps expanded, to more closely reflect the emerging course design. Semester competencies are analyzed to identify those pertinent to the course. Then, course competencies are written to include concepts and context particular to that course. Formulation of course competencies centers on the queries listed below.

- What semester competencies should be addressed in this course?
- Which aspects of the semester competencies seem best suited for this course?
- Which core curriculum concepts and professional abilities should be most evident in the course competencies?
- What is the context in which achievement of the competencies will be evident?

Determining Content

Educators might pose the following questions when selecting content for each course:

- Which core curriculum concepts are to be included in this course? What is important content through which to address these concepts?
- What portions of the possible content will contribute most meaningfully to learners' achievements of competencies?
- What is a reasonable depth and scope of content at this stage of the nursing curriculum?

- How can the content be organized and sequenced to emphasize philosophical approaches and facilitate students' achievement of the course competencies?

Deciding on Classes

Classes are created through the division of the content into conceptually meaningful and logically sequenced units. Course designers could review:

- The number of class sessions there will be
- How the content can be meaningfully and logically sequenced to match the number of class sessions
- Key professional abilities that should be emphasized through the content
- Which titles could be assigned to each class and whether these titles reflect the philosophical approaches, core curriculum concepts, professional abilities, and/or context of care; if the class titles present a picture that conveys unity within the course and within the curriculum.

Selecting Teaching-Learning Strategies

Selection of teaching-learning strategies is of vital concern to course designers since these define, in part, what faculty will do. As faculty members ponder the wide range of strategies and techniques available to them, they give thought to the following questions:

- What are the principal teaching-learning approaches identified in the curriculum nucleus? Which strategies are consistent with these approaches?
- What strategies best align with our philosophical approaches?
- Which strategies will best facilitate learner achievement of course competencies?
- Which are feasible within the course parameters?
- Which are suitable for our delivery method(s)?
- Which best suit students' learning needs and styles?

Creating Student Learning Activities

Formulating student learning activities for each class calls upon the creativity of course designers. Some questions they might ask are listed below:

- What types of student engagement with content will promote achievement of course competencies?

- Which curriculum possibilities, identified during analysis of the contextual data, would be suitable in this course?
- Which activities can facilitate learner achievement of course competencies?
- What readings and other resources will enhance student learning?
- What types of practice experiences will enable learners to achieve course competencies?
- Do our proposed learning activities match the principal teaching-learning approaches identified in the curriculum nucleus? Do they reflect adherence to the philosophical approaches of the curriculum?

Planning Opportunities for Students to Demonstrate Learning and Faculty Evaluation of Student Achievement

When considering how students might demonstrate learning in the course, faculty simultaneously give thought to how they will evaluate the evidence of learning. They are cognizant that both the evidence they are asking for, and the way they evaluate it, must be consistent with the curriculum philosophical and principal teaching-learning approaches, and course competencies. Decisions about evaluation methods, the nature and frequency of evaluation, learner choices, and provision of criteria to them, are among the decisions that faculty make when designing courses. Questions faculty should consider include:

- In what ways could learners demonstrate achievement of course competencies?
- Which are consistent with the philosophical and principal teaching-learning approaches, and course competencies?
- What are the advantages and disadvantages for students and faculty of the methods proposed?
- How and when might formative and summative evaluation be used?
- How will evidence of learning be weighted within the final course mark? Will learners have the option of determining their own weightings of different assignments?
- Should there be options from which students select the ways in which they demonstrate learning. If so, how can we plan this?
- Will learner self-evaluation be included?
- How can we fairly evaluate the learning evidence that students present? Should we develop specific criteria or marking rubrics? If so, will we share these with them, along with other course material information?
- What will be reasonable due dates for learners to submit their work? Could the dates be negotiated with the class?

Critiquing Course Design

As course design proceeds, faculty members engage in ongoing appraisal. Before finalizing the course design they critique it in a more holistic fashion, asking themselves questions such as:

- Does this course seem to fulfill its purpose in the curriculum?
- Is this course feasible within the design parameters?
- Is the course consistent with the curriculum nucleus?
- Will course processes and content lead learners to achieve course competencies?
- Are the expectations for learners reasonable? Are they feasible when considered in conjunction with other courses in the semester?
- Do written descriptions of course components reflect our intent in a way that will be meaningful to others?
- Have we taken learner diversity into account?
- Does this course result in a reasonable workload for faculty?
- Do the course components fit together in a unified fashion?

Preparing Course Packages

Once decisions have been made about the course design, a course package, or syllabus, can be prepared for learners. This compendium could be available for purchase or posted on a course Web site. Although the terminology and precise nature of the packages can vary, they generally include: an expanded course description; statement of course competencies; information about the opportunities for students to demonstrate their learning and their due dates; and the schedule, topics, and student guidelines for course sessions. As well, a compilation of journal articles and other materials can be prepared. While a reading package is convenient for learners, faculty must assemble it early enough for copyright permissions to be obtained, and for reproduction. Internet access to journal articles can minimize the size of this package and facilitate retrieval of readings.

Designing Individual Classes

The overall course design provides the framework for individual classes. Each class must contribute to the course purpose, with student learning activities particularized for each class. When planning classes, teachers might question:

- How can we title this class so that its relationship to the course is evident?
- How can the class be designed to clearly relate to course competencies?

- What should learners achieve in this class?
- What learning activities can be planned so that the class purpose is achieved? What should the students be doing? What should the teacher be doing?
- What is a reasonable sequence and time allotment for the activities?

If a traditional approach to course design is employed, lesson plans can be developed to organize each class. If a blended approach is used, class guidelines for learners can be beneficial. With either approach, class planning generally involves determining the following:

- Purpose learners should achieve
- Scope of content
- Teaching-learning strategies
- Learning activities to engage students
- Sequence and timing of class activities.

Within each class, there are a number of instructional events that teachers should arrange, according to Gagné, Briggs, and Wager (1992). Although the events are described in a behaviorist fashion, they have relevance for most classes. Table 10-5 lists the nine events with examples of how these could be enacted. It is important to note that one teaching activity can simultaneously encompass more than one instructional event. For example, questioning can be used to both elicit and assess performance. An understanding of these instructional events can help teachers plan classes in which student participation is required, learning is assessed, and transfer of learning is taken into account.

Many teachers like to obtain feedback about each class. Therefore, they plan a few minutes at the conclusion of each session to ask learners questions such as:

- What did you like about this class?
- What worked well for you?
- What might we have done differently, and how?

This information allows for refinement of the class if it is to be conducted in subsequent semesters. As well, if a pattern of responses emerges in reaction to the predominant teaching-learning strategies, it is possible to take this into account for later classes.

Faculty Development

Faculty development is directed towards facilitating members' knowledge and expertise in designing courses and classes. Depending on faculty needs, and following an initial review

Table 10-5   Examples of Teacher Activities for Instructional Events

Instructional Events	Examples of Teacher Activities
Gaining attention	State the focus of the class
	Provide or ask for a clinical example
Informing learner of objectives	Describe the purpose of the class
	State class goals
Stimulating recall of prerequisite knowledge	Ask for significant points from previous class or required reading
	Ask how required reading for present class relates to previous learning
Presenting the stimulus material	Lecture with audio-video augmentation
	Ask questions to initiate and stimulate group discussion
	Ask students to role-play
	Have students debate
	Have students do class presentation
	Use narrative dialogue
Providing learning guidance	Provide hints, non-verbal cues
	Ask additional questions
Eliciting student performance	Ask questions
	Pose problems
	Present cases for analysis
Providing feedback about performance correctness	Confirm responses
	Rephrase or redirect question
Assessing the performance	Ask questions
	Gauge quality of discussion
	Use directed paraphrasing
Enhancing retention and transfer	Summarize and synthesize
	Ask students for summary and synthesis
	Ask how understandings will influence practice
	Ask for one-minute papers

Source: Some data from Gagné, R.M., Briggs, L.J., & Wager, W.W. (1992). *Principles of instructional design* (4th ed.). Fort Worth: Harcourt, Brace, Jovanovich College Publishers.

session on the parameters involved, faculty development activities can include discussion about some or all of the course components.

Discussion about the approach to course design would be appropriate. This would help team members appreciate whether a traditional, contemporary, blended, or distance delivery approach would be most relevant to the curriculum's philosophical base, principal teaching-learning approaches, and outcomes. Mentorship for those less familiar with course and class design could be beneficial. Likely, some attention will have to be given to drafting course and class designs. This may be a first activity for some. Sharing, critiquing, and discussing can be facilitated by experienced faculty members. Faculty might also gain from microteaching sessions and peer learning of teaching-learning exchanges, to practice any new strategies proposed for courses. This could be followed by member critiques.

Chapter Summary

In this chapter, course components (title, purpose, and description; competencies, teaching-learning strategies, content; classes; opportunities for students to demonstrate learning and faculty evaluation of student achievement) are described and course design parameters detailed. Several approaches to course design are included. Attention is given to the process of course design, and ideas are presented for the design of individual classes. The intent is that courses incorporate the principal teaching-learning approaches, reflect the philosophical approaches, and are structured to facilitate learner achievement of course competencies, which will contribute to their accomplishment of intended curriculum outcomes. Activities for faculty development are offered.

⬩Synthesis
Activities ⬩●

Two case studies are presented below. The Ballard University case is followed by a critique. Discuss the situation and its analysis, considering additional ideas that arise. The second, Philmore University, is followed by questions to guide examination of the case. Finally, curriculum development activities are proposed for consideration in individual settings.

Ballard University

Ballard University School of Nursing has been offering nursing programs for 80 years. All undergraduate and graduate courses are offered on-campus. For several years, student evaluations of the RN-BSN program have indicated dissatisfaction with the traditional lecture approach. Students have stated that they would prefer a more contemporary approach with process-oriented courses. The small group of RN-BSN faculty has been reluctant to consider a more contemporary approach because valued content could be de-emphasized and there would be less reliance on their content expertise in classes.

The curriculum committee, which reviews course evaluations, has been unsuccessful in bringing about change in the teaching-learning approaches in the RN-BSN program. Committee members are mindful that the processes in these courses are inconsistent with those used in other programs in the school. They believe that all courses should conform not only to the university's mission to provide educational opportunities for learners throughout the region, but also to the school's mission to advance nursing practice through the provision of progressive nursing programs.

A resolution is endorsed by the School of Nursing Council to revise the teaching-learning approach in the RN-BSN program, in accordance with more contemporary approaches used in the school's other programs. Members of the RN-BSN faculty are distressed about this and unsure about how to begin redesigning courses for this new approach. Dr. Ioanna Adrastos, associate dean of undergraduate nursing programs, offers to help the group redesign their courses as needed, enlist the help of course designers from the university educational development department, and ensure that they receive support when they first offer their courses.

Critique

It is commendable that the school of nursing is modifying the teaching-learning approaches in response to learner feedback. Provision of support to faculty is essential as they consider course redesign and when they implement their courses.

Of concern is the fact that faculty members teaching in the RN-BSN program do not endorse the idea of changing their approach. It would be worthwhile for Dr. Adrastos to explore this reluctance with them. Do they believe that they might have to change their courses completely? Do they not understand integrated learning? Do they believe they will need considerable preparation to learn how to facilitate students' construction of understandings and meanings? Do they feel they will lose the essence of teaching if lectures are de-emphasized? Their hesitation should be taken into account and appropriate strategies implemented.

Considerable faculty development will likely be necessary so this group can learn about interactive approaches and how to implement them effectively. Also important will be dedicated time and assistance for course design. Instructional designers from the university educational development department and other faculty versed in this approach will be extremely helpful, as well as peer support during course implementation. Dr. Adrastos has promised assistance, but she should anticipate that the needed changes may not come easily for this group. It should be recognized that full implementation of a completely new approach to teaching and learning will likely take several years.

Philmore College

Situated in a small, non-industrial town, Philmore College was originally a "hilltop" college established in 1818 as a school for boys, and later, for boys and girls. The school has evolved into a 4-year, privately endowed, non-sectarian, post-secondary institution. Since the 1960s, programs leading to baccalaureate degrees in psychosocial and physical sciences have been offered.

A decision has been made to offer a 12-month accelerated BSN program, in response to the nursing shortage and the demand by applicants with prior degrees. This program will be additional to the upper division BSN degree currently offered.

The nine master's-prepared and four PhD full-time nursing faculty each have combined nursing practice and teaching experience ranging from 4–18 years. The director, Dr. Agnes Philmore, a direct descendant of the founder, joined Philmore College in 1996. All nursing faculty, including the director, engage in classroom and clinical teaching. The practice experiences for the upper division BSN students are offered in one local 200-bed community hospital, a 224-bed tertiary care hospital in a neighboring city, and a 76-bed long-term and residential care facility. Students also have community nursing experience, which is coordinated and supervised by a primary care nurse practitioner with an adjunct faculty appointment. Approximately 85 students graduate annually and have been consistently successful in the licensure examinations and in obtaining employment.

The director, faculty, several students, and a local nurse practitioner, who compose the curriculum committee, have been meeting to design the 12-month program. The curriculum nucleus has been determined and the curriculum outcomes written. The principal teaching-learning approaches are focused on active and constructed learning. Courses for the discipline-specific, accelerated 12-month program have been identified. The committee is ready to begin course design.

Questions for Consideration and Analysis of the Philmore College Case

1. What parameters must the curriculum committee consider when designing the courses?
2. In what way will a commitment to active learning influence course design?
3. Which components should be included in the courses?
4. What classroom and clinical experiences could be incorporated into the courses?
5. What would sample clinical and classroom courses look like for this accelerated baccalaureate nursing program?

Curriculum Development Activities for Consideration in Your Setting

Use the following questions to guide thinking about your course design.

1. How will the parameters influence our decisions about course design?
2. Which approach(es) to course design will we choose, and why?
3. What should be the purpose, description, and outcomes of the courses?
4. What is the scope of content for the courses?
5. What learning activities should we consider to facilitate students' achievement of course outcomes?
6. Which teaching-learning strategies could be used?
7. Which opportunities for students to demonstrate learning should we consider? How will we evaluate the learning evidence that students present?
8. How can we ensure that the requirements of all courses in a semester are manageable for learners?
9. What are faculty learning needs related to course design?

References

Bevis, E. O. (1982). *Curriculum building in nursing: A process* (3rd ed.). St. Louis, MO: C.V. Mosby.

Bevis, E. O. (2000a). Teaching and learning. The key to education and professionalism. In E. O. Bevis & J. Watson (Eds.), *Toward a caring curriculum. A new pedagogy for nursing* (pp. 153–188). Boston: Jones and Bartlett.

Bevis, E. O. (2000b). Nursing education as professional education: Some underlying theoretical issues. In E. O. Bevis & J. Watson (Eds.), *Toward a caring curriculum. A new pedagogy for nursing* (pp. 67–106). Boston: Jones and Bartlett.

Bowe, F. G. (2000). *Universal design in education: Teaching nontraditional students.* Westport, CT: Bergin & Garvey.

Bowles, D. J. (2006). Active learning strategies . . . not for the birds! *International Journal of Nursing Education Scholarship, 3,* Article 22. Retrieved February 18, 2008, from http://www.bepress.com/ijnes/vol3/iss1/art22

Bryson, C., & Hand, L. (2007). The role of engagement in inspiring teaching and learning. *Innovations in Education and Teaching International, 44*(4), 349–362.

DeYoung, S. (2003). *Teaching strategies for nurse educators.* Upper Saddle River, NJ: Prentice Hall.

Diekelmann, D. (2001). Narrative pedagogy: Heideggerian hermeneutical analyses of lived experiences of students, teachers, and clinicians. *Advances in Nursing Science, 23*(3), 53–71.

Erikson, H. L. (2007). *Concept-based curriculum and instruction for the thinking classroom.* Thousand Oaks, CA: Corwin Press.

Gagné, R. M., Briggs, L. J., & Wager, W. W. (1992). *Principles of instructional design* (4th ed.). Fort Worth, PA: Harcourt, Brace, Jovanovich.

Goldenberg, D., & Iwasiw, C. L. (1992). Reciprocal learning among students in the clinical areas. *Nurse Educator, 17*(5), 27–29.

Great Quotes.com (n.d.). Retrieved February 13, 2008, from http://www.great-quotes.com/cgi-bin/db.cgi?&uid=default&Author_First_Name=Joseph&Author_Last_Name=Joubert&mh=10&sb=4&so=ASC&view_records=View+Records&nh=4

Heinrich, C. R., Karner, K. J., Gaglione, B. H., & Lambert, L. S. (2002). Order out of chaos. The use of a matrix to validate curriculum integrity. *Nurse Educator, 27*(3), 136–140.

Ironside, P. M. (2003). New pedagogies for teaching thinking: The lived experiences of students and teachers enacting narrative pedagogy. *Journal of Nursing Education, 42*(11), 509–513.

Ironside, P. M. (2004). "Covering content" and teaching thinking: Deconstructing the additive curriculum. *Journal of Nursing Education, 43*(1), 5–12.

Ironside, P. M. (2005). Teaching thinking and reaching the limits of memorization: Enacting new pedagogies. *Journal of Nursing Education, 44*(10), 441–449.

Iwasiw, C. L. (1987). The role of teacher in self-directed learning. *Nurse Education Today, 7,* 222–227.

Iwasiw, C. L., & Goldenberg, D. (1993). Peer teaching among students in the clinical area: Effects on student learning. *Journal of Advanced Nursing, 18,* 659–668.

McAlpine, L. (2004). Designing learning as well as teaching. *Active Learning in Higher Education, 5,* 119–134.

Moore Schaefer, K., & Zygmont, D. (2003). Analyzing the teaching style of nursing faculty: Does it promote a student-centered or teacher-centered learning environment? *Nursing Education Perspectives, 24*(5), 238–245.

Oermann, M. H. (2004). Using active learning in lectures: Best of "both worlds." *International Journal of Nursing Education Scholarship, 1.* Retrieved February 28, 2004, from http://www.bepress.com/injes/vol1/iss1/art1/

Oermann, M. H. , & Gaberson, K. B. (2006). *Evaluation and testing in nursing education* (2nd ed.). New York: Springer.

Ridley, R. T. (2007). Interactive teaching: A concept analysis. *Journal of Nursing Education, 46*(5), 203–209.

Saunders, S., & Kardia, D. (2004). *Creating inclusive college classrooms.* Center for Research on Learning and Teaching, University of Michigan. Retrieved April 20, 2008, from http://www.crlt.umich.edu/gsis/P3_1.html

Seaton-Sykes, P. (2003). Teaching and learning in Internet environment in Australian nursing education. Unpublished doctoral dissertation, Griffith University, Queensland, Australia.

Sutinen, A. (2008). Constructivism and education: Education as an interpretative transformational process. *Studies in Philosophy and Education, 27*(1), 1–14.

Van Hoozer, H. L., Bratton, B. D., Ostmoe, P. M., Weinholtz, D., Craft, M. J., Gjerde, C. L., et al. (1987). *The teaching process: Theory and practice in nursing.* Norwalk, CT: Appleton-Century.

PART IV

Curriculum Implementation and Evaluation

CHAPTER 11

Planning Curriculum Implementation

Chapter Overview

Planning for implementation of a redesigned curriculum requires thought and effort throughout the curriculum development process so that the curriculum will be actualized as conceived. Making implementation plans public includes keeping stakeholders informed as the curriculum is developed and introduced. In this chapter, marketing and publicity are described, as are contractual agreements with healthcare and community agencies, and other educational institutions. The logistics of curriculum implementation are discussed, including personnel, scheduling, and phasing out the existing curriculum. Following a discussion of ongoing faculty development, synthesis activities conclude the chapter.

Chapter Goals

- Appreciate the planning necessary to implement a redesigned curriculum.
- Consider means to inform others, publicize, and market the curriculum.
- Review contractual and logistical arrangements essential in curriculum implementation.
- Recognize the value of ongoing faculty development for successful curriculum implementation.

Purpose of Curriculum Implementation Planning

The purpose of implementation planning is to ensure that the curriculum can be actualized as it was conceived, meaning that there will be *fidelity of implementation.* This term comes from the idea of *fidelity of intervention* in service programs and is defined as ". . . how well an intervention is implemented in comparison to the original program design . . ." (O'Donnell, 2008, p. 33). Criteria for assessing intervention fidelity, and which are relevant for curriculum implementation planning, are related to structure and process.

The structure criteria are: (1) adherence, whether the components are being delivered as designed; and (2) duration, or the number, length, and frequency of sessions implemented. The process criteria are: (1) quality of delivery, that is, the style in which the program is delivered through use of the approved techniques and processes; and (2) program differentiation, or the presence of critical features of the program that differentiate it from others (O'Donnell, 2008).

When a curriculum itself is the intervention, achievement of these criteria is referred to as *fidelity of implementation,* or more simply, *implementation fidelity.* To attain implementation fidelity, faculty members forecast the conditions that must be in place for the curriculum to be operationalized as conceived, and then they make the arrangements for these conditions to be realized. Therefore, simultaneous curriculum development, implementation planning, and faculty development increase the likelihood that implementation fidelity will be achieved.

Making Curriculum Plans Public

Implementation of a redesigned curriculum should not be a surprise to the community because relevant stakeholders have been included in the data-gathering that leads to a context-relevant curriculum. They have participated in curriculum development and served on advisory committees. All who have been involved in, and will be affected by, the curriculum redesign ought to be thoroughly prepared for its implementation. Informing others of evolving plans, and attending to details of implementation, must occur simultaneously with curriculum development.

Informing Stakeholders

Stakeholders' involvement in the creation of a context-relevant curriculum result in a sense of curriculum ownership and a desire to ensure its successful implementation. To this end, stakeholders can become regular and effective messengers, keeping others apprised of forthcoming changes and their rationale. The stakeholders help shape the path for a smooth transition from one curriculum to another.

Students Current students should be informed about ongoing curriculum development since they are naturally interested in the planned curriculum changes and what the changes will mean for them. This information-sharing can be accomplished by faculty and by students who are involved in the curriculum development process. Students can be very helpful in explaining and promoting the developing curriculum to their peers. Faculty must also be diligent in these efforts.

The Educational Institution As curriculum development proceeds, consultation with senior administrators and chairpersons of relevant institution-wide committees is ongoing. Keeping these people informed of the developing curriculum will expedite approval. As well, negotiations about non-nursing courses and their scheduling must occur before the curriculum is finalized.

Similarly, arrangements for financial resources, student services, library resources, technological support, and so forth must be made before curriculum approval is requested. Assurance about these matters is gained by engaging administrators and directors of relevant services in discussion early in the curriculum development process. In this way, they can alert the dean/director of the school of nursing, or the curriculum leader, about any anticipated problems, as well as attend to financial and personnel implications within their units.

Healthcare and Community Agencies Involvement and support of stakeholders outside the educational institution are foundational to a curriculum with a practice component. Steering committee members serve as ambassadors for the new curriculum to clinical and community agencies. However, support from these and other nursing leaders, while essential, may not be sufficient to ensure successful implementation in clinical sites.

Personnel with whom students will be working must be informed of the curriculum redesign. This can be accomplished, in part, through formal presentations and the provision of written materials. More detailed, small group meetings are also necessary to orient nursing and other staff to new learning outcomes, activities students will pursue, scheduling, and any plans related to placing students who are completing a different program level on a unit, from those who would normally be there. Faculty whose work intersects with clinical personnel have a critical role in this latter activity. Answering questions and allaying any apprehensions that might surface about the curriculum will be helpful in reducing misconceptions and subsequent misaligned expectations.

If placements are planned in agencies or units where students have not had previous clinical experiences, curriculum orientation will be particularly important. Discussion should focus on course competencies and activities, the nature of student interactions with clients and staff, and logistical details. Interpreting the role of nursing education and explaining how nursing students will contribute to the agency mission and client well-being are particularly important.

Ongoing Communication

As curriculum development proceeds, regular meetings with students, nurses, and others interested in knowing about the curriculum will serve to maintain open dialogue and facilitate a feeling of inclusion. Similarly, an electronic newsletter or a regularly updated Web site outlining progress and responses to frequently asked questions make the process transparent and keep interested parties informed about curriculum development progress and implementation plans.

Once implementation of the redesigned curriculum begins, follow-up meetings at placement sites, to review and discuss learner experiences, will promote ongoing successful implementation. These meetings can address:

- What is working well
- Concerns expressed by staff and/or students
- Appropriate actions to resolve concerns and capitalize on successes.

As well as facilitating learning experiences for students, these meetings can:

- Demonstrate the educational institution's interest in the views of practitioners.
- Provide an avenue to express appreciation for practitioners' involvement in student learning.
- Bring to light learning experiences not previously considered.
- Build commitment to student learning.

Marketing

Marketing of the redesigned curriculum to prospective students is fundamental for successful implementation. Many avenues can be used to make the program known and appealing. For example, professionally designed pamphlets and brochures can be sent to secondary school counselors and to academic counseling services within the educational institution. As well, face-to-face meetings can be planned with secondary school counselors to inform them about the curriculum and provide opportunities to clarify and update understandings of the profession and changes within.

An attractive, current, and simple-to-navigate Web site about the school of nursing, the curriculum, and the faculty will market the nursing curriculum to prospective applicants. Nursing students and faculty can provide valuable advice about important information to include. Within the site, there should be an e-mail link and a telephone number to contact the school. A prompt, accurate, and friendly response maintains potential applicants' interest in the school.

Other effective marketing tools are videos, DVDs, or CD-ROMs that capture attention by portraying the nursing profession and its varied career opportunities, the school of nursing, and the curriculum, in a dynamic, positive light. Although there are associated costs, these initiatives could stimulate trans-professional linkages by drawing on the expertise of faculty from other disciplines such as journalism, business, dramatic and visual arts, and information technology.

University and college academic fairs, nursing education fairs, open-houses at the school of nursing, and visits to secondary schools by nursing faculty, students, and recent graduates, will interest prospective students. Community outreach clinics by students and faculty, and spotlights on the school through press, radio, or television, could keep communities informed of the nursing curriculum. As well, posters on buses, subways, and billboards would place the school of nursing in the public eye.

Co-op opportunities for secondary school students that include attending some nursing classes or laboratory sessions could stimulate interest in the profession for individuals making career decisions. Job shadowing informs prospective applicants about the profession and the nursing curriculum. Additionally, short summer programs designed for middle and secondary school students to "be a nurse for a week" would plant the seeds for developing future nurses.

When trying to appeal to prospective applicants, the inclusion of nursing students and recent graduates who are similar to the target audience is useful. Applicants are more likely to identify with them than with members of an aging professoriate. Without doubt, potential applicants will be attracted only if the curriculum matches their expectations and personal aspirations (Walker, 2007).

Contractual Agreements

Healthcare and Community Agencies

Nursing programs are usually required to have formal agreements with agencies in which students have clinical experience. Administrators in the educational institution, on behalf of faculty and students, negotiate these affiliation or contractual agreements. Signed copies of the agreements are retained in the nursing school and the agencies providing learning experiences.

Developing working relationships with agency personnel begins with an initial contact with agency staff. During early meetings, the nature and expected outcomes of the practice experience can be explored and clarified. Agency personnel can explain the requirements of the setting and their expectations for students and faculty. These first meetings provide the basis for establishing a contract or formal agreement, later negotiated by administrative and legal personnel of both settings. The nature of the experience will influence whether a letter of agreement or formal contract is necessary, or if a letter with general terms could be followed by a contract with arrangements specified.

Meetings of faculty and agency staff are also necessary to complete the arrangements and discuss details of the learning experiences, such as:

- Intended outcomes and nature of the experience
- Numbers and level of students
- Students' schedules and roles
- Faculty members' roles
- Staff expectations and roles
- Other details important in the experience

These discussions confirm the appropriateness of faculty members' prior decisions about agencies and units to be used for clinical placements. These choices are linked to intended learning outcomes, nature of available learning experiences, clients, compatibility of school and agency philosophies, practice model in use, staff, and resources and support for students (Chaffer, 1998; Dolbear, 2005; Gaberson & Oermann, 2007; Goldenberg & Iwasiw, 1988; Hopkins, 2000).

Legal Areas of Concern   Nurse educators are concerned about issues related to student-educational-institutional relationships and their own professional liability if students make an error in their care activities. The calendar (bulletin) and other school documents, such as the student handbook, represent an agreement between students and the educational institution and should include a policy about safe clinical practice. In the practice setting, these documents have legal implications as they guide student and faculty behavior. Both should be familiar with the intended outcomes for the clinical experience, guidelines for clinical evaluation and grading, and policies relevant to clinical practice.

The responsibility and accountability of the educational institution, clinical or community agency, faculty, students, and agency staff should be clarified. All matters related to the legal aspects of clinical education are addressed when contracts are negotiated and arrangements made for student practice.

Insurance   Contracts with community and healthcare agencies generally stipulate that the educational institution must have insurance for student practice. The insurance policies should be made known to faculty and students and address matters, such as harm to clients, faculty and student liability, student injuries, and equipment loss or breakage. Additionally, the educational institution might require that students have malpractice insurance; faculty generally have professional liability insurance.

Additional Considerations Other matters may be addressed in discussions, formal contracts, or letters of agreement between the school of nursing and the healthcare or community agency. These might include considerations listed below:

- Whether full names of all students and instructors be specified prior to the experience (O'Connor, 2001)
- The maximum number of students who can be supervised by one instructor (O'Connor)
- An orientation of faculty and students to agency policies and procedures
- Health requirements, CPR, and first-aid certification of faculty and students
- Whether student experiences will proceed if faculty are absent
- Patients' or clients' rights with respect to care by students
- Responsibilities of staff in relation to student learning.

Other Educational Institutions

Formal arrangements made with other educational institutions depend on the nature of the relationship. Purchased courses on a fee-for-service basis offered at other institutions may not require a formal contract. Rather, a letter of agreement specifying the arrangements might suffice. However, for partnerships (such as collaborative or consortium), contractual agreements are typical. Responsibilities of all partners for developing, approving, and implementing the curriculum, and for financing, are specified.

Logistics

Planning for successful implementation of the nursing curriculum necessitates attention to certain logistics. Success requires a commitment by all stakeholders to the mission of the institution, purpose of education in general and nursing education in particular, and the curriculum philosophical approaches and outcomes. Additionally, there must be sufficient finances and human resources to mount and implement the curriculum, matters that should be attended to while the curriculum is being developed. Attention must be also given to course scheduling and phasing out the existing curriculum.

Personnel

Faculty Sufficient numbers of qualified faculty to teach the courses is of paramount importance. Nursing deans/directors will need to plan whom to retain, recruit, and appoint. Characteristics of suitable faculty include knowledge of relevant content, teaching skills, practice competence (especially those clinical teaching in practice courses), effective interpersonal relationships, and personal attributes of effective teachers. Faculty should be assigned to courses on the basis of their expertise and preferences, and in accordance with faculty workload agreements.

Some faculty will probably be required to teach in the existing and redesigned curricula simultaneously, and they may feel overstretched as they strive for excellence in both. The dean/director must be cognizant of suitable teaching assignments for individuals and ensure that not too much is expected. Conversely, some faculty may be faced with the prospect of a lightened teaching assignment, or even with no obvious teaching responsibilities for a semester or an academic year, as the redesigned curriculum is being introduced. The dean/director is responsible for ensuring that teaching loads are consistent with workload agreements, that there is a perception of fairness, and that faculty and students are well served in the process.

In the event that additional faculty will be required, they must be hired if available. As well, adjunct faculty could be engaged for some of the teaching. Inevitably, this would necessitate planning and organizing faculty orientation and development sessions that would require experienced and willing faculty to conduct these activities. When curriculum implementation is being planned, attention should be given to faculty shortages, turnover, retention, retirement, and renewal.

It is also possible that fewer faculty, or faculty with different expertise than the current faculty will be required. This could result in the loss of valued members who do not hold permanent appointments. It is incumbent upon the dean/director to minimize the pain to these individuals and their teaching colleagues.

Support Staff Administrative, secretarial, and clerical services must be in place to implement the curriculum successfully. Personnel such as an administrative assistant and/or secretary to the dean or director, secretaries for undergraduate and graduate programs, and staff to manage student practice placements, are to be aligned with the redesigned curriculum.

Scheduling

Most educational institutions require scheduling requests for classrooms, laboratories, and practice experiences far in advance of the term in which they are needed. In view of increasing enrollments in post-secondary institutions, and commensurate with budget limitations to fund new classrooms and buildings, equitable and careful planning and allocation of space and equipment are necessary. Administrators in the school of nursing, therefore, must have such data prepared in accordance with institutional deadlines so courses can be timetabled. This may entail some negotiation before classroom and laboratory schedules are finalized.

Similarly, healthcare and community agencies have deadlines for placement requests. Scheduling for student experiences requires joint planning with personnel from other programs and institutions. Learners in other nursing programs, medicine, physical therapy, occupational therapy, psychology, and social work, also need practice experiences. Therefore, placement schedules for all these groups must be coordinated within each healthcare or community agency where learning experiences occur.

Phasing out the Existing Curriculum and Introducing the Redesigned Curriculum

The process of phasing out the existing curriculum and introducing the redesigned one requires careful attention. It is common for experiences in a changed curriculum to be sequenced differently than in the previous one. Accordingly, learners in both curricula may require similar classroom courses, and access to the same practice sites, at the same time. This curriculum overlap must be accounted for so that neither group feels disadvantaged and practice sites are not overwhelmed by student numbers.

In addition to considering faculty workload during curriculum change, thoughtful attention must be given to the sensitivities of learners in both the existing and redesigned curriculum. References by faculty to the 'old' and 'new' curriculum can heighten negative feelings. Learners in the existing curriculum might feel that their program is outdated and that faculty interest lies with the altered curriculum. Special attention should be given to this group so they do not harbor resentment. In contrast, the first students admitted to the redesigned curriculum often feel that they are 'guinea pigs,' an experimental group on which new educational approaches are being tested. This perception may be reinforced by the fact that curricular refinements will occur for the second class. Faculty should consistently demonstrate confidence in both curricula and convey their belief that all students are receiving an education that will lead to competent nursing practice.

Further, faculty must think about how much overlap from the redesigned curriculum into the existing one is permissible. Understandably, as faculty members become immersed in altered philosophical and teaching-learning approaches, and emphasize different concepts, they begin to introduce these into the current curriculum. As well, they are influenced by altered curriculum outcomes and can unintentionally modify their expectations of learners in the curriculum that is being phased out. It is worthwhile for faculty to discuss this overlap and come to agreement about alterations (if any) that will occur so that a suitable balance is achieved between introducing learners to new perspectives and maintaining the integrity of the existing curriculum.

Faculty Development

Faculty support of the redesigned curriculum is foundational to success, and this support develops as the curriculum is being shaped. As Scales (1985) commented, "Faculty [who have] developed the curriculum . . . will own, honor, and respect the curriculum and will aggressively and actively implement it" (p. 108). The foregoing notwithstanding, active support of faculty is necessary as the redesigned curriculum is introduced. In particular, faculty development activities can support new teaching-learning and evaluation processes that are consonant with the philosophical approaches and outcomes of the changed curriculum. Faculty development should be an ongoing process, not merely a short-term orientation to the curriculum.

For faculty members who have not been involved in curriculum development, such as part-time clinical instructors, planned faculty development is vital. If the implemented curriculum is to have intervention fidelity, then all members with a responsibility for facilitating and evaluating student learning must be fully immersed in its tenets.

In a study linking professional development activities and program fidelity in a science curriculum, teachers' adherence to the curriculum was positively related to professional development about a number of faculty development concerns:

- Attention to implementation, such as alignment of the curriculum to standards and use of inquiry methods in their classrooms
- Content of the science curriculum
- Presence of ongoing, meaningful professional development within the schools
- Availability of equipment and technical support (Penuel, Fishman, Yamaguchi, & Gallagher, 2007).

These findings support the idea that faculty development related to the curriculum nucleus and how it is expressed and implemented is obligatory for successful implementation of the nursing curriculum.

Chapter Summary

Planning the details of curriculum implementation requires focused attention concurrently with curriculum development to ensure implementation fidelity. The logistics of curriculum implementation involve planning for personnel, scheduling, and phasing out the existing curriculum while introducing the redesigned one. Curriculum plans should be public, and this requires intentional efforts to keep all stakeholders informed. Marketing is important, as are contractual agreements with healthcare, community, and other educational institutions. Ongoing faculty development is key to implementation consistent with the curriculum design.

‸‿Synthesis
Activities:‸

In this chapter, two cases are again presented, one with a critique and the second followed by questions to guide analysis. Then, questions are presented to stimulate thinking when planning curriculum implementation.

Hercal Community College

The faculty of the Hercal Community College associate degree nursing program have been successful in enrolling increased numbers of first-year students. Attention to student recruitment and retention has been ongoing for the past 2 years in response to state and national nursing shortages. A revised curriculum, just completed, is to be implemented in the fall for 95 incoming students.

Active advertising for four additional faculty members to accommodate the increased enrollment has proven unsuccessful. There are no additional faculty to augment the existing pool of 15 full-time members. With classes to resume in 2 months, the director of the school has called a meeting of faculty to discuss workloads for the forthcoming academic year. Responsibilities for classroom and clinical teaching are to be allocated, with the goal of distributing workloads evenly while remaining within the union contract.

Local agencies have been contacted for practice experiences. These include one 300-bed, acute-care hospital and one 150-bed chronic and rehabilitation institution, where first- and second-year students have had practice experiences caring for senior, middle, and young adults, as well as children. Directors of these agencies are satisfied with previous arrangements, and further discussion was not deemed necessary.

However, to accommodate the increased number of students needing practice experiences, the director and faculty agreed that an experience with healthy school-aged children could be included for first-year students, in addition to caring for adult clients. Because of the limited time to plan for this experience, the director of the school telephoned the community health nurse manager responsible for school health. The manager agreed to the director's request for student placement.

Plans for implementation of the revised curriculum are in place. Faculty are determined to demonstrate respect for all learners and both curricula. They agreed not to refer to the two curricula as 'old' and 'new'. Faculty expressed commitment to assist all students to meet curriculum outcomes and attain professional standards. With the revised curriculum planned, and the existing curriculum ongoing, the faculty are ready to implement the revised curriculum.

Critique

The director and faculty of Hercal Community College associate degree program have done well to complete their revised curriculum. They have increased enrollment in response to the need for more nurses. The faculty have also met to adjust their workloads to 'cover' classroom and clinical teaching within the boundaries of their contract. It is apparent that they are a unified, caring group, as exemplified by their commitment to implement the revised curriculum, complete the existing one, treat all learners equally, and help them reach curriculum outcomes. Also noteworthy is the successful working relationship the director has with the public health nurse manager.

The agreement by the faculty to share the workload, while honorable on the surface, may not, however, be feasible. Increased teaching responsibilities in both curricula could prove onerous over time, and lead to dissatisfaction, if not to ineffective teaching. It would be wise for the director to hire part-time instructors and clinical teachers, at least for the forthcoming year, and use the 2 summer months for faculty development activities for teachers who may be inexperienced and/or unfamiliar with the curriculum. This investment could motivate such faculty to consider a full-time appointment. Active faculty recruitment efforts should be also undertaken to accommodate future enrollment.

Selecting a new experience for first-year students could be appropriate because of increased numbers. However, there has been no meeting with the community health manager and staff to discuss the purpose of the experience (where students have not been previously placed), scheduling, number of students, or roles and responsibilities of staff, faculty, and students. Scheduled meetings to discuss these matters, as well as contractual arrangements between the college and community health agency, should be planned. Further, if any of the clinical placements are to occur within the local city schools, involvement of the school principals (and possibly school board legal staff) is necessary.

Jasmine University School of Nursing

Faculty of Jasmine University School of Nursing have worked diligently to develop a new curriculum. Although they considered the advantages of an upper-division nursing program, they decided to continue with their 4-year integrated curriculum. The new curriculum is based in phenomenology, feminism, and humanism, with a strong emphasis on community-based nursing. However, hospital-based practice remains a feature of the curriculum. Concurrent with the introduction of the new curriculum will be a 50% increase in the class size from 100 to 150.

For more than 35 years, university students have had on-campus classes from Monday to Wednesday, with hospital and community practice on Thursday and Friday, during the day. Other nursing programs in the city have had clinical experiences at other times.

As they discuss phasing out the existing curriculum and introducing the redesigned one, faculty members identify a significant problem with clinical placements. Currently, fourth-year students have an experience on maternal-infant units in the fall semester. In the changed curriculum, this experience is scheduled in the fall and winter semesters of the second year (75 students in each semester). Both groups have 2 days of practice each week. This means that for 2 consecutive years, 100 fourth-year students and 75 second-year students require placements on the same units on the same days in the fall semester. In addition, the popularity of home births, hospital discharges 8–24 hours after delivery, and city-wide hospital restructuring, will lead to a 40% decrease in the number of beds for labor and delivery, and post-partum care.

Questions for Consideration of the Jasmine University Case

1. What are the logistical considerations in this case?
2. What options are possible to address this situation?
3. What are the likely implications for students, faculty, and clinical agency personnel for each of the options proposed?
4. Should faculty reconsider the design of the new curriculum? Justify whether or not they should.
5. In what ways can faculty prevent situations such as this when a revised curriculum is being planned and implemented?

Curriculum Development Activities for Consideration in Your Setting

The questions below are intended to guide thinking as you plan curriculum implementation.

1. What planning steps are critical for successful curriculum implementation?
2. How can stakeholders be informed of the developing curriculum and implementation plans?
3. How can a smooth transition to the changed curriculum in practice sites be ensured? How can clinical faculty inform practitioners of the proposed curriculum changes? How else can agency stakeholders be informed?
4. Who will be responsible for exploring learning opportunities in new practice sites? For initiating contract discussions? For orienting staff to the curriculum and course competencies?
5. Which marketing strategies could be used? Who will be responsible for them? Who could help with marketing?
6. How can necessary human, physical, and financial resources be ensured to implement the curriculum?
7. Who will be responsible for apprising administrative personnel of the scheduling needs within the new curriculum?
8. What strategies might alleviate student concerns about being learners in a redesigned curriculum? Similarly, how might concerns of learners in an existing curriculum be alleviated?
9. What are the plans for phasing out the existing curriculum?
10. Which ongoing faculty development activities could be planned?

References

Chaffer, D. (1998). Places please. *Nursing Standard, 12*(40), 25.

Dolbear, G. (2005, August). Clinical placement: Capacity and quality. *Synergy,* 19–22.

Gaberson, K. B., & Oermann, M. H. (2007). *Clinical teaching strategies in nursing* (2nd ed.). New York: Springer.

Goldenberg, D., & Iwasiw, C. (1988). Criteria used for patient selection for nursing students' hospital clinical experience. *Journal of Nursing Education, 27*(6), 258–265.

Hopkins, S. (2000). Support for students. *Nursing Management, 7*(7), 36–37.

O'Connor, A. B. (2001). *Clinical instruction and evaluation. A teaching resource.* Boston: Jones and Bartlett and National League for Nursing.

O'Donnell, C. L. (2008). Defining, conceptualizing and measuring fidelity of implementation and its relationship to outcomes in K–12 curriculum intervention research. *Review of Educational Research, 78*(1), 33–84.

Penuel, W. R., Fishman, B. J., Yamaguchi, R., & Gallagher, L. P. (2007). What makes professional development effective? Strategies that foster curriculum implementation. *Educational Research Journal, 44*(4), 921–958.

Scales, F. S. (1985). *Nursing curriculum development, structure, function.* Norwalk, CT: Appleton-Century-Croft.

Walker, K. (2007). Fast-track for fast times: Catching and keeping generation Y in the nursing workforce. *Contemporary Nurse: A Journal for the Australian Nursing Profession, 24*(2), 147–158.

CHAPTER 12

Planning Curriculum Evaluation

Chapter Overview

Planning curriculum evaluation is an ongoing process, which begins simultaneously with curriculum design. Nursing faculty and administrators are not only responsible for ongoing internal appraisal of the curriculum, but also preparation for program evaluation by external organizations. The definition, overview, and purposes of curriculum evaluation, as well as the benefits for faculty, are described. Evaluation models are overviewed and categorized. Planning evaluation, establishing standards, and determining data-gathering approaches are then addressed. Contained as well is more specific information about planning evaluation of curriculum components. Evaluation of curriculum outcomes, human and physical resources, learning climate, and policies are also addressed. Attention is given to judging curriculum quality, reporting results, and reflecting on the process. Finally, a brief discussion of faculty development activities related to planning curriculum evaluation is followed by the chapter summary and synthesis activities. These include two cases for discussion and questions to guide evaluation planning in individual settings.

Chapter Goals

- Appreciate evaluation planning as a component of curriculum development.
- Understand the purposes of internal and external curriculum evaluation.
- Gain insight into models of curriculum evaluation.
- Consider evaluation of individual curriculum components.
- Recognize the value of faculty development for curriculum evaluation.

Definitions of *Curriculum Evaluation* and *Program Evaluation*

Curriculum evaluation is an organized and thoughtful appraisal of those elements central to the course of studies undertaken by students, as well as graduates' abilities. Curriculum evaluation involves establishment of standards, systematic data gathering, application of the standards, and formulation of judgments about the value, quality, utility, effectiveness or significance of the curriculum (Fitzpatrick, Sanders, & Worthen, 2004). The aspects to be evaluated include the philosophical approaches, foutcome statements, design, courses, and teaching-learning and evaluation strategies. Also assessed are actual curriculum outcomes, implementation fidelity [the extent to which the curriculum is operationalized as it was conceived (see Chapter 11)], human and physical resources, learning climate, and policies.

In contrast, *program evaluation* encompasses a wider scope of elements. In addition to all aspects of curriculum evaluation, program evaluation includes attention to institutional support for the school; administrative structure of the school; faculty members' teaching, research, and professional activities; the school's relationships with other academic units; student support services; relationships with healthcare and community agencies; and so forth.

Curriculum evaluation is *utilization-focused evaluation,* that is "the focus [is] on the intended use by the intended users" (Patton, 1997, p. 20). Therefore, the evaluation questions and processes include matters that are significant to the users, most notably students and faculty. The knowledge generated and the appraisal or judgment (evaluation) attached to the data are context-specific and applicable for a particular point in time (Alkin & Taut, 2003). Moreover, curriculum evaluation is dependent on participatory and collaborative approaches. Curriculum developers, implementers, evaluation designers, evaluators, and evaluation users are all faculty members who work together, along with other stakeholders, to achieve the evaluation purposes.

Overview of the Curriculum Evaluation Process

The first, and possibly the most important step in curriculum or program evaluation, is to decide the purposes of the evaluation. Why is the curriculum being evaluated, and how will the evaluation data be used?

Agreement about the purposes leads to the selection of a suitable evaluation model. This choice is influenced by the curriculum's philosophical orientation, family members' familiarity with various models, match between the evaluation purposes and models, and the time span in which the evaluation must be completed and subsequent decisions made. Then, evaluation questions based on the purpose and model are formulated. From this, the precise elements to be evaluated are determined and standards defined.

An overall curriculum evaluation framework must be designed, with participants, accountabilities, required data, data sources, data-gathering methods, and timelines defined. Also included in the evaluation design are a system to manage data, plans to analyze and interpret data, and procedures to report results. An evaluation of the overall process is the final step (Fink, 2005; Fitzpatrick et al., 2004; Jacobs & Koehn, 2004; Killion, 2003a, 2003b; Patton, 1997). In addition to evaluating the process, participants can identify the learning they have gained from the process.

Purposes of Internal Curriculum Evaluation and External Program Evaluation

Purposes of Internal Curriculum Evaluation

Internal curriculum evaluation is conducted by members of a school of nursing to determine the curriculum strengths, weaknesses, merits, and deficits. Additionally, identification of possible future directions for the curriculum is typically an outcome of the evaluation process (Chen, 2005). As a quality control mechanism, the intent of curriculum evaluation is to assure that the curriculum, its courses, the processes undertaken, and student achievement of intended outcomes are meeting the required standards.

More specifically, the purposes of curriculum evaluation in nursing education are to determine the extent to which:

- The curriculum is relevant for its context
- It is internally consistent
- Implementation fidelity is maintained
- Outcomes are congruent with the curricular intent and demands of the external context
- Students, faculty, graduates, and employers are satisfied.

Two other reasons for curriculum evaluation are: (1) to obtain data that will influence decisions about curriculum maintenance, refinement, modification, reorganization, or discontinuance and replacement; and (2) to ensure that the curriculum is meeting defined standards.

Furthermore, curriculum evaluation results can be used to justify fiscal and other resource requests and allocations, determine faculty development needs, and fulfill approval and/or accreditation requirements.

Formative evaluation is carried out at regular intervals during curriculum implementation. The purpose is to provide evidence about the feasibility and effectiveness of a portion of the curriculum so that ongoing revisions and improvements can be made. As such, formative evaluation is more than mere *feedback*; it is feedback in relation to a standard (Taras, 2005). Formative evaluation involves purposeful data-gathering, comparison of the data to a standard, and rendering of a judgment about a gap (if any exists) between the data and the standard. Therefore, standards must be in place so that a judgment can be made about feasibility and effectiveness. The principal data sources are teachers and students, and along with administrators, they are the main audience for formative curriculum evaluation (Oermann & Gaberson, 2006).

Summative evaluation is carried out at the completion of a portion of, or the total curriculum. The purpose is to judge the effectiveness of the curriculum, and this becomes the basis of recommendations about maintenance, revision, or discontinuance. Evidence is obtained from faculty members, learners, graduates, administrators, employers, and other stakeholders. Audiences for summative evaluation results are those who provide evidence, as well as regulatory bodies, funders, and consumers (Oermann & Gaberson, 2006).

Whether data are collected for formative or summative evaluation, there is an implicit expectation by those providing the data that curriculum alterations will be forthcoming. Therefore, in all internal curriculum evaluations, often unstated and possibly unrecognized purposes include assuring stakeholders:

- Faculty are committed to ensuring curriculum quality
- The curriculum is responsive to influences within and beyond the school of nursing
- Learners will graduate from a dynamic and context-relevant curriculum.

Purposes of External Program Evaluation

External curriculum evaluation is undertaken as part of a more extensive program evaluation conducted for approval or accreditation by an outside agency. State or provincial approval and national accreditation are processes by which an external organization evaluates and recognizes an institution or program of study as meeting certain predetermined criteria.

Approval Nursing program approval is a compulsory evaluation or review process concerned primarily with the protection of public interests. This protection is accomplished by ensuring that a program has met prescribed minimum standards set by a body designated in state or provincial legislation, or according to regulations authorized by that legislation. Every nursing program leading to licensure examinations must meet the standards of the body authorized to regulate nursing. Approval indicates that a nursing program is of a quality sufficient for graduates to be allowed to write the licensing examination. The schools cannot operate without approval, since graduates would not be eligible to write the licensing examination.

In the United States, approval by state boards of nursing is required for all nursing education programs. In Canada, approval is granted by provincial nursing regulatory bodies. However, in some provinces national accreditation of baccalaureate programs is required by the provincial body, and accreditation may replace a separate approval process.

Accreditation   Accreditation is an endorsement of a nursing program by a nongovernmental agency concerned with nursing education; national accreditation is understood to connote excellence. The accreditation process is voluntary (although mandatory in Ontario). It is a rigorous appraisal of the program to determine the extent to which it meets standards set by the profession. Nursing programs undergo accreditation to demonstrate their quality to the consumers of their products (students, alumni, employers (Heydman, 2006). Accreditation can be important in attracting students and faculty, and it can influence a school's eligibility for outside funding, graduates' entrance to subsequent programs, and students' ability to obtain grants or loans.

The major accrediting organization for licensed practical, diploma, and associate degree nursing programs in the United States is the National League for Nursing Accrediting Commission (NLNAC). Baccalaureate and graduate nursing programs are accredited by the NLNAC and the Commission on Collegiate Nursing Education. In Canada, accreditation exists only for baccalaureate programs. The Canadian Association of Schools of Nursing (CASN) is the accrediting body. These organizations are authorized to make accreditation decisions within their established policies.

Benefits of Curriculum Evaluation for Faculty Members

Because it is the faculty who plan and undertake curriculum evaluation, determine recommendations from the evaluation data, and agree on subsequent actions, the value of curriculum evaluation extends beyond improvements to the curriculum itself. The process has rewards. For example, faculty members may experience benefits such as pride in being part of a progressive, dynamic program, or the social rewards and empowerment that accrue from engaging in important activities with colleagues and stakeholders. Curriculum improvements may yield increased learner satisfaction, resulting in a more congenial environment.

Individually and collectively, faculty members may increase their awareness and appreciation of curriculum evaluation and its value. They may expand their capacity to design and implement curriculum evaluation processes, and this will have relevance throughout their careers. Importantly, through curriculum evaluation, some members may modify or develop deeper conceptual understandings of some aspects of the curriculum (Alkin & Taut, 2003), and this could inherently improve their teaching. Finally, the curriculum evaluation process may extend faculty members' capability to develop practical curriculum recommendations based on systematically collected data, and this in turn, could augment their sense of empowerment. These benefits are independent of the evaluation findings (Robinson & Cousins, 2004).

Curriculum Evaluation Models

A curriculum evaluation model is a framework that guides the evaluation of a curriculum. Variations in models arise from differing conceptions and definitions of *evaluation*. Accordingly, they differ in the emphasis placed on the curricular aspects to be examined, the approaches to data-gathering, and the basis of judging the quality of the curriculum. The models provide a path for planning and conducting evaluation, not a detailed roadmap.

Evaluation models and approaches range from checklists and suggestions to comprehensive appraisals. In nursing education, evaluation of the total curriculum is comprehensive, since a holistic evaluation is most appropriate for a unified curriculum. It is typically based on standards of quality and incorporates both quantitative and qualitative approaches.

Predetermined structure and criteria generally employ quantitative approaches, although not exclusively. Examples are Scriven's Goal-Free Model, Provus' Discrepancy Evaluation Model, and program logic models. Questionnaires are typically used for some data collection. In contrast, qualitative models are more open. For example, the constructivist (fourth-generation) evaluation model addresses the concerns, claims, and issues of stakeholders, and the methods to examine these are negotiated with stakeholders (Guba & Lincoln, 2001). If the appreciative inquiry model is used, the focus is to discover what is working well and then to build on the positive through dialogue (Cooperrider & Whitney, 2005). In qualitative approaches, data are obtained through direct observations and interviews.

Typology of Evaluation Models

Evaluation models have been categorized into many typologies. Each classification system presents a different perspective on educational and service program evaluation, even though many of the same models are included. For instance, Stufflebeam, Madaus, and Kellaghan (2000) labeled models as questions/methods-oriented, improvement/accountability-oriented, and social agenda (advocacy)-oriented. Fitzpatrick et al. (2004) identified them as: objectives-, management-, consumer-, expertise-, and participant-oriented. Guba and Lincoln's (1989) typology classified models as to first, second, third and fourth generations, according to the evaluation focus. See Table 12-1 for a summary of the four generations of evaluation models.

Many curriculum and program evaluation models used in nursing education and service are third-generation models. Several are summarized in Table 12-2. Increasingly, however,

Table 12-1 Summary of First, Second, Third, and Fourth Generation Evaluation Models

First Generation (technical)	**Measurement** (Prior to WWI): Students were targeted for evaluation. Tests were developed to measure variables of interest. Student scores were used to determine curriculum success.
Second Generation (description and technical)	**Description** (Post WWI): Curriculum was targeted for evaluation in an objectives-oriented (Tylerian) description approach (patterns, strengths, and weaknesses related to specific objectives). Congruence between student performance and described objectives was assessed. The program, materials, teaching strategies, organizational patterns, and "treatments" were evaluated. Measurement was redefined as one of several tools to use.
Third Generation (judgment-based, description, and technical)	**Judgment** (Post 1967): Program goals and performance were targeted for evaluation. Judgments about merit and worth were based on standards. Information collected depended on the evaluation model, e.g., decisions (decision-oriented models); experienced "effects" (goal-free models); internalized guideposts (connoisseurship models).
Fourth Generation (holistic and inclusive)	**Responsive, Constructivist, Naturalistic** (Post late 1970s): Took into account the claims (values), concerns, and issues of those involved in the evaluation (students, faculty, clients, administrators). It is a *responsive* (determines parameters and boundaries through an interactive, negotiated process that involves stakeholders), *constructivist* (interpretive, hermeneutic, relates to the methodology employed), *naturalistic* (sociopolitical, diagnostic, change-oriented, education process) and rejects the controlling, manipulative, experimental approach. Results in a constructed understanding of needed improvements and changes, based on consensus of all stakeholders.

Source: Some data from Guba, E., & Lincoln, Y. (1989). *Fourth Generation Evaluation*. Newbury Park, CA: Sage.

elements of third- and fourth-generation models are combined to yield richer evaluations. For example, use of program logic models in evaluation is built on concepts underlying Provus's Discrepancy Evaluation Model (Fitzpatrick et al., 2004). This is primarily a third-generation model, since the focus of the evaluation and the indicators are known in advance. However, attention to stakeholders' concerns, claims, and interests may also be negotiated, more like fourth-generation evaluation.

Rationale for Choice of an Evaluation Model

Each evaluation approach has particular strengths that illuminate different aspects of the curriculum. Therefore, selection of a curriculum evaluation model, or evaluation approach, should be contingent upon the purpose of the evaluation, the questions to be addressed, the issues that

Table 12-2 Summary of Several Third Generation Evaluation Models

Models in Chronological Order	Description
Scriven's (1967, 1972) goal-free	Measures all outcomes/effects of program, regardless of program goals or objectives. There are no pre-specified objectives. May be applied to total or sections of the curriculum.
Donabedian's (1969) quality assurance	Measures efficiency and effectiveness of courses or units of study. Component parts include trial, structure, purpose and output.
Stufflebeam's (1971) CIPP	Involves decisions about planning (**C**ontext); structuring (**I**nput); implementing (**P**rocess); and recycling (**P**roduct). Investigates: what needs to be done; how it should be done; if it is being done; and if it succeeded. Assesses and reports on merit, worth, probability, significance.
Provus' (1971) discrepancy evaluation	Compares performance with standards, to determine if a discrepancy exists between the two. Includes 5 stages: definition of program, installation of program, process, product or outcomes, and cost-benefit analysis. Involves intended vs. actual outcomes, and effects.
Stake's (1972) (countenance) congruence-contingency	Involves congruence (agreement between desired and actual outcomes), and contingency (relationship among variables). Takes into account: *antecedents* (characteristics of students, teachers, curriculum, facilities, materials, organization, community); *transactions* (all educational experiences); *outcomes* (abilities, achievements, and attitudes resulting from educational experience).
Renzulli's (1972) key features	Considers major concerns of groups who have a direct or indirect interest in the program. Key features are prime interest groups and time.
Parlett & Hamilton's (1972) illuminative evaluation	Proposes that understanding of the curriculum is possible only in its wider contexts and in the biography of each course. The approach is not pre-determined but develops as issues or problems are identified. It is an ethno-graphic approach with two core concepts: instructional systems (courses) and learning milieu.
Stenhouse (1975)	Discloses meaning of curriculum, purposes of courses, problems amenable to solutions, influence of context on curriculum, and whether the evaluation contributes to theory development. Includes five criteria: meaning, potential, interest, conditionality, and elucidation.
Eisner's (1977, 1985) connoisseur/critic	Premise is that experts (connoisseurs) can understand and appreciate subtle qualities of the classroom or program, and merits of the teacher and curriculum.
Starpoli and Waltz (1978)	Includes specific questions of concern to varied audiences, depending on what is being evaluated. Specifies decision-makers for each question, i.e., who should be responsible for evaluation activities, and how evaluation will proceed. There are four distinct, interrelated levels of evaluation: school, program, sub-program, course level; and three frames: input, operations, output.

Table 12-2 continued

Model	Description
Stufflebeam's (1983) educational decision	Educational decision-making model which addresses four concerns: a) *context*: setting, mission, community, philosophy, internal/external focus; b) *input*: resources, support systems; learners, program plan; c) *process*: implementation, teaching/learning strategies and transactions, learning materials, efficiency and effectiveness; d) *product*: learner outcomes and satisfaction; all to facilitate decision-making.
Wholey's (1983) Program logic model (based on Provus's model)	Compares program progress against pre-determined indictors. Assesses logical linkages (as described by the program model) among parts of the program, such as resources and activities, program processes, outcomes, outputs, and impact.
Stake's (1991) education	Is organized around issues and concerns of stakeholders (students, faculty, administrators, parents, employers); goal is to discover merits and weakness of the program. Data generated to respond to identified issues and concerns.

Source: Some data from Herbener & Watson, 1992; Stufflebeam, Madaus, & Kellaghan, 2000; Stufflebeam, 2007; Valley of the Sun United Way, 2006; Wholey, 1983.

must be taken into account, available resources, and faculty preference for one model over another. Applegate (1998) suggests the chosen model should be based "on the faculty's beliefs about education [and] the political and institutional context in which the program exists" (p. 183).

Whichever model(s) can provide the best evidence to answer the evaluation questions deemed important within the resource constraints, would be a good choice for evaluating a curriculum. If no one model seems sufficient, a combination of relevant concepts from different models can be used. This eclectic approach, while not an evaluation model as such, might offer more scope than one model, as well as mature, diverse, and sophisticated evaluation strategies (Fitzpatrick et al., 2004). Within a *dynamic evaluation approach,* elements from different models are selected (eclecticism), with the additional feature that ongoing attention is given to assessment and refinement of processes, even as the evaluation is being conducted (Grammatikopoulos, Koustelics, Tsigillis, & Theodorakis, 2004).

As an alternate to choosing one model or using elements from several models, faculty members can design their own models and derive the subsequent evaluation framework so that local purposes are fully incorporated. For example, the Relevance-Congruence-Adequacy-Reasonableness (RCAR) Framework (Iwasiw, 2008) was designed specifically to address curriculum evaluation priorities of the Western–Fanshawe Collaborative BScN Program. The model is presented in Figure 12-1, and Table 12-3 depicts a portion of the evaluation framework derived from the model.

This evaluation model is premised on a philosophy of pragmatism and a belief in the ability of experienced nurse educators to make sound, evidence-based judgments about curriculum quality. From the model, a framework of evaluation questions, indicators, data sources, and data collection methods has been derived. Four dimensions are encompassed in the model, and these provide the criteria and framework for curriculum evaluation:

1. *Relevance* of the:
   - Curriculum for the context in which it is offered and in which graduates will practice nursing
   - Outcomes for the context

2. *Congruence* of the:
   - Curriculum design with the philosophical approaches and curriculum outcomes
   - Implementation with the curriculum nucleus and design (implementation fidelity)
   - Actual outcomes with the curricular intent

3. *Adequacy* of resources to deliver the planned curriculum

4. *Reasonableness* of the curricular demands on students and faculty

Notes:
Relevance   = applicability to, or suitability for current and anticipated contextual circumstances
Congruence   = logical consistency, agreement
Adequacy   = sufficiency
Reasonableness = the state of being possible or sensible

Figure 12-1 Relevance-Congruence-Adequacy-Reasonableness (RCAR) Curriculum Evaluation Model

Source: © C. L. Iwasiw 2008 (used with permission).

In accordance with the premises of utilization-focused evaluation, the model or methods selected and the evaluation design created, should achieve the purposes determined by the prime users of the evaluation results. The approaches used should be practical, cost-effective, and ethical (Patton, 2002).

Table 12-3   Relevancy Dimensions of the Relevancy-Congruency-Adequacy-Reasonableness (RCAR) Curriculum Evaluation Framework

Dimension	Main Questions	Indicators	Data Sources	Data-Gathering Methods	Accountability for Activity
Relevancy	1. To what extent do the philosophical approaches reflect a clear connection with the:				
	• mission and philosophy of the educational institution?	Correlation between the mission and philosophy of the educational institution and curriculum philosophy	Institutional documents	Document review	Faculty task group 1
	• present and anticipated context of nursing practice?	Correlation between philosophical approaches and context	See Chapter 6	See Chapter 6	Faculty task group 2
	2. To what extent do the curriculum outcomes or goals reflect a clear connection with the:				
	• philosophical approaches	Philosophical approaches explicitly evident in outcomes or goals	Curriculum documents	Document review	Faculty task group 1
	• present and anticipated context of nursing practice?	Outcomes or goals are relevant to trends emanating from contextual data	External contextual data and trends	See Chapter 6	Faculty task group 2

Source: © C. L. Iwasiw 2008. Used with permission of the author. The contribution of the Western–Fanshawe Collaborative Program Evaluation Committee is appreciated in the refinement of this document.

Planning Curriculum Evaluation

Planning curriculum evaluation is a dimension of curriculum development that should occur simultaneously with curriculum and course design. Curriculum evaluation is a participatory process with faculty and other stakeholders involved in the planning and implementation. Consensus and shared understanding about the purposes and procedures of the evaluation might lead to more willing acceptance of recommendations that result from the evaluation (De Valenzuela, Copeland, & Blalock, 2005).

Since curriculum evaluation is only one aspect of a school's activities, this undertaking must be confined to that which is necessary to achieve the purposes of the evaluation. Decisions are made about:

- Purposes and audiences of the curriculum evaluation
- How closely the internal curriculum evaluation will reflect the requirements for external approval or accreditation
- Individual or committee responsible for coordinating the curriculum evaluation process
- Evaluation model to be used
- Evaluation questions to be addressed
- Standards and criteria to be used
- Data essential to answer the evaluation questions
- Methods and timing of data-gathering
- Persons responsible for obtaining or providing data
- Repository for the data
- Individuals who will interpret and judge the evidence, and formulate recommendations
- Process to report evaluation results to relevant audiences
- Deadline for completion.

Resolution of these matters in advance of curriculum implementation will allow for organized formative and summative evaluation. The ongoing accumulation of data, and subsequent curriculum refinements, evidence commitment to continuous curriculum improvement. Moreover, if data-gathering for curriculum evaluation is viewed as a regular, expected, and normal part of curriculum implementation, then the stress associated with intermittent internal and external evaluations is markedly lessened.

The decisions outlined above are not made separately. Rather, they are based on iterative discussions that arise from the following questions:

- What are faculty's beliefs and values about curriculum evaluation?
- Why is curriculum evaluation being undertaken?
- What learning is anticipated about the curriculum? What are the evaluation questions to be answered?
- Which evaluation model(s) is/are consistent with the curriculum's philosophical approaches?

- What will constitute quality?
- Which aspects of the curriculum should be evaluated?
- How often and when should the curriculum be evaluated?
- What data are required? How can it be obtained?
- How will evaluation results be used?
- Who will be responsible for managing the evaluation process?

Generally, curriculum evaluation activities are shared among all faculty members. Yet, the overall responsibility must rest with an individual or group, such as the program chair, a curriculum committee, or curriculum evaluation committee, so that efforts are coordinated and complete. Documenting the evaluation efforts and recording results and subsequent curriculum modifications will provide information important for later internal and external curriculum and program evaluations. Inevitably, evidence of systematic and ongoing evaluation, and the results of these appraisals, are required for accreditation.

Establishing Standards, Criteria, and/or Indicators

Decisions about curriculum effectiveness and quality depend on a clear understanding of the standards against which the curriculum is being judged and the criteria used to determine if the standards are being attained. *Standards* are the "authoritative or recognized exemplar[s] of correctness, perfection, or some definite degree of any quality" (Oxford English Dictionary Online, n.d.). *Criteria* are distinguishing characteristics used to judge whether a standard has been achieved. Standards and criteria should be delineated as much as possible. As well, agreement must be reached about whether the standards are absolute or relative (Fitzpatrick et al., 2004).

Delineation of precise standards and criteria for all curriculum components is not possible, necessary, nor feasible. Therefore, it may be more appropriate to define *indicators*, that is, *observations or calculations that show the presence or state of a condition*. For example, the nature of faculty questions during classroom interactions is an indicator of how well class activities assist students to achieve intended course competencies.

Faculty members rely, in part, upon guidelines, standards, and/or criteria for program approval and accreditation when establishing curriculum standards. They might also write standards particular to the school of nursing. As an illustration, one school determined that graduates' success rates on NCLEX will exceed national standards (Jacobs & Koehn, 2004). Consideration should also be given to standards for various curriculum components. For some, such as teaching-learning strategies, the literature is replete with criteria for effective teaching. These can be invaluable in reaching an agreement about school-specific standards. For other components, faculty may have to develop their own standards. *Context-relevance, internal consistency, logical flow*, and *implementation fidelity* are criteria that faculty might choose for both the curriculum design and individual courses.

The specification of standards, criteria, and/or indicators allows faculty to answer the questions: Is this a quality curriculum? On what basis can we say so? The standards, criteria, and indicators must be specific enough to be understandable and provide direction for gathering data and making evaluative judgments, while not being too extensive or overly time-consuming to create. These can be refined in the future, if necessary. As well, experienced and knowledgeable nursing faculty are generally able to recognize the merits and deficits of a curriculum; they are connoisseurs. Faculty might ask themselves questions such as:

- Are the standards, criteria, and/or indicators consistent with the curriculum intent and with those used by external evaluating agencies?

- Do the number and nature of the standards, criteria, and/or indicators seem reasonable?

- Will we be able to exercise reasonable economy of data-gathering effort in assembling evidence about the standards and criteria?

Planning Data-Gathering about the Curriculum

The standards, criteria, and indicators that have been formulated give direction about which data are necessary for curriculum evaluation. Although a wealth of data might be pertinent, only the most significant should be assembled. The same data could provide evidence of the effectiveness of several aspects of the curriculum. For example, learners' reflective journals can indicate the extent to which intended course competencies are being achieved, as well as provide evidence of the appropriateness of the methods by which students demonstrate their achievements. In planning data-gathering, faculty should consider what is reasonable and feasible.

Data-Gathering Methods

Data-gathering methods are linked to the evaluation purposes, model selected, evaluation questions, and predetermined standards. Typically, both qualitative and quantitative methods are employed. The methods and tools should allow for a comprehensive evaluation, be understandable and easy to use, cost- and time- efficient, valid and reliable (if quantitative), and credible (if qualitative).

Quantitative and qualitative data-gathering methods and procedures with which most faculty are already familiar can be employed for curriculum evaluation. Surveys can be used to assess teachers' and students' satisfaction with the curriculum, their views about specific teaching-learning strategies, infusion of the philosophical approaches into the curriculum, aspects of implementation fidelity (such as quality of delivery), and so forth. Interviews (individual or focus groups) can uncover qualitative data from students, faculty, or graduates for similar purposes. Interviews and surveys are also effective in obtaining data from clinicians and employers.

Unstructured observations, and annotations about them, can be useful early in the evaluation process. From these, structured observation based on criteria can be planned. For example, observations of learners in the clinical area can lead to criteria related to students' clinical abilities, attitudes and values, and subsequently to guidelines for structured observations and the acquisition of more specific data. *Anecdotal notes* can be used to record observations related to course competencies, and when accumulated, provide evidence for evaluations of student performance. The evaluations are indicators of whether course competencies are being achieved (Bourke & Ihrke, 2005; Fitzpatrick et al., 2004). Similarly, *peer or expert observation* can provide insights into classroom and clinical teaching-learning encounters and implementation fidelity.

Rating scales, checklists, and *self-reports* are other means of obtaining data for curriculum evaluation. Rating scales could be used to measure abstract concepts, while checklists identify expected behaviors or competencies and related student performance. *Attitude scales* can measure how students and faculty feel about a particular subject or situation, such as a clinical placement or a teaching-learning activity. Faculty could use *self-reports* or *journals* to record their ideas and insights as they implement the curriculum. Similarly, *student narratives* can provide information about their reflections, thoughts, fears, progress, successes, actual outcomes, and ideas for curriculum improvement.

Data Sources

Data sources can include faculty, students, graduates, administrators, clinicians, employers, and nursing leaders, as well as curriculum and course documents. Test scores, essays, journals, and other assignments lead to valuable insights about learners' knowledge, attitudes, and experiences. Records, such as student grades, attrition rates, or success rates on licensure examinations and other external tests, are useful for curriculum evaluation. As well, data can be used from formal evaluation processes already in place, such as institution-wide teaching or course evaluations. Multiple sources produce a fair and balanced system, with the combination making up for the shortcomings of each (Appling, Naumann, & Berk, 2001).

Data-Gathering Schedule

The timing of data-gathering is important. It should begin with the introduction of the first courses so that formative evaluation is undertaken concurrently with curriculum implementation. In this way, early decisions arising from formative evaluation can stabilize the curriculum and prevent problems that might occur in courses yet to be implemented.

Some scheduling seems self-evident. Student evaluation of courses typically occurs at the completion of each course. However, formal course evaluation mandated by educational institutions is unlikely to address all the questions to which curriculum evaluators seek answers. Additional data-gathering should be scheduled when learners are likely to provide opinions about courses without fear of penalty for unfavorable comments, or relinquishing time they feel would be better spent on assignments or studying. Similarly, it is evident that data-gathering about graduates' abilities cannot occur until there are graduates, but timing and frequency must be determined.

A reasonable schedule for gathering pertinent data should be developed. It might be decided that some data do not require annual collection, such as a survey of graduates. This could be undertaken every 2 years. The intent is to ensure that data are obtained as frequently as necessary to provide an adequate basis for meaningful evaluation, yet not so often that the task becomes unduly burdensome.

Managing and Reporting Data

A decision should be made about who will be responsible for data-gathering and compiling, interpreting, and formulating judgments and recommendations. Additionally, there should be a system developed to store data and record evaluation decisions and subsequent actions. When regular reporting to external agencies is necessary, accountability for doing so must be established.

Agreement about reporting evaluation results to stakeholders is important. Reporting procedures and decisions about which information to provide varies among schools of nursing. Some might report a summary of all data and the subsequent curriculum decisions to all stakeholders. Others might emphasize data from a particular stakeholder group to that group. Understandably, stakeholders want to know how their data contributed to decisions and actions about the curriculum. Consequently, decisions are made about when and to whom data and recommendations should be reported. As full a disclosure as possible is desirable.

Finally, a decision is made about whether data gathered for curriculum evaluation will be used for other purposes. If so, who will have access to the data? If teaching or course evaluations beyond standardized institution-wide questionnaires are undertaken, discussion is necessary about how the results will be reported and used. If faculty journals or portfolios are requested, who will read them, and how will they be assessed in relation to the curriculum? Who will receive the results? Will school-specific teaching evaluations be public, if this is not mandated by institutional policies? Will school-specific teaching evaluations be used solely for curriculum evaluation, or will they also be used for promotion and tenure purposes? Agreement about these and similar questions is necessary before curriculum evaluation activities begin.

Deliberating about Data-Gathering Plans

Planning the data-gathering requires attention to the methods to be employed, the scope of data required, and logistics of the undertaking. When developing a plan for data-gathering, faculty might anticipate such questions as:

- What data are required to ascertain if standards are being attained?
- How can data be obtained expeditiously?
- When, how, and from whom will data be collected?
- Which established data-gathering tools could be used? Are they appropriate?
- Who will be responsible for developing, pilot-testing, and approving school-specific data-gathering tools?
- Who will be responsible for obtaining the data?
- Who will have responsibility for overseeing data-gathering and analysis?
- How often will data be collected, reviewed and interpreted, so that conclusions can be drawn and recommendations formulated? Who will participate in this process?
- How and to whom will evaluation results be reported?
- How will evaluation activities, results, and curriculum alterations be documented so that these records can contribute meaningfully to external summative evaluation?
- Will evaluation data be used for faculty evaluation or faculty development purposes?
- What resources are required to conduct these activities?

Planning Evaluation of Curriculum Components

Philosophical Approaches

The philosophical approaches are fundamental to the implementation of the curriculum and to students' beliefs about, and approach to, clients. For the purposes of curriculum evaluation, it is important to know if the philosophical approaches are operational. Essentially, evaluators want to learn the extent to which:

- The philosophical approaches are being enacted in teaching-learning encounters
- Processes used to assess student learning are congruent with the philosophical approaches
- The written description of the philosophical approaches is understandable to learners
- Learners can articulate the philosophical approaches and explain how they act in accordance with these approaches in classroom, clinical, and peer interactions.

Curriculum Outcome Statements

The outcome statements broadly identify the abilities of graduates and incorporate the philosophical approaches and major concepts of the curriculum. The complexity of the abilities should be appropriate for the educational level of the program and be consistent with (or exceed) criteria for approval and/or accreditation. The statements might include a reference to readiness to write licensure examinations.

When planning the evaluation of curriculum outcome statements, faculty want to determine if the outcomes are appropriate and reasonable, in other words, are these the *right* outcomes? More specifically, faculty are interested in the extent to which the curriculum outcome statements:

- Reflect the practice and standards of the educational institution, higher education, the nursing profession, state or provincial licensing bodies, and approval or accrediting organizations
- Are relevant to the healthcare context
- Are appropriate to the program level
- Reflect the curriculum nucleus.

Curriculum Design

When planning evaluation of the curriculum design, the scope of this component becomes evident. The design encompasses the curriculum outcome statements and the configuration of the program of studies (e.g., courses, their sequence, interrelationships, and mode of delivery). As well, it includes teacher and learner activities, and policies governing the curriculum. When planning evaluation of the curriculum design, faculty are interested in the extent to which:

- There is internal consistency (i.e., how well the curriculum elements fit together)
- The design reflects the philosophical approaches and is relevant to the context in which the curriculum is offered
- The configuration of courses supports student achievement of curriculum outcomes
- There is consistency, congruence, and organization among and within courses
- Non-nursing courses facilitate achievement of curriculum outcomes and contribute to a well-rounded liberal education
- Necessary prerequisites are included so learners can be successful
- Students and faculty believe that courses are appropriate and logically sequenced
- Course titles present an image of a conceptually unified curriculum
- The curriculum 'hangs together' as a unified whole.

Curriculum Outcomes

The purpose of all nursing curricula is to prepare graduates who will practice nursing competently in a changing healthcare environment, thereby contributing to the health and quality of life of those they serve. It is essential to determine if current students are progressing toward this outcome and if graduates are successful as they begin practice. Evaluation of actual student outcomes is viewed by some as the most important aspect of curriculum evaluation. The overriding question is whether students are being adequately prepared for professional practice. Success rates on licensure examinations, possibly in comparison to state, provincial, or national results, should be examined as well. Data about the extent to which:

- Students are achieving intended course competencies and curriculum outcomes.
- Students and faculty can articulate philosophical approaches, intended curriculum outcomes, major curriculum concepts, and key professional abilities.
- Students can explain how they use curriculum concepts and philosophical approaches in clinical experiences.
- Graduates feel ready to begin practice.
- New graduates are successful in their positions.
- Employers are satisfied with graduates' nursing practice.

Courses

Evaluation of courses is, in some measure, a microcosm of the total curriculum evaluation. All aspects of course design and implementation are considered. Faculty might determine the extent to which:

- Course competencies are appropriate and linked to curriculum outcome statements.
- Expectations of learners are reasonable
- Learning activities are consistent with the philosophical approaches, principal teaching-learning approaches, and intended course competencies
- Course activities contribute to learners' progress
- Course activities suit the delivery mode
- Teaching-learning strategies and technologies are effective in facilitating learning
- Content is current, evidence-based, related to other fields of study, and logically organized
- Core curriculum and key professional concepts are evident in course materials and classes
- Evaluation methods are appropriate in nature and number.

- Learners have achieved intended course competencies.
- Each course can be justified within the curriculum.
- Each course has been implemented as originally conceived (i.e., has implementation fidelity).
- There are redundancies or deficiencies among courses.

Teaching-Learning Strategies

When planning evaluation of teaching-learning, faculty can be guided by literature that describes effective teaching and desirable teacher competencies, behaviors, or characteristics for classroom and practice courses (Bevis, 2000a, 2000b; Elcigil & Sari, 2008; Gaberson & Oermann, 2007; Gignac-Caille & Oermann, 2001; Gillespie, 2005; Hanson & Stenvig, 2008; Johnsen, Aasgaard, Wahl, & Salminen, 2002; Vandeveer & Norton, 2005). These descriptions generally address the dimensions of professional competence, relationships with students, personal characteristics, evaluation practices, and teaching skills. Ideas from the literature can be adopted, adapted, or extended to suit the curriculum.

The National League for Nursing (2004) has recommended that ". . . evaluation practices do not inhibit . . . faculty efforts to be creative in their approaches to teaching" (p. 49). This implies that evaluation standards, procedures, and judgments should be flexible so that teaching strategies are not fixed and unchanging. In general, faculty seek to answer the following questions:

- What is the nature of student-faculty interactions?
- How do learners respond to the teaching-learning strategies?
- In what ways have faculty affected learners' growth as individuals and future practitioners?

Faculty will also want to know to what extent the following occurs:

- Are teaching-learning strategies congruent with the philosophical and principal teaching-learning approaches?
- Do teaching-learning strategies assist learners in their progress toward course competencies and curriculum outcomes?
- Do teaching-learning strategies respect learner diversity?
- Are learners satisfied with the teaching-learning approaches and strategies?
- Do faculty feel satisfied with the teaching-learning approaches and strategies they employ?

Strategies to Evaluate Student Achievement

Appraisal of strategies to evaluate student achievement is another important dimension of curriculum evaluation. The methods by which students are asked to provide evidence of their learning, and how that evidence is assessed, have great significance to them, and color their reaction to the curriculum. Questions that might be considered when evaluating these strategies are listed below:

- What student evaluation strategies are used throughout the curriculum? Is there diversity or do some strategies predominate?
- How do students and faculty perceive the evaluation strategies with respect to diversity, fairness, and flexibility?
- To what extent:
  - are student evaluation strategies congruent with the philosophical approaches and intended curriculum outcomes?
  - do the strategies provide for demonstration of all types of learning?
  - are evaluation strategies varied within a course, semester, and year to accommodate students': (1) diverse ways of knowing, (2) academic workloads, (3) need for formative and summative feedback, and (4) desire to have input into their evaluation?
  - do student evaluation strategies accommodate faculty members' academic workloads, expertise, and preferences?

Human and Physical Resources

An important dimension of curriculum evaluation is ascertaining if suitable and sufficient human and physical resources are present. When planning curriculum evaluation, faculty ask about the extent to which:

- Academic and clinical faculty are sufficient in numbers and academic preparation to maintain implementation fidelity
- Faculty teaching assignments are aligned with their expertise
- Staff numbers, roles, and functions are reasonable to support the curriculum
- Offices and meeting rooms are available and suitable
- Classrooms are satisfactory in size, structure, comfort, and appearance
- Classrooms and labs are equipped with appropriate and functional technologies
- Clinical placements and experiences match requirements in quality and quantity
- Library holdings are sufficient in number, scope, and quality
- Material resources are adequate.

Learning Climate

The learning climate consists of the social, emotional, and intellectual atmosphere that exists within the school, and within courses offered through distance delivery methods. It is a strong indication of one aspect of implementation fidelity, specifically, the congruence between the espoused philosophical approaches and the philosophical approaches in action. The learning climate strongly influences the satisfaction, psychological comfort, and empowerment of students, faculty, and staff. In planning evaluation of this aspect of the curriculum, faculty determine the extent to which faculty and learners are satisfied with:

- Learning opportunities available
- Settings in which learning occurs
- Flexibility in the curriculum
- Relationships with one another
- Perceived freedom to take intellectual risks and make mistakes without repercussions
- Support available when undertaking new challenges
- Variety of perspectives in course content, discussion, and readings
- Diversity of backgrounds of authors of required texts and readings (Saunders & Kardia, 2004)
- Fostering of responsibility and accountability
- Sense of belonging and feeling of community.

Policies

Curriculum policies are developed to support students' achievement of curriculum outcomes while ensuring that academic standards are maintained. Therefore, in reviewing and evaluating curriculum policies, faculty consider whether the policies are appropriate, reasonable, understood by faculty and learners, and applied consistently. Evaluators might also ascertain if there have been situations that might indicate a need for new policies.

Judging Curriculum Quality and Making Recommendations

Faculty members compare the evaluation data with the standards, criteria, and/or indicators previously defined. They then interpret the extent of correspondence or divergence between the data and the standards to reach a judgment about the quality of the total curriculum and its components. This comparison is more holistic than microscopic, although attention is given to problematic matters in the evaluation data. From conclusions drawn, recommendations are formulated about actions required to maintain or improve curriculum quality. Alternately, there could be a recommendation to discontinue the curriculum and begin afresh with curriculum development.

Reviewing and interpreting evaluation data, reaching a judgment, and making recommendations are typically the responsibilities of a committee. The recommendations are then generally considered by the total faculty group, and if accepted, the specified actions are implemented.

Reporting Evaluation Results, Recommendations, and Subsequent Actions

Many people are involved in providing data for internal curriculum evaluation, most notably learners, faculty, and external stakeholders. They are interested in knowing about the data they and other groups have provided, and what will happen as a result of the evaluation process. Will there be changes to the curriculum, and if so, what will they be, and when will they happen?

Most stakeholders appreciate a comprehensive view of the data and the rationale for curriculum recommendations. As broad a view of data as possible will allow individuals to see where their data fit into the big picture, and possibly to understand how their suggestions are integrated into the recommendations, or why their ideas are absent. The total faculty group, learners, and stakeholder representatives require an opportunity to discuss and possibly modify the recommendations before endorsement can be expected.

Although learners are involved in the curriculum evaluation process, and have a strong interest in its outcomes, they are sometimes forgotten when evaluation results, recommendations, and subsequent actions are reported. Hosting student forums and/or posting information on student Web sites could be effective ways of disseminating information about evaluation outcomes and endorsed recommendations. Students want to know if and how their ideas will influence the curriculum.

Results of internal curriculum evaluation and actions taken as a result of the evaluation should also be reported to appropriate administrators and incorporated into external evaluation reports. If curriculum revision is to be undertaken as a consequence of the evaluation, the evaluation results provide rationale for a request for resources.

Reflecting Back and Looking Forward

Although not always undertaken, a collective review of the curriculum evaluation process can be useful to identify which processes worked and should be retained for future curriculum evaluations, and which were not successful and should be modified or eliminated. A collective review of the curriculum evaluation process can also be useful to identify what might be added to future curriculum evaluations, and what might have been unnecessary or redundant and could be eliminated.

Another aspect of reflecting on the process is to identify the individual and collective learning that resulted from participating in curriculum evaluation. Some members might have a clearer sense of how course components should be linked; others may have more knowledge of curriculum evaluation processes. There could be a collective revisioning of the school as an organization that is progressively working to achieve excellence. Provision of an opportunity for faculty and other stakeholders to reflect on the curriculum evaluation processes, and share their learning, can increase the capacity and empowerment of all groups.

Faculty Development

Faculty development can initially focus on the purposes and processes of curriculum evaluation. Following this, information about evaluation models, approaches, standards, criteria, and indicators can be presented. Through discussion, faculty can formulate evaluation questions to be answered about each curriculum component, and determine data-gathering approaches. Published accreditation or approval guidelines can serve as exemplars during these activities. Through their involvement in curriculum development, novices will understand the curriculum components, but they may need assistance with defining standards and criteria, and limiting the extent of data-gathering. Provision of curriculum data will allow faculty to practice interpreting and judging data, and then deriving recommendations. After the curriculum evaluation is completed, methods to help members identify the learning that was gained could include reflective processes such as storytelling, descriptions of changes and progression in members' work, and group development of the meaning that could be derived from the curriculum evaluation process and results (Verdonschot, 2006).

Chapter Summary

In this chapter, the definition, overview, purposes of internal and external evaluation, and models of curriculum evaluation are presented, as well as benefits to faculty. These are followed by ideas about planning the overall curriculum evaluation: establishing standards, criteria, and/or indicators; and planning data-gathering. Then, evaluation of individual curriculum components is addressed, with emphasis on evaluation questions that might be considered for each. The curriculum components include intended and actual outcomes, design, and courses; teaching-learning and evaluation strategies; human and physical resources; learning climate; and policies. Ideas are offered about judging the quality of the curriculum, reporting evaluation results, and reflecting on the total process. Possible topics for faculty development activities are proposed.

⁘Synthesis Activities⁙

As in previous chapters, two cases are presented for review and discussion. The first is critiqued; the second is for analysis. Following the cases are questions for consideration when curriculum evaluation is planned in individual settings.

Parkview Community College Department of Nursing

The nursing faculty of Parkview Community College Department of Nursing have been revising their associate degree nursing curriculum for the purpose of updating, and for the forthcoming accreditation visit. Using their collected reports of periodic formative curriculum evaluations and the annual summative evaluation, faculty have been revising the curriculum over the past 8 months. They are satisfied with their progress. According to all stakeholders, the revised curriculum is complete. Relevant external and internal factors that impinge on the curriculum were taken into account. The reshaped philosophical approaches and outcome statements were aligned with the institution's mission and current healthcare requirements of the community. As well, supports to enhance student success and faculty members' beliefs were more clearly articulated.

The chairperson, faculty, and other stakeholders have worked together to redesign the overall curriculum and individual courses. This has been a time-consuming undertaking, and all have participated beyond their usual workload to complete the revisions for the incoming class. They are satisfied that the revised curriculum will enable students to achieve the outcomes, and feel prepared to submit the accreditation self-report in the autumn. The chairperson has reminded faculty that evaluation of the revised curriculum should proceed, once it is implemented in the fall term.

Critique

Parkview nursing faculty have progressed to the point that they feel they are ready to implement the revised nursing curriculum in the fall, and undergo program accreditation. They are to be congratulated for completing the work in 8 months, and for periodically evaluating the former curriculum. Furthermore, they appear to be a cohesive group, working collaboratively with the chairperson, and agreeing upon the curriculum revisions.

While there is evidence of curriculum evaluation, there is no mention of organized documentation, recording, or reporting of the evaluation results, nor of how the formative and summative evaluations have shaped the revised curriculum. It also does not appear that thought has been given to establishing a curriculum evaluation subcommittee, or to using a curriculum evaluation model appropriate for the curriculum. An evaluation plan for monitoring the revised curriculum is not evident. This would make one wonder what curricular components will be evaluated, who will do this, how and when it will be done, what tools will be used to collect the data, and whether the faculty realize the contributions these data can make to the curriculum, students, and themselves. Additionally, a curriculum evaluation subcommittee and/or the faculty should first develop evaluative criteria and indicators, based on an agreed-upon curriculum evaluation model. This approach would be useful in meeting approval and accreditation requirements.

Northern Lights University Department of Nursing

Northern Lights University is located in the circumpolar region at the border of the Yukon Territory in Canada and Alaska in the United States. It is an unusual institution, jointly administered by Canadian and American educators, with students from the northern regions of both countries. Many courses, even entire programs, are offered through distance delivery and, therefore, few faculty are present on campus. Face-to-face programs and courses are offered at the home site, or in communities in Alaska, the Yukon, and Northwest Territories. Courses requiring travel by faculty are typically not offered during the harshest months of November to March.

An upper-division baccalaureate nursing program was developed to meet the needs of the northern regions for nurses. There is a strong emphasis on community-based nursing care, community development, and traditional health practices and beliefs of indigenous peoples. The Northern Lights nursing program hopes to retain its graduates in the north, since students who leave to study in the 'south' generally do not return to their home communities.

Three masters-prepared and one PhD-prepared nursing faculty designed the curriculum to be responsive to the northern context, and to achieve the accreditation standards of the National League for Nursing Accreditation Commission and the Canadian Association of Schools of Nursing. Variations in the program take national differences into account. For example, there are two courses about healthcare systems, legislation, and policy: one addresses the American context, and the other, the Canadian. Students enroll in the course that matches their national origin.

All non-nursing courses can be completed by distance delivery from Northern Lights or through American and Canadian 'southern' universities contracted to provide courses. These courses are prerequisite to the upper division nursing courses.

The nursing courses are ready to be offered for the first time. In the junior year, nursing theory classes will be offered on campus, with concurrent community-based experiences. Hospital-based clinical experience will occur in blocks in May and June, and August and September following the junior year, and again in March of the senior year. A 1-month practicum in the site of each student's choice is scheduled for April of the final year. Students will graduate in June.

In addition to classroom courses, university faculty will provide direct practice teaching. Because some practice experiences are in geographically dispersed locations, local nurses will assume responsibility for clinical teaching. Practice teaching workshops have been planned, but only a few nurses are likely to attend because of teaching. Information is also provided through printed materials, on the school Web site, and by audio teleconferencing.

Twenty-five students will be admitted to the nursing courses every second year. Consequently, all nursing courses will not have to be offered simultaneously.

Faculty recognize that an evaluation plan should be in place, and that evaluation should be initiated concurrently with curriculum implementation. This seems like a daunting task as they busily prepare the first courses. Nonetheless, they have decided that they will use Stufflebeam's CIPP model, since they believe it will make evident the unusual context of the program.

Questions for Consideration and Analysis of the Northern Lights Case

1. Does Stufflebeam's CIPP model seem like a reasonable choice? Why? Which other models would be appropriate?

2. Which data will address each component of the model?

3. What would be a feasible data-gathering and management plan for this faculty?

4. How, when, and to whom should evaluation results be reported?

5. How does the number of faculty influence planning and conducting curriculum evaluation?

6. What features of the curriculum will likely be of particular interest to external reviewers? How can faculty take these into account in their evaluation plan?

Curriculum Development Activities for Consideration in Your Setting

Use the following questions to guide your thinking about your plans for curriculum evaluation, whether your curriculum is face-to-face or offered by distance education.

1. For what purposes should curriculum evaluation be undertaken?
2. Which evaluation model or approaches should be used, and why?
3. Which aspects of the curriculum will be evaluated?
4. How can we establish standards, criteria, and/or indicators?
5. What data should be gathered, and from whom?
6. How frequently should data be gathered?
7. How will data be recorded?
8. What is our plan for interpreting and judging the data, and making recommendations?
9. How will a record of our evaluation efforts and subsequent curriculum alterations be maintained?
10. When, how, and to whom will data, evaluation results, and recommendations be reported?
11. What are faculty learning needs in relation to curriculum evaluation?
12. Which individual or group will be responsible for planning and coordinating the curriculum evaluation?
13. How can we plan for a review of the evaluation process?

References

Alkin, M. C., & Taut, S. M. (2003). Unbundling evaluation use. *Studies in Educational Evaluation, 29*, 1–12.

Applegate, M. H. (1998). Curriculum evaluation. In D. M. Billings & J. A. Halstead (Eds.), *Teaching in nursing. A guide for faculty* (pp. 179–208). Philadelphia: W. B. Saunders.

Appling, S. E., Naumann, P. L., & Berk, R. A. (2001). Using a faculty evaluation triad to achieve evidence-based teaching. *Nursing and Health Care Perspectives, 22*(5), 247–251.

Bevis, E. O. (2000a). Teaching and learning: The key to education and professionalism. In E. O. Bevis & J. Watson (Eds.), *Toward a caring curriculum: A new pedagogy for nursing* (pp. 153–188). Boston: Jones and Bartlett.

Bevis, E. O. (2000b). Appendix I: Criteria for student-teacher-student interactions. In E. O. Bevis & J. Watson (Eds.), *Toward a caring curriculum: A new pedagogy for nursing* (pp. 379–381). Boston: Jones and Bartlett.

Bourke, M. P., & Ihrke, B. A. (2005). The evaluation process: An overview. In D. M. Billings & J. A. Halstead (Eds.), *Teaching in nursing. A guide for faculty* (2nd ed., pp. 443–464). St. Louis, MO: Elsevier Saunders.

Chen, H.-T. (2005). *Practical program evaluation.* Thousand Oaks, CA: Sage.

Cooperrider, D. L., & Whitney, D. (2005). *Appreciative inquiry.* San Francisco, CA: Berrett-Koehler.

De Valenzuela, J. S., Copeland, J. R., & Blalock, G. A. (2005). Unfulfilled expectations: Faculty participation and voice in a university program evaluation. *Teachers College Record, 107*(10), 2227–2247.

Elcigil, A., & Sari, H. Y. (2008). Students' opinions about and expectations of effective clinical mentors. *Journal of Nursing Education, 47*(3), 118–123.

Fink, A. (2005). *Evaluation fundamentals* (2nd ed.). Thousand Oaks, CA: Sage.

Fitzpatrick, J. L., Sanders, J. R., & Worthen, B. R. (2004). *Program evaluation: Alternative approaches and practical guidelines* (4th ed.). Boston: Pearson.

Gaberson, K. G., & Oermann, M. H. (2007). *Clinical teaching strategies in nursing.* New York: Springer.

Gignac-Caille, A. M., & Oermann, M. H. (2001). Student and faculty perceptions of effective clinical instructors in ADN programs. *Journal of Nursing Education, 40*(8), 347–353.

Gillespie, M. (2005). Student–teacher connection: A place of possibility. *Journal of Advanced Nursing, 52*(2), 211–219.

Grammatikopoulos, V., Koustelics, A., Tsigillis, N., & Theodorakis, Y. (2004). Applying dynamic evaluation approach in education. *Studies in Educational Evaluation, 30*(4), 255–263.

Guba, E. G., & Lincoln, Y. S. (1989). *Fourth generation evaluation.* Newbury Park, CA: Sage.

Guba, E. G., & Lincoln, Y. S. (2001). *Guidelines and checklist for constructivist (a.k.a. Fourth Generation) evaluation.* Retrieved June 13, 2007, from http://www.wmich.edu./evalctr/checklists/cpnstructivisteval.pdf

Hanson, K. J., & Stenvig, T. E. (2008). The good clinical nursing educator and the baccalaureate nursing clinical experience: Attributes and praxis. *Journal of Nursing Education, 47*(1), 38–42.

Herbener, D. J., & Watson, J. E. (1992). Evaluating nursing education programs. *Nursing Outlook, 40,* 27–32.

Heydman, A. M. (2006). Planning for accreditation. In S. B. Keating (Ed.), *Curriculum development and evaluation in nursing* (pp. 297–315). Philadelphia: Lippincott Williams & Wilkins.

Iwasiw, C. L. (2008). Relevancy-congruency-adequacy-reasonableness model of curriculum evaluation. Unpublished manuscript.

Jacobs, P. M., & Koehn, M. L. (2004). Curriculum evaluation: Who, when, why, how? *Nursing Education Perspectives, 25*(1), 30–35.

Johnsen, K. O., Aasgaard, H. S., Wahl, A. K., & Salminen, L. (2002). Nurse educator competence; A study of Norwegian nurse educators' opinions of the importance and application of different nurse educator competence domains. *Journal of Nursing Education, 41*(7), 295–301.

Killion, J. (2003a). 8 smooth steps. *Journal of Staff Development, 24*(4), 14–21.

Killion, J. (2003b). Steps to your own evaluation. *Journal of Staff Development, 24*(4), 22–26.

National League of Nursing. (2004). NLN statement: Innovation in nursing education: A call to reform. *Nursing Education Perspectives, 25*(1), 47–49.

Oermann, M. H., & Gaberson, K. B. (2006). *Evaluation and testing in nursing education* (2nd ed.). New York: Springer.

Oxford English Dictionary Online. (n.d.). *Standard.* Retrieved April 1, 2008, from http://dictionary.oed.com/cgi/entry/50236067?query_type=word&queryword=standard&first=1&max_to_show=10&sort_type=alpha&result_place=1&search_id=2FgD-TLRyCD-11881&hilite=50236067

Patton, M. Q. (1997). *Utilization-focused evaluation* (3rd ed.). Thousand Oaks, CA: Sage.

Patton, M. Q. (2002). *Utilization-focused evaluation checklist.* Retrieved March 31, 2008, from http://www.wmich.edu/evalctr/checklists/ufe.pdf

Robinson, T. T., & Cousins, J. B. (2004). Internal participatory evaluation as an organizational learning system: A longitudinal case study. *Studies in Educational Evaluation, 30*(1), 1–22.

Saunders, S., & Kardia, D. (2004). Creating inclusive college classrooms. Center for Research on Learning and Teaching, University of Michigan. Retrieved April 21, 2008, from http://www.crlt.umich.edu/gsis/P3_1.html

Stufflebeam, D. L. (2007). CIPP evaluation model checklist. Retrieved June 13, 2007, from http://www.umich.edu/evalctr/checklists/cippchecklist_Mar07.pdf

Stufflebeam, D. L., Madaus, G. F., & Kellaghan, T. (Eds.). (2000). *Evaluation models: Viewpoints on educational and human services evaluation* (2nd ed.). Boston: Kluwer Academic.

Taras, M. (2005). Assessment—summative and formative—some theoretical reflections. *British Journal of Educational Studies, 53,* 466–478.

Valley of the Sun United Way. (2006). *Logic model handbook 2007.* Retrieved Apr 26, 2008, from http://www.vsuw.org/site/DocServer/Logic_Model_Handbook_Updated_2007.pdf?docID=801

Vandeveer, M., & Norton, B. (2005). From teaching to learning: Theoretical foundations. In D. M. Billings & J. A. Halstead (Eds.), *Teaching in nursing: A guide for faculty* (2nd ed., pp. 231–281). St. Louis, MO: Elsevier, Saunders.

Verdonschot, S. G. M. (2006). Methods to enhance reflective behaviour in innovations processes. *Journal of European Industrial Training, 30*(9), 670–686.

Wholey, J. S. (1983). *Evaluation and effective public management.* Boston: Little, Brown.

PART V

Flexible Delivery of Nursing Education Curricula

CHAPTER 13

Flexible Delivery of Nursing Education Curricula

Chapter Overview

In this chapter, the inclusion of flexible delivery in nursing education curricula is discussed. First *distance education* and *flexible delivery* are differentiated. Described are requirements for the use of flexible delivery methods. The source of decisions to employ flexible delivery and consequent curriculum implications are outlined, as are values and beliefs inherent in their use. Curriculum design is briefly overviewed. The section on course design includes pedagogical frameworks for course design, and integrates pedagogy and technology, teaching-learning strategies, and opportunities for students to demonstrate learning and faculty evaluation of student achievement. The section also covers deciding on course design and evaluating course design. Faculty development for flexible delivery and a chapter summary follow. Then, synthesis activities include two cases and questions for readers to consider in individual settings.

Chapter Goals

- Understand the influence of flexible delivery methods on curriculum and course design, implementation, and evaluation.

- Appreciate how flexible delivery methods offer new possibilities for nursing education.

- Consider how the choice of flexible delivery methods influences course implementation and evaluation.

- Reflect on faculty development activities pertinent to flexible delivery.

Distance Education and Flexible Delivery

Distance education is a commonly used term that suggests forms of study where a geographic distance exists between and among students (individually or collectively), the instructor, and program of interest. The instruction can be synchronous or asynchronous.

Although *distance education* may be used synonymously with *online learning* and *e-learning*, it is more encompassing. Distance education includes print-based correspondence study, and audio, video, and computer technologies. Distance education provides an opportunity to access learning opportunities for individuals who cannot or prefer not to be on campus (Larreamendy-Joerns & Leinhardt, 2006).

The concept of *flexibility* suggests suppleness, elasticity, and nimbleness, adjectives that capture the idea of non-linearity, a concept consistent with teaching-learning processes. The term *flexible delivery* is used to contrast it with *traditional face-to-face delivery*, which is time- and place-dependent. *Flexible delivery*, therefore, implies single or combined use of delivery methods that are adaptable to a wide variety of learners and expected learning outcomes. There is flexibility in the delivery methods employed, in addition to when and how they are used.

The technologies used for flexible delivery can be Web-based, multifaceted learning platforms with provision for private, as well as 2-way communication between and among teachers and students. Other technologies include local podcasts, access to learning objects, and so forth, some without communication avenues. However, in all instances, the 'delivery' of the teaching and subsequent student learning occur when teachers and learners are not physically together. Although not strictly distance education, flexible delivery methods can be employed as convenient and effective adjuncts to on-campus, face-to-face courses.

With the introduction and expansion of technology to support education, geographic distance, by itself, is no longer an obstacle to education. Nonetheless, there are individuals for whom computer ownership is not possible, Internet access absent or slow, and efficacy with technology lacking. Accordingly, technology-based distance education is not a universal solution for advancing the education of nurses.

Requirements for the Use of Flexible Delivery

Flexible delivery can be incorporated into a nursing curriculum only if suitable supports are in place. Without them, the desire of nursing faculty to provide courses through flexible delivery will be unfulfilled. Because individual nursing faculty members are unlikely to influence any of these supports quickly, the nature, quality, and extent of the supports become parameters for curriculum and course design.

Technological Infrastructure

The structural features, processes and procedures of the infrastructure selected, developed, or upgraded by the institution should meet specified criteria and quality standards related to adaptability, responsiveness, security, capacity, and cost-effectiveness (Jairath & Stair, 2004). Institutional resources (hardware, multimedia and authoring tools, graphic design and course software) must be available, reliable, and secure with password protection, encryption, and backup systems to ensure quality and validity of information (Billings, 2000; Institute for Higher Education Policy [IHEP], 2000; Jairath & Stair). Essential are an institutional technology plan and a centralized system to support maintenance and growth of distance delivery (IHEP), including costs associated with upgrading hardware and software. Technological and instructional design support and resources (e.g., modem speed, mail accounts, help desk support, security of assignments, copyrights, and intellectual property protection) are fundamental requirements (Jairath & Stair).

Resources to Support Teaching and Learning

Library System and Services Access to learning materials is vital to support course-related work for faculty and students unable to visit or be physically present in the on-campus library. They require reliable alternate access to library materials, reference services, and resources (Zhu, McKnight, & Edwards, 2006), as well as assistance to navigate and troubleshoot online library systems with ease.

Faculty Development and Support The institution is obligated to provide support to faculty members while they learn to use the course delivery and management system, and to develop and implement courses. This entails faculty development before, during, and after the transition to flexible delivery. Technical support and instructional design assistance during course development and implementation make flexible delivery possible. Without these, faculty cannot create engaging courses, nor can they feel secure during course implementation.

Student Support Students also require assistance to learn to use the technology and processes that will form their learning environment. Orientations to technology can be accomplished through on-site sessions, provision of written material or instructional Web sites before they begin courses, peer-tutoring systems, and so on. Prompt assistance from personnel at 24-hour technical and library help desks, and from faculty members about course matters, will reduce stress and build confidence. The importance of technical assistance during exam periods cannot be over-emphasized. Learner frustration and discouragement, as well as negative instructor ratings, can be consequences of lack of timely assistance when students experience technological problems (Tallent-Runnels et al., 2006).

Other Student Services Learners also require the student services that are available on campus, such as assistance with course registration and study skills, financial aid, and personal counseling. Access to all should be online. Similarly, academic counseling is important, and this will likely be provided by the school of nursing rather than the wider institution.

Policies

Workload adjustments to compensate for the time required to build courses in a different medium are desired by many faculty, yet this may not be a provision of faculty contracts. Additionally, guidelines related to class size and examination processes to ensure safety, security, and rigor should be in place (Vaughn, 2007). Policies for online instruction are available in some institutions, but policies related to support course development and evaluation usually have not been established, nor is there research to substantiate that "Universities have established comprehensive policies to guide distance education for online courses" (Tallent-Runnels et al., 2006, p. 115). It has been noted that institutions suffer from "policy vacuums" (Smith & Oliver, 2000, p. 135).

Decisions to Employ Flexible Delivery and Consequent Curriculum Implications

A decision to employ flexible delivery methods in a curriculum can arise from three different circumstances. Each has implications for subsequent curriculum development and course development.

First, during curriculum development, the analysis of contextual data can lead to the logical decision that principal teaching-learning approaches should include flexible delivery for all or part of a curriculum. In this situation, the total faculty group has endorsed the use of flexible delivery methods, and this decision will be a significant parameter in *de novo* curriculum and course development.

Secondly, apart from a formal curriculum development process, faculty members can decide to initiate or expand the use of flexible delivery within existing programs in response to student characteristics, desire to increase enrollment or access, conviction that quality learning outcomes can be achieved, and so forth. This choice will result in modifications in course design and implementation, within the existing curriculum design. The number of courses involved will determine the extent of necessary development activities. One curriculum design change could be the addition of an orientation to technology-based learning.

Thirdly, there can be a strategic decision by the educational institution to increase access to educational programs through flexible delivery. As a consequence, the school of nursing is obligated to support the institution's strategic plans. This situation can result in the development of a completely reconceptualized curriculum, or modifications within the existing curriculum.

Values and Beliefs Inherent in the Use of Flexible Delivery

Use of flexible delivery reflects faculty members' values and beliefs about themselves, nursing education, and the nursing curriculum: acceptance and openness to advances in educational methods and technology, readiness to learn new pedagogical skills, willingness to engage students in non-traditional learning environments, and belief in the importance of accessible education for nurses. It also suggests openness to non-traditional ways of offering curricula, and implies an appreciation that the curriculum will incorporate approaches to teaching and learning consistent with the selected medium.

Values and beliefs about teaching, learning, and learners are inherent in the use of any delivery approach. Prominent among those related to use of flexible delivery are:

- Dedication to the development of learning communities and supportive class cultures
- Trust in learners' autonomy and desire to learn
- Confidence in students' ability to achieve course competencies without the teacher's physical presence
- Respect for diverse learning styles
- View of active participation as an essential characteristic of learning
- Support of a constructivist view of learning (Martens, Bastiaens, & Kirschner, 2007)
- Integration of guidance and support to provide opportunities for scaffolded learning (Larreamendy-Joerns & Leinhardt, 2006).

The widespread use of flexible delivery methods to extend nursing programs beyond campus boundaries is evidence of the demise of behaviorism and its associated tenets as the foundation of nursing curricula. Adoption of flexible delivery methods reflects nurse educators' changed values and beliefs, and compels them to continue to strive for equity in all areas of nursing education. Many flexible delivery methods 'blind' students and faculty, that is, participants generally can neither see nor hear one another. Consequently, all are equal, and can engage fully without pre-conceived ideas arising from appearance or voice.

Curriculum Design Incorporating Flexible Delivery

Curriculum design, explicated as the configuration of a program of studies, includes the courses selected, their sequencing and delivery, relationships between and among them, as well as associated curriculum policies. The *curriculum design process* entails all activities and decisions that result in the creation of the actual program of studies, that is, the completed curriculum. The design process for curricula with flexible delivery parallels that for traditional, campus-based, face-to-face delivery.

The starting point for curriculum development is the context in which the curriculum will be offered and in which graduates will practice nursing. The goal is to develop a curriculum that is context-relevant, feasible, and supported by stakeholders; provides opportunities for students to achieve intended outcomes; is congruent with the curriculum nucleus; and has internal consistency and logical flow. There should be planning to maximize implementation fidelity and to prepare for formative and summative evaluation of the curriculum components and outcomes. These fundamental considerations are necessary in all curriculum development, regardless of discipline or delivery method.

Designing Courses for Flexible Delivery

Designing courses for flexible delivery includes planning all components of traditional courses: title, purpose, and description; outcomes, teaching-learning strategies, and content; classes; opportunities for students to demonstrate learning and faculty evaluation of student achievement, and the relationships between and among these components. A defining aspect of course design for flexible delivery is the confluence of pedagogy and technology. Achieving a satisfactory convergence can require assistance from instructional design experts.

Course designers are mindful of parameters that influence all course design, such as characteristics of learners, the curriculum nucleus, curriculum outcomes, placement of courses in the curriculum, and so forth. When preparing courses for flexible delivery methods, they are cognizant that the available technology is a major parameter of course design.

Developing fully online or hybrid courses with an online component, is more than placing course notes or power-point slides on Web sites (Oblinger & Hawkins, 2006; Ryan, Hodson Carlton, & Ali, 2005; Tallent-Runnels et al., 2006). It is a transformative rather than translational process (Halstead, 2005; Torrisi & Davis, 2000), requiring "deliberate instructional design that hinges on linking learning objectives to specific learning activities and measurable outcomes" (Oblinger & Hawkins, p. 14). The key is careful integration of pedagogical and technological knowledge and skill (Oblinger & Hawkins). Design activities are facilitated by collaboration with instructional designers, consultation with experts, and access to materials that capture best practices.

Xu and Morris (2007) studied faculty and instructional designer roles and curricular decisions during team development of an online humanities course. Berge's online facilitator roles (pedagogical, social, managerial, and technological) and Stark and Lattuca's framework on academic plans (purpose, content, sequence, learner, instructional resources, instructional process, evaluation, and adjustment) (as cited in Xu & Morris) were used to guide analysis. During course development, faculty members emphasized content and materials for individual classes, although attention was given to all course components, as described by Stark and Lattuca. The design expert provided significant input into curricular decisions and facilitated the design process through social, managerial, and technological roles. Role overlap between faculty and the design expert brought cohesiveness, yet caused some conflict when curricular decisions were involved. Faculty felt constrained by the 'same look and feel' principle for all classes. The authors suggest that faculty might benefit more from working with a same-discipline colleague who is an expert in online course development, rather than with an instructional designer.

Pedagogical Frameworks for Course Design

Once the course purpose, description, and competencies have been prepared, the next logical next step is to use an instructional design framework to guide development decisions (Jeffries, 2005). Two frameworks are described for course design. Both emphasize the processes within courses, rather than attention to specific course components, such as methods for students to demonstrate learning. Course components, however, remain essential considerations when designing courses.

Seven Principles of Good Practice in Undergraduate Education   Chickering and Gamson's (1987) seven principles of good practice in undergraduate education can be used as a framework for course design. Proposed, is that faculty should:

- Encourage contacts between students and faculty
- Develop reciprocity and cooperation among students
- Use active learning techniques
- Offer prompt feedback
- Emphasize time on task
- Communicate high expectations
- Respect diverse talents and ways of learning (p. 2).

These principles were used by Jeffries (2005) when creating an online, clinical, critical care nursing course. Incorporated were variables such as sequencing and continuity of content; interaction; and attention to students' diversity and multiple ways of knowing. The following features were included:

- Accommodation of a variety of learners (in academic programs, critical care practice, or pursuing career development). Learners would focus on modules in the order of interest to them and at the depth they required. Course content was organized into a core didactic component, a clinical practicum, a virtual center for best practices, and access to clinical experts and the course instructor. Completion of components was based on learning and professional needs.
- Use of a triad model of learner, faculty member, and preceptor to enhance students' clinical competencies.
- Access to a virtual center of best practices with evidence-based practice protocols, current research, and other materials
- Access and flexibility for learners with opportunities for interaction with faculty, students, and other professionals, as well as patients and families
- Educational mobility to attract and inspire nurses to continue their education.

3 'C' Model Bird's (2007) 3 'C' model for flexible delivery includes: *content* (knowledge associated with the course), *construction* (social construction of knowledge that occurs through interaction and engagement with authentic learning activities), and *consolidation* (development of new understandings through reflection). Emphasized in this model is the critical link among assessment, learning activities, and learner engagement. The following are the key components of this model:

- Social constructivism
- Active rather than passive learning
- Attention to content, construction, and consolidation
- Intentional integration of dialogue and discussion
- Collaborative learning activities integrated with assessments
- Appropriate online facilitation
- Sufficient "scaffolding" and student support
- Access to learning resources.

Application of Bird's (2007) model is described in three iterative stages: a module analysis grid, a module activity map, and a week-by-week program. This iterative approach to module development focuses course designers' attention on content in concert with process, as well as the level of learners. The pedagogical reasons for design decision selection are evident. This model provides academics with ". . . a methodology for mapping out online educational experiences which are pedagogically sound, constructively aligned, and maximize the learning opportunities afforded by electronic connectivity" (Bird, p. 166).

Integrating Pedagogy and Technology

When designing courses for flexible delivery, learning platforms such as Blackboard Learning Systems, Moodle, Desire2Learn, and Knowledge Hub provide an organizational template for course materials and teaching learning processes, although individual flexibility is possible (Halstead, 2005; Nelson, Meyers, Riozzolo, Rutar, Proto, & Newbold, 2006). A standardized *look* across courses facilitates students' familiarity with and timely access to more commonly used course elements such as syllabi, discussion groups, timetables, handouts, and Web links (Halstead). The appearance should be welcoming, and navigation in the course site should be readily transparent.

Consistency in the 'look and feel' of templates does not preclude creativity in designing individual modules and learning activities that stimulate and maintain learners' interest and attention. The range of possible learning activities is determined by the convergence of course competencies, features of the learning platform, faculty members' creativity, pedagogical framework, and instructional designers' support. Skillful integration of pedagogy and technology give vitality to courses.

However, there exists a potential with some interactive learning environments and intelligent tutoring systems (such as Director, Authorware, and Toolbook) that pedagogical aspects of course development may take a back seat to technology (Janicki & Liegle, 2001). There is a risk that learning is linear and lacks congruence with expert teaching and active learning processes that promote divergent thinking and social interaction.

Since some aspect of technology is integrated into courses designed for flexible delivery, the delivery method's user-friendliness, learner control, accessibility, support when problems arise, as well as faculty strengths and preferences, are necessary considerations when designing courses (Zhu et al., 2006). Pedagogy underpins every decision, regardless of the medium. If the pedagogical bases are lacking, no degree of technical wizardry, in itself, will be sufficient to create meaningful learning experiences.

Teaching-Learning Strategies

The teaching-learning strategies must, of course, move students toward achievement of course competencies in a way that is assisted, not hampered by, the technology in use. Strategies can encompass all those normally used in a classroom, and more. An advantage is that all, or nearly all, can be available simultaneously so learners can access course information and strategies pertinent to them at any time.

Since use of flexible delivery methods is premised on a belief in the value of active learning and constructed knowledge, learning processes comprise divergent thinking, discussion, and debate. Consequently, embedded opportunities within courseware for social interaction, synchronous and asynchronous discussion, and collaboration on practice issues or case studies perceived as authentic by learners, will promote disciplinary discourse and allow learner engagement with the content and the process of knowledge construction (Dunlap, Sobel, & Sands, 2007; Larreamendy-Joerns & Leinhardt, 2006; Martens et al., 2007). With large classes, small groups can be formed and their discussion segmented from other groups' discourse. Access to each group discussion could be open to all class participants, or only to designated group members.

With courses delivered through learning platforms, didactic material and links to other learning resources can be posted electronically. These presentations can be designed with technological enhancements to overcome limitations of written text and static presentations. The learning resources could consist of videos, journal articles, material posted on other Web sites, supplementary notes, and so on.

 Other teaching-learning strategies might be an online live discussion or a real-time virtual classroom with lectures and demonstrations (Cornelius & Smith Glasgow, 2007), if these features are part of the learning platform. Such strategies are convenient for guest lecturers and practice experts, and add immediacy and authenticity to the learning. Student presentations are also possible in this way, or through didactic postings. Full use of learning platform components allows for a wide range of teaching preferences and response to a variety of learning styles.

Countless combinations and permutations of teaching and learning strategies and media are possible, and are limited only by faculty members' imagination, creativity, time, and expertise, and the institution's technology infrastructure and support. In an expanding technological world, most critical is to select strategies to maximize achievement of curriculum outcomes, and to respect learner diversity and multiple ways of knowing.

Opportunities for Students to Demonstrate Learning and Faculty Evaluation of Student Achievement

Whether a course is offered traditionally or through flexible delivery modes, students will be expected to demonstrate, and faculty to evaluate, achievement of course competencies. The choice of methods for students to demonstrate learning is related to consistency with philosophical approaches, teaching-learning approaches, course competencies, and the like. As always, a variety of methods is preferred. The appropriateness of giving grades for participation remains controversial.

When deliberating about methods for students to demonstrate achievement, faculty members examine factors such as:

- Compatibility with the delivery medium
- Student access to the necessary resources and supports to demonstrate learning
- Potential for timely feedback
- Scheduling of synchronous evaluation sessions (e.g., examinations)
- Security and ease of assignment submission system.

Deciding on Course Design

Decisions about course design are similar for traditional courses and those offered through flexible delivery, with the added feature that an instructional designer may be part of the process. Recursive and integrated discussion occurs about course competencies, content, teaching-learning strategies, and possibilities within the delivery medium. Some matters that faculty members and course designers should consider are:

- The 'look and feel' of the course. Will it be similar to other courses in the curriculum? Will there be variation among classes in the course?
- The convergence between the course competencies and the medium. Is it possible for learners to achieve the competencies through the technological environment? Which features of the technology would best advance achievement of which course competencies?
- Teaching-learning strategies: Which are possible via technology? How much variation is reasonable? Which can be incorporated while maintaining ease and transparency of navigation within the technology?
- Moderating discussion: Will faculty and teaching assistants do this entirely, or will learners also be expected to be discussion moderators?
- Methods for students to demonstrate learning: Which match the course competencies and are possible and reasonable within the technology?
- Release of course components: Will all components be available at the beginning of the course, or will some be accessible as the course progresses? Why?
- Provision of guidelines, rubrics, and self-assessment tools to help students develop confidence in their learning progress (Dunlap, 2005)
- Faculty preferences and efficacy with the medium

- Anticipated learner comfort with the medium
- Course etiquette: Should this be explicitly described? Negotiated? Not addressed unless a problem arises?
- Teacher availability to respond to learner e-mail messages.

Discussion points for hybrid courses incorporating flexible delivery could be:

- Choice of delivery mode(s) in addition to face-to-face delivery
- Selection of learning activities to be conducted in the face-to-face setting or online (Teeley, 2007)
- Provision of lectures, preparatory and/or supplementary materials via a Web component, podcasts, streaming media, and so on. Which material? Which media?

A finalized course design will result when nursing faculty members and instructional designers are satisfied that they have achieved a reasonable convergence of pedagogy and technology. The result should be a course that engages learners and moves them toward achievement of curriculum outcomes within a technological environment whose navigation is smooth and transparent.

Evaluating Course Design

Faculty members continually engage in appraisal of curriculum and course design, an activity also encompassed in flexible delivery. The design of the course evaluation should be completed before the course is implemented and be consistent with the evaluation plan, model, and procedures in use in the full curriculum.

There may be a need to clarify the purpose of course evaluation specific to flexible delivery, if the entire curriculum is not offered in this way. Criteria or standards specific to flexible delivery courses could be necessary, if not already part of the overall curriculum standards. Reporting of evaluation results may extend beyond the school of nursing and its usual stakeholders to instructional designers, who are now stakeholders.

All aspects of course evaluation, described in Chapter 12, should be included in the evaluation of courses delivered via technology. Useful information specific to the pedagogy-technology interaction include learners' feedback about specifics such as:

- Time on task
- Ease of navigation (Doutrich, Hoeksel, Wykoff, & Thiele, 2005)
- Fit between specific learning activities and technology
- Reasons why learners did or did not engage in specified activities (TLT Group, n.d.)

- Ease in using communication features of the system, such as e-mail and submission of completed assignments
- Suitability of technology for learning about a person-centered, practice discipline
- Authenticity of activities (Bird, 2007; Dunlap et al., 2007; Larreamendy-Joerns & Leinhardt, 2006; Martens et al., 2007)
- General satisfaction with course delivery.

Additionally, faculty members' and instructional designers' feedback should be obtained. Included is information about scheduling of their collaborative activities, satisfaction with their collaborative processes, and use of integrated course resources (Juntunen & Heikkinen, 2004).

Billings (2000) proposed a comprehensive framework for assessing outcomes and practices in Web-based nursing courses. The framework encompasses the following five major concepts and accompanying operational variables:

- Outcomes: Learning, recruitment, retention, graduation, access, convenience, connectedness, preparation for the real world, computer tool proficiency, professional practice socialization, satisfaction
- Educational practices: Active learning, time on task, feedback, student–faculty interaction; interaction and collaboration among peers, respect for diversity, high expectations
- Faculty support: Faculty development, orientation to technology, ongoing technical support, workload recognition, rewards
- Student support: Information, orientation to technology, ongoing technical support, learning resources, student services
- Use of technology: Accessible and reliable infrastructure, use of hardware/software promotes productive use of time (p. 61).

The results of organized and regular course evaluations contribute to ideas about subsequent course refinement or revision. When offering courses by flexible delivery modes, it is incumbent on nurse educators to expand ideas of course evaluation to explicitly include features of the delivery mode and its intersection with learning about nursing.

Summary of Curriculum and Course Design Process for Flexible Delivery

Curriculum and course design for flexible delivery share many of the same processes as traditional delivery. The difference lies in the influence of the delivery medium on the design. Involvement of an instructional design expert is usually necessary until faculty develop expertise in creating courses that incorporate flexible delivery modes. Nonetheless, all decisions and deliberations take into account the curriculum nucleus and curriculum outcomes. Important to remember is that the process of design is iterative, with the intent of achieving an internally consistent course with a harmonious blending of pedagogy and technology.

Faculty Development

The overall goal of faculty development as it relates to curriculum and course design for flexible delivery is to advance members' appreciation, understanding, and knowledge of alternate delivery methods and their intersection with pedagogy. Faculty development can range from individual, micro-level assistance with course development, based on faculty members' comfort, knowledge, and expertise with these methods, to more system-wide or macro-level academic guidance related to curriculum planning (Power, 2008; Smith & Oliver, 2000).

If the adoption of flexible delivery methods involves a change in faculty members' perspectives about learning and the role of teachers and students, they could require new skill sets whereby they are able to:

- Understand how to develop activities that promote learner engagement.
- Appreciate what the course looks and feels like from the learner`s point of view.
- Recognize emotional needs of learners.
- Grasp the nuances of flexible delivery so that teaching-learning strategies are congruent with a coherent and integrated learning experience (Cotler & Matthews-DeNatale, 2005).
- Accept that course redesign involves conceptualization of learning outcomes, content, teaching, learning, and evaluation processes to suit flexible learning environments (Ryan, Hodson Carlton, & Ali, 2004).

According to Tallent-Runnels et al. (2006), faculty desire timely and ongoing training and support for alternate delivery methods, and assistance to solve technological problems. Provision of technological support relieves stress and is emotionally encouraging (Doutrich et al., 2005). Technological support should be available from a central help desk, but the value of immediate help from a colleague is underscored. Help from a peer with expertise makes the undertaking seem possible.

Learning opportunities with a wider scope might include centrally offered workshops to address strengths and limitations of selected delivery media, or informal 'lunch and learn' dialogue among faculty about successes and frustrations with specific delivery media. Sharing circles with novice and more experienced faculty could encourage discussion among those who are tentative about the effectiveness of flexible delivery and those who are convinced of its value. Such perspectives and experiences might provide a balance between positive and negative views about specific applications.

Guided workshops for faculty converting courses to flexible delivery could include brainstorming about course reconfiguration to suit different media. As well, novices might be observers in courses being offered, and mentored by experienced peers as they develop their own courses for flexible delivery.

In addition to learning how to design courses for flexible delivery, faculty must be able to conduct them effectively. Online facilitation is a skill that involves knowing when to intervene; where to intervene (in the public discussion forum or privately by e-mail); how to phrase ideas so the intent is conveyed without benefit of paralanguage and non-verbal behavior; and when to observe without comment. Examples of online discussion (used with participants' permission) provide opportunities for practice. Faculty experienced with flexible delivery can readily lead these sessions.

Chapter Summary

In this chapter, *distance education* and *flexible delivery* are differentiated. The source of decisions to employ flexible delivery and consequent curriculum implications, as well as values and beliefs associated with flexible delivery are described. Considerations for course design are offered, including pedagogical frameworks, convergence of pedagogy and technology, teaching-learning strategies, opportunities for students to demonstrate learning and faculty evaluation of student achievement, deciding on course design, and evaluating course design. Two key points to be recalled are that the choice of delivery medium is a prominent influence on design course, and that pedagogy must underpin every decision regardless of the medium. Finally, ideas for faculty development activities are offered.

▸Synthesis
Activities ⚹

> Below are two case studies. The Plato University case is followed by a critique. Determine if additional ideas should be considered in the analysis. The second case, Pinnacle College, is followed by questions to guide examination of the case. Finally, questions are presented related to flexible delivery in individual situations.

Plato University Faculty of Nursing

The Plato University Faculty of Nursing has a long-standing history of offering high-quality undergraduate and graduate nursing education in a research-intensive university. Like Plato's Academy in Athens, the university is devoted to research and instruction in philosophy and the sciences. A recent institutional strategic direction is to provide access to education through integration of alternate delivery methods. The faculty of nursing's new strategic plan is aligned with the university plan; however, concrete, organized activities have not been initiated. Nonetheless, several faculty members have experimented with various technologies and are eager to try new ways of offering courses.

At the faculty of nursing council meeting, Dean Rachelle reported about government funding to modify nursing curricula so students could complete their BSN programs one semester sooner than the current pattern. The intent is to ready graduates for the nursing workforce earlier, and thereby address the nursing shortage in the city and region. Reducing the program length would require, in part, that final semester courses be reconceptualized for flexible delivery.

Dean Rachelle supported the idea and asked for faculty members' views. Deliberations concluded with consensus to participate in the initiative. Four faculty members offered to form a task group to investigate possibilities for flexible delivery. Dean Rachelle proposed that an instructional designer from the university faculty development and support center join the task group. One faculty member suggested that a colleague from the faculty of science experienced with several delivery modes be invited as well. Dean Rachelle stated that she had resources to support a faculty retreat focused on flexible delivery.

The task group met several times to plan the retreat and discussed design principles they believed important for faculty members to consider in advance of a change in delivery methods. Task group members proposed that the first retreat focus on design principles. They felt that a fulsome discussion and consensus on ideas such as learner control, interactive dialogue, active learning, metacognition, and reflective analysis, would set the philosophical stage from which to move forward. They recommended to Dean Rachelle that a facilitator with expertise in flexible delivery be engaged.

Critique

The alignment of the faculty of nursing strategic plan with the university plan reinforces the idea that the initiative is a positive one to pursue. Presenting the government initiative as being open for discussion permitted dialogue among faculty about their concerns and questions. The presence of faculty members eager to explore flexible delivery options was an asset. Formation of a task group provided them with an opportunity for synergy and development of workshop plans. Knowledge of university services to support course development for flexible delivery and expertise in the faculty of science was valuable as these resources could be involved in discussions about flexible delivery options. Providing financial resources for a faculty retreat focused on flexible delivery was a wise decision on Dean Rachelle's part, as it demonstrated tangible support for the anticipated direction. This was also strategic as she recognized the value of faculty development.

Identifying key design principles upon which to focus was a shrewd suggestion from the task group. They believed that if faculty recognized that core design principles are relevant to all courses regardless of medium, the facilitator could help them conceptualize the congruence of these principles with alternate delivery methods. In this way, faculty might more readily appreciate the parallels between campus-based and flexible delivery courses, and prepare themselves for future course development.

Pinnacle College School of Nursing

Pinnacle College School of Nursing is planning to offer an online, 2-year primary healthcare nurse practitioner master's degree, using WebCT as the delivery platform. Students must be registered nurses with a BSN and have a minimum of 2 years of full-time practice experience before they are eligible to enroll. The program is expected to be intensive. Part-time enrollment is possible, with 3 years allowed for completion. Thirty students will be admitted annually. All courses will have a practice component. The theoretical components will be organized in modules that combine synchronous and asynchronous interaction among participants, as well as monthly face-to-face tutorials and labs. The modules will have a similar organizational structure but module elements will vary according to specific courses. The final course will be an 8-month internship with PhD-prepared nurse practitioners. It is expected that students will be successful on certification examinations and will be in high demand after graduation.

Faculty members decided to use Bird's (2007) analysis framework to guide module development. However, rather than using Bird's term, *consolidation* (interpreted as *static fusion of information*), they are employing the word *integration* to indicate dynamic knowledge synthesis. The first course to be developed is a 6-credit hour course called Health Assessment for Nurse Practitioners. Course competencies will include integration of theory and physical assessment skills into comprehensive health assessments, and incorporation of knowledge of normal physiology and health assessment techniques into written case analyses. The course will be offered over two, 12-week semesters. Learners are expected to dedicate 12–15 hours per week to this course. The analysis grid is as follows:

Health Assessment for Nurse Practitioners

Module elements	Content (receiving, seeking, discussing information)	Construction (active learning opportunities)	Integration (individual reflective anal-yses; group discussions)	Total hours
	Anticipated hours of student effort			
Pre-induction	2		2	4
Face-to-face induction	2	3		5
Online induction	1	2	1	4
Researching content	30		30	60
Guided reading	30		30	60
Group work	10	20	10	40
Weekly online dialogue	10	20	10	40
Individual reflection	5		10	15
Simulation activities	12	24	12	48
Client assessments	8	12	24	44
Final examination			4	4
Total hours	110	81	133	324

Questions for Consideration and Analysis of the Pinnacle College School of Nursing Case

1. Does the balance between content and process seem reasonable? How might the balance shift to reflect sound pedagogy?

2. What module elements are missing or redundant?

3. Should more attention be focused on any particular element?

4. To what extent do the elements prepare learners to achieve course competencies?

5. Might students perceive learning activities as authentic?

6. What expertise will faculty require to develop and implement this course?

7. What might be the demands on faculty if there are 20–25 students in this course at any one time?

Curriculum Development Activities for Consideration in Your Setting

Use the following questions to guide thinking about flexible delivery:

1. Which flexible delivery method is most appropriate for the curriculum and courses we are developing?

2. What factors particular to our context will influence the choice of delivery method(s)?

3. Does our setting have the infrastructure to support the integration of flexible delivery approaches?

4. What institutional policies are in place to support flexible delivery initiatives?

5. What course development model might best suit our context?

6. What faculty development activities might be effective to support faculty movement towards experimenting with or integrating flexible delivery?

References

Billings, D. M. (2000). A framework for assessing outcomes and practices in web-based courses in nursing. *Journal of Nursing Education, 39*(2), 60–67.

Bird, L. (2007). The 3 'C' design model for networked collaborative e-learning: A tool for novice designers. *Innovations on Education and Teaching International, 44*(2), 153–167.

Chickering, A. W., & Gamson, Z. F. (1987). Seven principles for good practice in undergraduate education. *AAHE Bulletin, 3*, 3–7, ED282491.

Cornelius, F., & Smith Glasgow, M. E. (2007). The development and infrastructure needs required for success–one college's model: Online nursing education at Drexel University. *Techtrends, 51*(6), 32–35.

Cotler, D., & Matthews-DeNatale, G. (2005). Faculty as authors of online courses: Support and mentoring. Academic commons. Retrieved April 21, 2008, from http://www.academic commons.org/commons/essay/matthews-denatale-and-cotler

Doutrich, D., Hoeksel, R., Wykoff, L., & Thiele, J. (2005). Teaching teachers to teach with technology. *Journal of Continuing Education, 36*(1), 25–31.

Dunlap, J. C., Sobel, D., & Sands, D. I. (2007). Supporting students' cognitive processing in online courses: Designing for deep and meaningful student-to-content interactions. *TechTrends, 51*(4), 20–31.

Dunlap, J. C. (2005). Workload reduction in online courses: Getting some shuteye. *Performance Improvement, 44*(5), 18–25.

Halstead, J. A. (2005). Promoting critical thinking through online discussion. *Annual Review of Nursing Education, 3,* 143–164. Retrieved April 21, 2008, from ProQuest Nursing & Allied Health Source database (Document ID: 842569121).

Institute for Higher Education Policy (IHEP). (2000). Quality on the line: Benchmarks for success in Internet-based distance education. Retrieved April 21, 2008, from http://www.ihep. org/assets/files/publications/m-r/QualityOnTheLine.pdf

Jairath, N., & Stair, N. (2004). A development and implementation framework for web-based nursing courses. *Nursing Education Perspectives, 25*(2), 67–72.

Janicki, T., & Liegle, J. O. (2001). Development and evaluation of a framework for creating web-based learning modules: A pedagogical and systems perspective. *Journal of Asynchronous Learning, 5*(1), 58–84. Accessed March 27, 2008, from http://www.sloan-c.org/publications/ jaln/v5n1-janicki.asp

Jeffries, R. P. (2005). Development and testing of a hyperlearning model for design of an online critical care course. *Journal of Nursing Education, 44*(8), 366–372.

Juntunen, A., & Heikkinen, E. (2004). Lessons from interprofessional e-learning: Piloting a caring of the elderly model. *Journal of Interprofessional Care, 18*(3), 269–278.

Larreamendy-Joerns, J., & Leinhardt, G. (2006). Going the distance with online education. *Review of Educational Research. Winter, 76*(4), 567–605.

Martens, R., Bastiaens, T., & Kirschner, P. A. (2007). New learning design in distance education: The impact on student perception and motivation. *Distance Education, 28*(1), 81–93.

Nelson, R., Meyers, L., Riozzolo, M. A., Rutar, P., Proto, M. B., & Newbold, S. (2006). The evolution of educational information systems and nurse faculty roles. *Nursing Education Perspectives, 27*(5), 247–253.

Oblinger, D. G., & Hawkins, B. L. (2006). The myth about online course development. *Educause Review, 41*(1), 14–15.

Power, M. (2008). A dual-mode university instructional design model for academic development. *International Journal for Academic Development, 13*(1), 5–16.

Ryan, M., Hodson Carlton, K., & Ali, N. S. (2004). Reflections on the role of faculty in distance learning and changing pedagogies. *Nursing Education Perspectives, 25*(2), 73–80.

Ryan, M., Hodson Carlton, K., & Ali, N. S. (2005). A model for faculty teaching online: Confirmation of a dimensional matrix. *Journal of Nursing Education, 44*(8), 357–365.

Smith, J., & Oliver, M. (2000). Academic development: A framework for embedding learning technology. *International Journal for Academic Development, 5*(2), 129–137.

Tallent-Runnels, M. K., Thomas, J. A., Lan, W. Y., Cooper, S., Ahern, T. C., Shaw, S. M., et al. (2006). Teaching courses online: A review of the research. *Review of Educational Research, 76*(1), 93–135.

Teeley, K. H. (2007). Designing hybrid web-based courses for accelerated nursing students. *Educational Innovations, 46*(9), 417–422.

TLT Group: Teaching, Learning and Technology. (n.d.). The Flashlight approach to evaluating educational uses of technology. The TLT Group. Retrieved April 21, 2008, from http://www.tltgroup.org/Flashlight/ Handbook?flashlight_approach.pdf

Torrisi, G., & Davis, G. (2000). Online learning as a catalyst for reshaping practice—The experiences of some academics developing online learning materials. *International Journal for Academic Development, 5*(2), 166–176.

Vaughn, N. (2007). Perspectives on blended learning in higher education. *International Journal on E-Learning, 6*(1), 81–94.

Xu, H., & Morris, L. V. (2007). Collaborative course development for online courses. *Innovative Higher Education, 32*(1), 35–47.

Zhu, E., McKnight, R., & Edwards, N. (2006). *Principles of online design.* Retrieved April 21, 2008, from http://www.fgcu.edu/ onlinedesign/index.html

PART VI

Future Perspectives

CHAPTER 14

The Future of Curriculum Development in Nursing Education

Curriculum development and evaluation in nursing education will continue to evolve in accordance with changing demographics and in response to the internal and external factors that influence nursing curricula. Dedicated and competent nursing faculty and administrators will make nursing knowledge and dynamic curricula relevant to changing times. Nursing education will be accessible and transparent to students whose aspirations, goals, and ambitions are to practice nursing skillfully as graduate professionals in a changing global healthcare environment, and thereby contribute to the health, well-being, and quality of life of diverse individuals, families, groups and communities, nationally and internationally.

Influences on Curriculum Development in the Future

A significant aspect of the external context is the nursing shortage. Of concern may be that as nursing shortages grow, expediency in the production of healthcare workers could become more highly valued by politicians and healthcare employers than the preparation of educated professionals. Pressure may arise to refocus existing nursing curricula to emphasize job readiness at the expense of a person-centered nursing perspective, in the erroneous belief that graduating adequate numbers of nurses to fill empty positions should be the goal of nursing education (Iwasiw, Goldenberg, & Andrusyszyn, 2005).

The shortage of nurses and practice placements has an impact on nursing education. In some situations, nurses are feeling stressed, over-stretched, and unable to assist students with their learning. As well, the high acuity of hospitalized patients has resulted in reduced access to acute care placements for nursing students, even though acute care settings are the employment choice for most baccalaureate graduates (Hartigan-Rogers, Cobbett, Amirault, & Muise-Davies, 2007). A curricular concern is that learners sometimes feel that practice experiences are not aligned with future practice requirements, particularly community and long-term care placements where a professional nursing presence is limited or absent. Insufficient numbers of preceptors, some staff nurses' unwelcoming attitude, and at times, lack of clarity about the nursing role, may leave students feeling inadequately prepared for practice, and/or reconsidering their career choice. The potential is that some will be lost to the profession. Therefore, the availability and nature of practice learning environments will continue to influence nursing curriculum development into the future.

A focus on interprofessional education, and acceptance of flexible delivery for all levels of nursing education, are growing. Use of flexible delivery methods may overcome the logistical barriers presently facing the introduction of interprofessional education into health professional programs. Each separately, and the two in combination, will be significant influences on nursing education.

Occurring concomitantly with the growing nursing shortage is the impending retirement of large numbers of experienced nurse educators. Seventy-five percent of the faculty population in the United States is expected to retire from their positions by 2019 (National League for Nursing, 2007). The loss of nursing faculty, particularly those with degrees in nursing education, will have a profound effect on the development and delivery of nursing curricula. This nurse educator cohort, for whom curriculum development and teaching may have taken precedence over research, has been responsible for the development, progress, growth, and solidity of undergraduate and graduate programs. Moreover, because faculty members with more recent PhD degrees may prefer to concentrate on the development and expansion of their research careers, it is possible that this strength in curriculum development, implementation, and evaluation will be compromised. The result could be that nursing curricula will be less cohesive, and graduates may have less comprehensive and integrated perspectives of the vast scope of professional nursing. Accordingly, faculty numbers, their individual experiences and priorities, as well as the mission of schools of nursing, will continue to affect the nursing curricula that will be developed.

Coupled with a rebalanced emphasis in many schools of nursing toward research, is a reluctance of many master's and PhD nursing graduates to consider a career in academia. These graduates may have witnessed the many responsibilities inherent in the professorial role, and what professors must do to attain tenure and be perceived as successful (i.e., secure research grants, publish, teach, supervise graduate students, fulfill community service obligations, and possibly remain clinically active). As well, they might have seen or speculated about the cost to family life, and may conclude that they prefer a career that allows for a more equal balance between the professional and personal dimensions of their lives. Many will decide that such a balance cannot be achieved in an academic career. Moreover, assistant professor salaries may be no higher than those of staff nurses. Quality of work life, requirements for success, faculty support programs, and remuneration will be increasingly important factors in attracting faculty members, and thus, in the development of nursing curricula.

In spite of a nursing faculty shortage, the importance of evidence-based practice in nursing education continues to grow, as does the prominence of nursing education research. The importance of this is reflected in the Excellence in Nursing Education Model developed by the National League for Nursing (NLN) (2006). *Evidence-based programs* and *teaching/evaluation models* are among the eight components of excellence. This model, along with accreditation standards, will continue to influence nurse educators and nursing curricula in the future.

Curriculum Development in the Future

Nurse educators are, and will be, obligated to respond to the need for nurses in the healthcare context nationally and abroad, despite a shortage of faculty members within the internal context of nursing schools. They have been meeting this responsibility through increased enrollments, collaborative programs, accelerated programs, distance education (Oermann, 2004), and provision of international clinical experiences. However, as the demand for more nursing graduates continues to grow, we, as nursing faculty, ought not to succumb to assertions that the main goal for nursing education is to produce more and more graduates, or that *numbers* are the most important measure of a program's success. Rather, we should be firm in our conviction about the *type* and *quality* of professional nurse graduates necessary to respond to the health situations of growing populations locally, nationally, and internationally. These graduates are required to be knowledgeable, careful thinkers with excellent interpersonal, assessment, intervention, health promotion, and delegation skills. We should be adamant that these attributes are acquired in educationally-focused programs, and not in those that merely emphasize training. Therefore, it is incumbent upon nurse educators to continue development of sound evidence-based curricula whose graduates will respond to the need for well-educated and competent professional nurses, able to work with graduates from other countries and other health professions, and motivated to provide skillful, ethical, and compassionate care.

Necessary to successful nursing curriculum development in a future with insufficient numbers of nurses, will be increased involvement of clinical and healthcare stakeholders throughout the process. Greater participation in curriculum development by those who will employ graduates could serve several purposes:

- Increased understanding and acceptance of the goals of nursing education programs by external stakeholders
- Lessening of the education-practice gap in the preparation of future nursing practitioners
- Enhanced clinical learning environments for students
- Stronger sense of a joint mission in the preparation of nurses.

Although the goal of a nursing education program should not merely be to have graduates 'job-ready' for local employers, stakeholders' deeper and sustained collaboration in curriculum development could lead to increased employer satisfaction with new graduates.

In addition to expanding the view of curriculum development to include active and continuing participation by stakeholders, nurse educators should ensure that curricula in master's and doctoral nursing programs contain some focus on nurse educator competencies (e.g., teaching, evaluation of learning, course design), since these abilities are relevant for all areas of nursing. Then, nurses with graduate degrees will have some preparation relevant for curriculum development and implementation, as well as enhanced abilities to support student learning.

Within the context of a nursing and nursing faculty shortage, it is essential that nurses in clinical practice nurture students and newcomers to the professions. Support of student learning is a standard of nursing practice in some jurisdictions, and should be a value held by all members of the nursing profession. Accordingly, it would be judicious for nurse educators to give attention to the values they explicitly teach and enact with learners, colleagues, and clinicians. Specifically, as nurse educators develop curricula, they and stakeholders should consider how to ensure that faculty and clinicians "consciously and consistently inculcate students with the conviction that they have a responsibility for the well-being and success of future nursing colleagues" (Iwasiw, Andrusyszyn, & Goldenberg, 2007, p. 1).

After a period of decline in the 1990s, the field of nursing education is again gaining prominence. Increasing numbers of graduate programs addressing nursing education, growth in continuing nursing education, the National League for Nursing's Certification in Nursing Education, and the adoption of Boyer's (1990) model of scholarship (which includes the scholarship of teaching) by many universities, are indicators of the respect and renown that have been accorded to nursing education as a field of study and practice. Faculty members whose graduate education has a nursing education focus, and who concentrate on this in their research and publications, will be the leaders in nursing curriculum development in the future.

As always, nursing curricula will be only an inert collection of words unless brought to life by forward-thinking, knowledgeable, dynamic faculty, willing to lead, take risks, respond to significant contextual influences, and thereby, collectively, prepare new graduates for the future. The continuing challenge will be to design context-relevant curricula that engage students, excite them about nursing, and position them for productive, far-reaching careers in nursing. The future of curriculum development in nursing education is now.

References

Boyer, E. (1990). *Scholarship revisited. Priorities for the Profession.* Princeton, NJ: Carnegie Foundation.

Hartigan-Rogers, J. A., Cobbett, S. L., Amirault, M. A. & Muise-Davies, M. E. (2007). Nursing graduates' perceptions of their undergraduate clinical placement. *International Journal of Nursing Education Scholarship* 4(1), Article 9. Retrieved April 10, 2008, from http://www. bepress.com/ijnes/vol4/iss1/art9

Iwasiw, C., Goldenberg, D., & Andrusyszyn, M. A. (2005). Extending the evidence base for nursing education. *International Journal of Nursing Education Scholarship*, 2(1), Editorial. Retrieved March 30, 2008, from http://www.bepress.com/ijnes/vol2/iss1/editorial1

Iwasiw, C., Andrusyszyn, M. A., & Goldenberg, D. (2007). Fostering future nursing professionals: It's a matter of values. *International Journal of Nursing Education Scholarship*, 4(1), 1. Editorial. Retrieved March 30, 2008, from http://www.bepress.com/ijnes/vol4/iss1/editorial1

National League for Nursing. (2006). *Excellence in nursing education model.* New York: Author.

National League for Nursing. (2007). Nurse faculty shortage fact sheet. Retrieved April 11, 2008, from http://www.nln.org/governmentaffairs/pdf/NurseFacultyShortage.pdf

Oermann, M. H. (2004). Reflections on undergraduate nursing education: A look to the future. *International Journal of Nursing Education Scholarship*, 1(1), Article 5. Retrieved April 7, 2008, from http://www.bepress.com/ijnes/vol1/iss1/art5

Index

B

baccalaureate programs, 203
Ballard University School of Nursing (case study), 256–257
beginning curriculum development, 16–18
behavioral change, 82, 86–87
behaviorism, 174, 179
beliefs. *See also* philosophical approaches; values
  as area of conflict, 92
  cultural differences, 111
  in current curriculum, 89–90
  of educational institution, 104, 105
  of flexible curricula delivery, 315
  nursing philosophies, 175–178
Bellemore University School of Nursing (case study), 130–131
Bird's 3 "C" model, 318–319
blended course design strategies, 244, 253
blended curriculum delivery, 197–200, 236
block pattern for course sequencing, 211
boards of nursing, curriculum outcome statements for, 185
brainstorming curriculum possibilities, 139–140
branching design for curriculum, 205
broad-fields curriculum design, 204
broadcast television, 198, 237
budget. *See* financial considerations
building blocks design for curriculum, 204, 205
buzz groups, as teaching-learning strategy, 236

C

career development of curriculum leaders, 40–41
change, resistance to, 11
  addressing with faculty development, 80, 83–92
  changing perspective on curriculum, 74–75
    reframing resistance to change, 88–89
  development timeframe and, 20
  initial objections to curriculum development, 23–25
change theories, 81–83
changing between curricula, 79–92
  change theories, 81–83
  how to respond to resistance, 83–92
  implementation of, 271
  supporting faculty during, 83
charismatic leadership, 36
Charlevoix University School of Nursing (case study), 27–29
checklists for evaluation curricula, 293
CIPP curriculum evaluation model, 286
classes (sessions), 238–239, 250
  designing, 252–253
classical philosophies, 174
climate for learning. *See* environments for teaching
clinical courses, content of, 238
clinical teaching-learning strategies, 235, 336

clinicians, curriculum outcome statements for, 184–185
co-op opportunities for secondary school students, 267
code of student conduct, devising, 221
cognitive abilities
  defined, 136
  inferring need for, 139, 153
cognitive apprenticeship, 175, 179
collaboration. *See also* beliefs; communication; values
  behavioral change, 82, 84–87
  changing roles and relationships, 75
  in course design, 243, 246, 252, 321–323
  on curriculum design, 215–217, 222–223
  on curriculum evaluation, 281, 289–291, 294–295
  curriculum nucleus, validating, 148–149
  in faculty development, 79
  feedback loops in curriculum development, 10
  on flexible curricula delivery, 314–315
  formulating outcome statements, 185–186
  informing stakeholders of curriculum development, 26
  interpersonal aspects of curriculum development, 11. *See also* culture of educational institution
    adoption of innovation, 81–82
    course design, 244
  leadership. *See* leadership styles; leading curriculum development
  on philosophical approaches, 9
  philosophical approaches, agreeing on, 181
  responding to resistance. *See* resistance to change
  selection of formal development leader, 36–37, 40
  widening of, 335–336
Collaboration for Academic Education in Nursing (CAEN), 202
collaborative inquiry, 176, 179
collaborative partnerships for curricula delivery, 200–203
  course design and, 247–248
  curriculum implementation planning, 267–269
colleagues. *See entries at* faculty
collecting data for research, 116, 127
collective appeals for faculty support, 22–23
commitment, 20
communication. *See also* collaboration
  in adoption of innovation, 81–82
  informing learners of objectives, 254
  informing of curriculum development, 26
  publicizing curriculum plans, 264–266
  reporting on curriculum evaluation, 294, 301
  responding to resistance. *See* resistance to change
community environment, 114–115
  contractual arrangements, 267–269
  informing agencies of curriculum development, 265
competencies (to learn). *See* professional abilities
competency statements for courses, 234, 249
  evaluation of student achievement, 240

view of curriculum, changing, 74–75
   reframing resistance to change, 88–89
virtual reality, as teaching-learning strategy, 237
vision, of educational institution, 104, 105
voice tools in Web-based courses, 199

W

Web-based learning platforms, 199. *See also* flexible
   curricula delivery
Web-based surveys, 120

Web marketing of redesigned curriculum, 266–267
Web searches, 119
work cycle of school, 19–20
working together. *See* collaboration
workload considerations, 24, 91, 107–108, 270
written assignments
   to evaluate student achievement, 239
   as teaching-learning strategy, 237
written curriculum, 5